A. Taft

THE

HOMŒOPATHIC THEORY AND PRACTICE OF MEDICINE.

BY E. E. MARCY, M. D.

Similia similibus curantur.

NEW-YORK:
WILLIAM RADDE, 322 BROADWAY.

1850.

H. Ludwig and Co. Printers, N.Y.

PREFACE.

The profession of the art and science of renewing and preserving health has, in all periods and in all nations, been held to be of the highest dignity, for the devotion and bravery necessary in those who adopt it, as well as for its association, as ameliorator, with almost every form of human suffering. In its widest and justest acceptation, it may be said to be the sum of logic, since nearly all knowledge, in metaphysics as well as in physics, is necessary to the thorough understanding and the illustration of its various principles and phenomena.

In an age preëminently distinguished for intellectual as well as for physical activity, the theories of disease and cure have shared the general advancement, and the new doctrines that have obtained, for their elucidation and practical application, demand a new literature. Since the discoveries of the Newton of Medicine, old treatises, founded upon erroneous and soon to be obsolete hypotheses, are, for the most part, comparatively valueless, except for purposes of history. Everything is to be reconstructed. Much has indeed been done in Europe and in this country, since the announcement of the true laws of cure, yet so little in proportion to the necessity, that no apology will be required for this attempt to occupy one of the chief places of dethroned but still unsilenced Error.

At the beginning of a system of Theory and Practice, produced under such circumstances, and for such purposes, it is appropriate to disclose briefly its leading characteristics, and especially the positions it occupies in relation to points which may be considered still unsettled and debateable. The grand proposition, *similia similibus curantur*, is not only the basis of the homœopathic method, but is also, we believe, the hitherto unknown law of the most successful treatment by the allopathists. Whether we advocate the use of high or low attenuations, or believe in the topical and material, or the dynamical and immaterial action of drugs, are matters of proportionably little importance, while we abide by this fundamental doctrine in the practical application of remedies. The physician of the old school, who cures delirium tremens with a large dose of opium, acts as strictly in accordance with the theory of Hahnemann, as he who cures it with a high attenuation of the same drug, but with this difference—that the treatment of the former is attended with danger, and the restoration is slow, tedious, and defective, while the primary specific impression by the philosophical process is slight, and the curative reaction of the organism speedy, complete, and permanent.

Although the question of doses is of considerable importance in individual cases, yet too much stress has been laid upon it by the advocates of both high and low attenuations. We are constantly presented with well-authenticated cures by the undiluted tinctures and low dilutions, and have also as thoroughly understood and successfully practised the high attenuations. We occasionally see, too, that strong preparations afford prompt relief where the weaker have failed, and *vice versa*. Some constitutions may be powerfully acted on by a thirtieth, while others will not respond to any weaker than a first dilution. The different conditions of the tissues likewise offer the most varied and important modifications with reference to the effects of agents. How absurd, then, to fix upon this or that attenuation, and to make use of the term *high* or *low* dilutionist, when we have to deal with organisms of every possible grade of delicacy and susceptibility, and with morbid conditions which, in some instances, may be modified by even a mental emotion, and in others only by the strongest tinctures.

We say, therefore, to the true homœopathist, let the grand maxim of HAHNEMANN, *similia similibus curantur*, be our prime and constant rule of medical faith and practice ; but never attempt to confine our doses within the narrow limits of the ultraists of either party, for the unanswerable reason, that *the susceptibilities of the tissues to medicinal impressions vary in precise accordance with the degrees of inflammation and nervous erethism.* From a condition of health, or a slight irritation of the textures, up to a high point of inflammatory action, or nervous excitability, there are almost innumerable gradations of impressibility ; and he who would prescribe wisely and successfully, must select his attenuations, and order his repetitions with strict regard to these degrees. Of this subject we have treated at some length in chapter VII.

In our observations on general pathology and therapeutics, we have endeavoured to explain what we believe to be the true nature of inflammation, and have pointed out some of the more general means of avoiding and counteracting the causes of inflammatory action. In forming many of our inferences, we have been indebted to the recent labours of Liebig, Müller, Matteucci, Flourens, Majendie, and Philip. Although the views advanced have no material bearing upon the homœopathic doctrine of cure, yet if they illustrate this most important of the subjects connected with the morbid conditions of the economy, we shall have done well for medical science. We are aware that Liebig has carried some of his chemical hypotheses farther than facts or logic warrant, but admit that many of his positions, as to the production of animal heat, the metamorphoses of the tissues, the supply and waste of the constituents of the structures, and the phenomena of inflammation, are in the main correct. If he errs in supposing that *all* the phenomena of life are attributable to *chemical action*, that the human body is subject to the same laws as *inert* matter, and that the mass of blood may be contaminated by contact with substances in decomposition with a similar kind of degeneration, he has also shown truly that chemical action has at least an important influence in the operations of the functions. Let not, therefore, his mistakes prevent a rigid scrutiny of his opinions, that we may reject the untenable, and appropriate the true.

Believing and advocating the doctrine of *absorption* and the *topical action* of drugs, we have derived numerous arguments for our views from the recent experiments of Matteucci, Flourens, Rau, Müller, Blake, and Majendie. These profound investigators have demonstrated that most medicinal substances possess well defined *specific* properties, and that it is necessary to their legitimate effects, that they be *absorbed* and conveyed by the blood—as a medium merely—to the tissues for which they have affinity, there to operate (probably upon the sentient nerves), by actual contact. The very numerous and accurate experiments with almost every known drug, instituted by these physiologists upon animals, are quite conclusive as to the point of the absorption and topical action of remedies. We have repeated many of their experiments, and have made a great variety of new ones for the therapeutical illustration of the subject, and have thus formed from facts alone, the conclusions we have here announced, as to the manner in which remedial agents operate. The scope and design of this treatise will not permit a detail of these interesting experiments and their results, but we hope hereafter to submit them to the public. In the meanwhile, attention is invited to the chapter in which we have treated of this subject.

There is another doctrine now entertained by a majority of the physicians of *both* schools, but in no way connected with our theory of cure, to which we have devoted special attention; we mean that so often advanced respecting what are called "*vital properties*" of parts—a *nervous fluid*—a *dynamic influence*, different from the soul. We object to these terms because they are merely arbitrary, and are used to designate properties which have no real existence; because, as Matteucci well observes, they may have no meaning, or may mean everything. The vitalists define disease to consist in an alteration of the *vital properties* of parts. But what are these vital properties? Are they material or spiritual? something or nothing? What is the nature and what are the processes of their influence? We are told that miasmata act dynamically or spiritually upon the vital properties of the tissues; but what are miasmata but minute particles of vegetable matter, subdivided by heat and moisture, and so diffused in imponderable forms through the air? Have these atoms really lost their *material* form or weight, and become *annihilated? Can* a material substance, by any means, be reduced into an *immaterial* nothing, and retain its identity or individuality? In other words, can *matter* be transformed into *spirit?* Surely, no; but we may subdivide substances so minutely as not to be able, by our most delicate tests, to detect them; yet they may have affinities, and be capable of combinations with other atoms, and of producing other *material* effects when brought into contact with certain tissues of the organism. When these material (not *dynamic* or *spiritual*) particles have reached the structures to which they have specific relations, they impress the sentient extremities of the nerves, so that the capillaries and other parts over which these nerves preside, respond to their impression, and there are chills, followed by inflammations. It is evident, then, in this and other analogous instances, that a *material* agent operates *topically* upon the tissues, thus impairing the normal integrity of the parts, but not *dynamically* upon certain (assumed) *vital properties.*

The general principles of allopathy we have briefly considered and compared with those of homœopathy; but want of space has prevented such elaborate discussion of these subjects as was demanded by their interest and importance. We trust, however, that what we have written may attract attention, particularly to the real points at issue between the schools, and that the shafts of our antagonists may hereafter be directed against our distinctive principle of cure, rather than against our doses, and the exhibition of our remedies.

Hahnemann, and some other writers of eminence, have expressed doubts respecting the utility of the common classifications of diseases, since descriptions must necessarily be general and imperfect. In a therapeutical point of view, this distrust of classifications is reasonable, and it has probably arisen from the custom with the old school, of bringing the symptoms of every disease under some one general head, and prescribing for the congeries, however diverse the separate elements, under a particular name. For example, the allopathist called to a patient with febrile symptoms, finds a rapid pulse, a hot and dry skin, headache, pains in the back and loins, oppression at the præcordia, restlessness and irritabilility, foul tongue, thirst, scanty and high-coloured urine, confusion of ideas, and nightly delirium. He is now to arrange these symptoms under one of the general heads of his classification, but is at a loss whether to call it typhus, bilious, or inflammatory, sthenic or asthenic. The case, however, admits of no delay, and he arbitrarily decides that it is *bilious*, and bleeds, vomits, and purges, well knowing that if it proves a *typhus*, he can persuade himself and the patient's friends that it has *degenerated* from one type into another. He forgets to make known that copious venesection, emetics, and cathartics, are deemed by many of the most intelligent of his own school, to be fatal in typhus, and attributes all evils to the versatile and intractable nature of the malady, while complacently appropriating to himself whatever credit may chance to accrue from favourable symptoms. On the other hand, if he had regarded the disease as a *typhus*, and pursued the expectant or tonic treatment sanctioned in his school, and it had proved an *inflammatory* fever, lesions might have taken place, and the patient might have succumbed from the inefficiency of his remedies. Objections of a similar nature apply in a majority of the classifications treated by the allopathist. But while it is unquestionable that all these are useless as guides in the application of remedies, it must be conceded that they enable us to concentrate groups of symptoms under appropriate heads, and thus to arrive more conveniently at just conclusions respecting the nature of diseases. Accordingly, in this treatise, we have adopted a classification varying little from those usually employed, which we believe will facilitate the true apprehension of disordered conditions. We have described the diseases of the separate systems under the same head, instead of treating of *acute* varieties in one part of the work, and of *chronic* in another. This course has been deemed proper on account of the difficulty, in many cases, of fixing the line of demarcation between acute and chronic affections, and for convenience of reference to, and of comparison of the different diseases of the same system.

In arranging the symptoms which demand particular medicines, we have adopted the following classification:

I. External indications, or what have been designated by

Marshall Hall as *physical signs* of disease. Under this head are included all those signs which belong to the external or visible appearance of the patient, and over which he has little or no control, as the expression of countenance, colour and temperature of the skin, pulsations of the heart and arteries, respiration, breath, condition of the digestive and genito-urinary organs, attitude, appearance of the eyes, and of the nose, lips, tongue, mouth, and throat, the secretions, excretions, surface of the body, swellings, (in relation to size, hardness, softness, elasticity, fluctuation, &c.,) the condition of the muscles, (in relation to contractility, strength, debility, and motion,) the voice, mode of expression, and appearance of discharges from the stomach, intestines, bladder, uterus, vagina, nose, ears, eyes, mouth, and from abscesses, ulcers, &c.

These phenomena may always be observed without any descriptions by the patient or his friends, and, in many instances, without the patient's consciousness; and, as we have elsewhere shown, they often indicate with much certainty the character of a malady. In infants and children, and adults, who, from injury or disease, become incapable of communicating their sufferings, they are of the utmost importance, and will frequently be sufficient for our direction in the exhibition of remedies.

II. Physical sensations, including most of those symptoms which are commonly described as *rational signs* of disease. These comprise pains of all descriptions, weaknesses, irritations, oppressions, obstructions, and all other uneasy or unnatural feelings, and all circumstances connected with the approach, continuance, aggravation, or remission of the patient's sufferings. For a knowledge of them, we must rely for the most part upon verbal descriptions; for the best method of procuring which, with truth and exactness, we refer to Hahnemann's Organon, pages 125 to 133, where our venerated teacher has pointed out with great minuteness the necessary directions upon the whole subject of such investigations.

III. Mental and moral symptoms, including the condition of the mental faculties, the disposition, temper, and all variations of the intellectual and moral sentiments, from the normal standard. This arrangement has been adopted with reference to convenience in investigation, and in the selection of remedies. As some diseases are characterized by manifestations of one or more of the external indications, and others by internal pains, or a perversion of the mental and moral faculties, so different drugs develope correspondences in the organism. As it is an object that our remedies should have as exact an affinity as possible to the symptoms, and to these alone, the advantage of this classification of symptoms will be readily perceived.

In descriptions of special symptoms created by different remedies, and presumed to indicate their therapeutical properties, we have drawn freely from all reputable sources, whether European or American. In some instances, we have not hesitated to rely upon drug-symptoms as described by accurate practitioners of the other school, in cases of poisoning. Although little confidence can be placed in their ordinary observations upon the diseased organism in relation to this point, yet symptoms are occasionally recorded during the operation of poisonous doses upon the healthy, which could not well be obtained in any other manner, and which undoubtedly form an important addition to our knowledge of pure drug-symptoms.

A difference of opinion exists in the philosophical school respecting the most suitable form for the exhibition of remedies. Some, entertaining a dread of medicinal aggravations, and believing that the minutest quantity of an appropriate medicine is sufficient to induce a curative reaction, employ, for the most part, pellets that have been saturated with the drug. Others, having less fear of these aggravations, and preferring to know with certainty the precise quality and quantity of their doses, make use of triturations, given dry, in small powders, and dilutions, either mixed with pure water or dropped on sugar.

We have preferred powders and dilutions for the following reasons :

I. A large number of medicinal substances evaporate so quickly, that, after a time, many of their active particles must necessarily escape.

II. Very small quantities of many drugs, when exposed a few weeks to the action of the oxygen of the air, either become entirely neutralized, or so altered in their properties as to be no more identical with the original drug. On this account, it is better to impregnate larger quantities of the medium that less surface may be exposed to the air, and thus to render it certain that a portion of it retains particles of the drug unimpaired.

III. The importance of using our medicines in a form that shall be certain to produce the requisite impressions upon the disordered structures. We deem it an evil of much less magnitude to risk the occasional induction of some temporary medicinal symptoms,—thus being sure that the remedy has reached the affected tissue,—than to administer it in such a form as to produce no visible effects, leaving us in doubt for a time whether an impression has or has not been made upon the affected parts. We do not deny that pellets, in many instances, may prove entirely efficient and satisfactory, and for non-professional use, perhaps they are the safest ;

but since we have it in our power to select forms which are certain to contain the active properties of drugs, and which enables us to prescribe with greater exactness, we think that such forms should be generally adopted by the profession. We are compelled, therefore, with deference to many distinguished cotemporaries, to regard the ideas which have so often been promulgated respecting medicinal aggravations, as altogether exaggerated and unworthy that serious consideration with which they have often been received. For further observation upon this subject, we refer to the chapter on "Attenuations of Drugs and Repetitions of Doses," page 111.

Finally, if some of our opinions clash with those of our homœopathic brethren, we have only to assure them that our only objects have been to ascertain *truth*, and advance our science, and that we shall always be willing to investigate facts, and to listen candidly to arguments, and whenever convinced of errors, to acknowledge and renounce them.

ERRATA.

On page 221, tenth line from the bottom, for "Inclination is also present," &c., read—"Inclination to vomit is also present," &c.

On page 239, Section XII., heading:—for "POPULAR," read—"PAPULAR."

In the Table of Contents, on page 13, Chapter XV is omitted, and Chapter XVI is substituted. Chapter XVII should read Chapter XVI.

On page 35, second line from bottom, read *medendi* for *modendi*.

On page 93, sixteenth line from top, read *attenuations* for *tenuations*.

On page 94, first line, read *Berzelius* for *Bergelius*.

On page 200, tenth line from top, *comma* for *period*, and small *w* for capital W.

On page 305, 24th, 27th, 29th, 30th, 32d, after first, second, third, fourth, and fifth, small letters for capitals.

HOMŒOPATHIC MEDICINES.

Wm. Radde, 322 Broadway, New-York, respectfully informs the Homœopathic Physicians, and the friends of the System, that he is the sole Agent for the Leipzig Central Homœopathic Pharmacy, and that he has always on hand a good assortment of the best Homœopathic Medicines, in complete sets or by single vials, in *Tinctures*, *Dilutions* and *Triturations;* also, *Pocket Cases of Medicines; Physicians' and Family Medicine Chests to Laurie's Domestic* (60 to 82 Remedies)—EPP'S (58 Remedies)—HERING'S (82 Remedies).—*Small Pocket-Cases*, at $3, with Family Guide and 27 Remedies.—*Cases* containing 415 Vials with Tinctures and Triturations for Physicians.—*Cases* with 260 Vials of Tinctures and Triturations to Jahr's New Manual, or Symptomen-Codex.—Physicians' *Pocket Cases* with 60 Vials of Tinctures and Triturations.—*Cases* from 200 to 300 Vials with low and high dilutions of medicated pellets.—*Cases* from 50 to 80 Vials of low and high dilutions, etc., etc. Homœopathic Chocolate. Refined Sugar of Milk, pure Globules, etc. *Arnica Tincture*, the best specific remedy for bruises, sprains, wounds, etc. *Arnica Plaster*, the best application for *Corns*, *Urtica urens*, the best specific remedy for *Burns*. Also, Books, Pamphlets, and Standard Works on the System, in the English, French, and German languages.

CONTENTS.

B

CHAPTER XX.

CHAPTER XXI.

CHAPTER XXII.

CHAPTER XXIII.

Diseases of the Respiratory Organs.

CHAPTER XXIV.

Diseases of the Heart and its Appendages.

CHAPTER XXV.

Diseases of the Brain and Nervous System.

CHAPTER XXVI.

Diseases of the Urinary and Genital Organs.

HOMŒOPATHIC

THEORY AND PRACTICE OF MEDICINE.

CHAPTER I.

A GLANCE AT SOME OF THE PROMINENT MEDICAL DOCTRINES OF THE PAST AND PRESENT.

In tracing the history and philosophy of medical science, from the earliest periods to the present time, we are presented with a singular spectacle. Commencing with those pioneers in medical art, the Asclepiades, we find that there has been a constant series of revolutions, in both the theory and practice of their noble profession, down to the present day. Hypotheses have been advanced and theories established by one generation, to be admired and followed for a time, only to be overthrown and superseded by others, which, in their turn, were doomed to a similar fate. Each generation has looked upon the generations which have passed, commiserating their errors and delusions, while the *present* doctrines have been complacently regarded as correct, and destined to stand unchanged before the investigations and discoveries of all future ages.

The grand cause of all this may be found in the fact that these theories have been based upon conjecture. Certain conditions have been assumed, and certain states of the system supposed to exist, without any real grounds for such assumptions or suppositions. Instead of bringing facts to bear—facts susceptible of demonstration—and raising thus their theories on a solid foundation, each writer has given himself to subtle and abstruse reasonings, taking for his data conjectural agencies and false positions in relation to the structures and functions of the economy.

Notwithstanding, however, the great errors which most of these doctrines have contained, the world has derived, from their promulgation, many useful hints and valuable suggestions. Indeed, as far as close and accurate observation of the phenomena of disease is concerned, the ancients were by no means inferior to the moderns. Nor should posterity depreciate their labours or detract from their fame: for when we bear in mind the paucity of anatomical and chemical knowledge, and the numerous disadvantages under which the earlier writers laboured, we cannot but admire their persevering industry, and behold with astonishment the amount of real truth which they discovered. Whether the moderns, with all their improvements in other sciences, have done as much for the advancement of medicine, is a question which we shall leave for others to decide.

In contemplating the earlier history of medical doctrines, we shall not fail to observe that many of the pathological opinions of Hippocrates have prevailed down to a very late period. Although the "father of medicine" drew largely upon his imagination, in establishing the humoral pathology, instead of trusting exclusively to known truths, yet so great was the influence which he acquired in the medical world, that almost implicit reliance was placed on his views, both pathological and therapeutical, for many centuries. Unfortunately for mankind, many of his most valuable ideas upon these subjects have been unappreciated and almost entirely neglected. During the time of Hippocrates, and even preceding his day, the importance of physical education was much dwelt upon, not only as a means essential for the perfect development and health of the body, but for the strength and activity of the intellect. To Herodicus, who appears to have been the inventor of the gymnastic treatment, ancient Greece was indebted for the superior physical culture which her sons enjoyed, and which conduced so materially to her glory. The principals of these gymnastic schools were men skilled in medicine, and their efforts were exerted to secure for their pupils the highest possible state of physical and mental vigour. Let us endeavour to emulate the practice of these wise men, in this now unappreciated branch of education, and thus, by perfecting the development of the body, in accordance with the dictates of nature, secure to mankind more uninterrupted health and a higher degree of intellectual power.

For some centuries subsequent to the death of Hippocrates, few real discoveries were made in medical science. Although several men like Praxagoras of Cos, Chrysippus, Herophilus, and Asclepiades, advanced new hypotheses, and introduced, from time to time, many innovations in practice, yet, in the main, they were all advocates of the humoral pathology. About a century before Christ, however, Themison, the founder of the methodic sect, made his appearance. Discarding the doctrines of Hippocrates, he advanced the opinion that all diseases arise from two morbid states of the system, which are contrary to each other—a state of *constriction* and a state of *relaxation*. To these he afterwards added a third state, compounded of the two former, which he termed the *mixed* state. The remedies which he considered applicable to these different conditions were relaxants and astringents.

After Themison came the classic Celsus. Without wedding himself to any particular theory, he made judicious selections from the doctrines of his predecessors, and thus instituted his method of practice. He conceived that diseases have a direct tendency to cure themselves, and that the measures of the physician should be so directed that the efforts of nature are not interfered with, and that the remedies applied shall be those which experience has shown to have a tendency to aid the operations of nature. He classified the different species of fever, and discarded the doctrine of Hippocrates in regard to critical days; and by clearing away many of the absurdities of his predecessors, contributed much to simplify and correct the prevailing doctrines. The expectant method of practice owes its origin to this distinguished man.

After Celsus, a few bright stars shone out in the medical firmament, shedding their rays of knowledge over the world, until the second century after Christ, when all were extinguished ; and medicine, in common with the other sciences, slumbered through the dark ages. Amongst those who were most conspicuous in this earlier period, may be mentioned Aretæus, Musa, Scribonius Largus, Andromachus, Rufus the Ephesian, and, finally, Galen. These were all advocates of the humoral pathology, but to the latter must be awarded the palm, not only for the able manner in which he amplified and explained the doctrines of Hippocrates, but for the immense number of practical facts which he gave to science.

At the commencement of the sixteenth century, the attention of physicians began to be more particularly directed to the study of anatomy and chemistry, for the purpose of elucidating the phenomena of disease, and the operations of medicines. About this time appeared Paracelsus, who boldly denounced all previous theories, and ushered into the world a new doctrine, founded upon chemical views. This celebrated person taught that all living bodies were composed of the same elements as other kinds of matter, and were subject to the same chemical laws. These elements were supposed to be sulphur, mercury, and salts; upon a due proportion of which the health of the body was believed to depend, and any variation from this proportion to constitute a cause of disease. He supposed that a certain intelligence which he calls "*archeus*," located in the stomach, presides over these elements, and causes their good qualities to be assimilated to the body, and the noxious principles to be rejected. This "archeus," like the "phusis" of Hippocrates, served an excellent purpose in filling the gap whenever no plausible explanation could be found for the establishment of his absurd propositions.

To Paracelsus, however, is due the credit of having first suggested the true therapeutical principle, to give those drugs for the cure of disease, which in health give rise to a train of symptoms *similar* to those of the malady. But the numerous erroneous notions which he entertained respecting physiology, pathology, and the specific effects of medicines, prevented the practical development of the magnificent idea which his mind had conceived.

The next reformer of note is Sydenham, who flourished about the middle of the seventeeth century. He also was a humoralist, and indulged largely in hypotheses; but he contributed much to the advancement of science. Until this period, the idea had prevailed that disease consisted in an altered state of the fluids. Whether disciples of Hippocrates and Galen, chemists, mechanicians, or metaphysicians, all believed in the humoral pathology. After Sydenham, however, Baglivi and Hoffman appeared, and effected a change of an important character. With Baglivi originated the doctrine that all morbid changes commenced in the solids, and that the fluids were acted upon secondarily. Hoffman embraced the views of Baglivi, but enlarged upon them, and introduced the hypothesis that the "muscular fibre is endowed with a certain degree of tone, which constitutes its healthy state; but from various circumstances, this action may be morbidly impaired, or increased, on the one hand, so as to generate spasm, or morbidly diminished, until it arrives at the opposite condition of atony."

Contemporary with Hoffman, was Stahl, who advanced the idea of the existence of an independent principle, which pervades the body, affording to it its vital energies, and upon which the operations of the economy depend. Not having acquired an accurate knowledge of the chemical operations which are constantly going forward in the body, or any just ideas in regard to the phenomena of life, it is not surprising that this great man confounded the operations of the intelligence with the vital principle. But however erroneous may have been many of the ideas of Stahl, his writings contain some entirely new and very valuable truths.

Stahl supposed that the superintending principle, the "*anima*," presides over the operations of the living organism, having no exclusive location, but pervading every part of the body, causing motion in the organs of motion, sensation in the organs of sense, and all the phenomena of life, by a direct operation or influence upon each particular part. Had he not been imbued with the prevailing absurdities respecting a "vital principle," a "nervous fluid," a "dynamic influence," &c., this idea might have led to splendid results; but instead of recognising in this *anima*, the *soul*, or *intelligence*, he confounded it with certain supposed spiritual or vital properties which pertained alone to the body, and which he supposed were annihilated on the death of the body. Elsewhere we shall again allude to this subject.

The brilliant intellect of Stahl also distinctly recognised the truth of *similia similibus curantur*, and pointed out its advantages over the then universal law of cure, *contraria contrariis opponenda*. Had he, or Paracelsus before him, adopted the course of Hahnemann in experimenting with drugs, in *health* and in *disease*, and by this means accumulated a sufficiency of facts—the incontrovertible arguments in sustaining any theory—homœopathy would long since have been the only system of medicine. Both these reformers were possessed of gigantic intellects—genius, indeed, of the highest order—and the most exalted moral courage, which enabled them to disregard the ex-cathedra dogmas of antiquity; but they lacked that patient and self-sacrificing devotion in pursuit of facts, and that unbounded benevolence and love of mankind, which so essentially characterized the career of Hahnemann. To the latter therefore should be rendered all the credit which attaches to this school of medicine.

Since the time of Stahl, physicians have formed their therapeutical opinions mostly by observation of phenomena, both in regard to the action of the organs and the effects of remedies. The rapid advancement in the knowledge of anatomy, physiology, pathology and chemistry, has conduced much to call into existence better ideas in the entire science, and to do away with the mass of hypothetical rubbish which had been accumulating for so many centuries. From the age of Stahl each man began to rely more upon his own observation in forming his views; and the influence of ancient names and ancient doctrines became less powerful. In the list of innovators may be placed the names of Haller, Sauvages, the "father of Nosology," Brown, Darwin, Bichat, Morgagni, Broussais, and many other writers with whose doctrines we are all familiar.

We have thus briefly alluded to a few of the more eminent men of the past, not to enter into an exposition of their peculiar doctrines, but to illustrate the numerous changes which have occurred in the theory and practice of physic. And how few of the views of all these great men are at this day deemed worthy of consideration! How little have modern writers been able to profit by this labour of centuries, in erecting a true and uniform system of pathology and therapeutics! Indeed, Allopathy at this moment, is entirely destitute of any recognised theory. Her followers, for the most part, are eclectics; each man, like Celsus of old, selecting one idea here and another there, as best suits his taste. Better far would it be for mankind, if they would follow their illustrious examplar still further, and trust more to the efforts of nature, and less to the violent and uncertain effects of their applications.

CHAPTER II.

GENERAL OBSERVATIONS ON PATHOLOGY.

We shall now lay before our readers some views in regard to general pathology and inflammation, which we trust may conduce somewhat to the advancement of our science. In offering these opinions to the public, we have not the presumption to suppose that we are about establishing any new theory; but if we succeed in throwing some new light upon the complicated operations of the human economy, our end will be attained.

We hold that it is the province of the physician not only to cure diseases, but to point out the surest methods of preventing them. In order to do this successfully, it is necessary that he appreciate those conditions which constitute health, so as to guard against the numerous causes of its disturbance. In all living bodies, certain states are essential to this condition. The most important of these states are—1st, a soundness of the organs and tissues; 2d, an adequate supply of nutritious food; 3d, pure air, that the blood in the lungs may be oxygenated; 4th, a calm activity of *mind*, so that the requisite stimulus of the intelligence shall produce its peculiar effects upon all parts of the body; 5th, an avoidance of the various causes which debilitate, overtask, or in any way impair the integrity of the nervous or muscular systems; 6th, the practice of those means which are calculated to ensure the due performance of all the functions, as exercise, amusements, the cultivation of a cheerful temper, bathing, and moderation and regularity in all the habits of life. Thus the functions will be performed in a certain definite and uniform manner, the requisite equilibrium between the *supply* and *waste* of the body be retained, and that state secured by which health is constituted.

It should be firmly impressed upon the mind, that the important offices of respiration, circulation, digestion, assimilation, absorption, secretion, &c., are dependent upon the chemical action which is constantly going forward within the body, between the elements of the tissues and the inspired oxygen on one hand, and a uniform supply, through the nerves, of spiritual stimuli on the other. When these elements are supplied in due proportion, from the food and the air, and no unnatural or injurious cause acts on the system, health must result.

But if the quantity of oxygen absorbed to unite with the elements of the tissues, is insufficient to generate the natural amount of animal heat and motion, or if the strength of one or more of the tissues becomes, from any cause, so impaired as to be incapable of offering the requisite resistance to the oxygen of the blood, *disease* ensues. In the latter case, the impaired state of the diseased structure does not offer sufficient contractile power to prevent the intromission of red globules into those parts which, in the normal state, contain only the ordinary products of the transformations of the tissues. The result is, that the pores are obstructed, the sweat is retained in the system—thus affording additional fuel for combustion, with the oxygen of the blood, and from the unnatural irritation which it causes, giving rise to accelerated respiration, circulation, and the other phenomena of fever. If the resisting power of the tissues continues impaired for a length of time, and the oxygen continues to act as usual, disorganization must follow.

It has been proved that 32½ ounces of oxygen enter the system of an adult daily, the whole of which goes into combination with the elements of the food, and is thrown off through the lungs and skin in the form of carbonic acid and watery vapour.

The same quantity of carbon and nitrogen is supplied to the blood from the elements of the food, to reproduce the organs, which is lost by the waste or exercise of the functions. According to Liebig, "the quantity of oxygen absorbed determines the amount of food necessary to be assimilated."

If then the food be properly digested and assimilated, a due quantity of pure air be respired, and the normal integrity of the organs remain unimpaired, all the structures will act with uniformity, and a healthy equilibrium will result. To ensure a continuance of such a condition, it is not only necessary to avoid all of those causes which are directly capable of disturbing this complicated series of functions, but to make use of those means which tend to invigorate the system, and aid nature in her operations. In civilized life, these sources of disturbance are almost innumerable; but in the progress of this work, we shall endeavour to point out some of the more prominent, and show in what manner they operate in causing disease.

In the healthy state of the system, certain structures possess the power of effectually excluding the red globules of the blood; thus preventing a too great change of matter, which an event of this kind would inevitably produce. This power is dependent, for its normal action, upon the presence of two conditions, viz., an adequate amount of resisting power in the muscular fibres, which modern writers term *contractility*, and an unimpaired state of the nerves, in order that the *intelligence* may communicate with the extreme parts, and thus afford the muscular fibres an additional stimulus or power of resistance. This *stimulus*, of which the nerves are the conductors, is an agent of immense importance in modifying and altering the functions of the structures. In the normal state, its effects are apparent during the various perceptions and emotions which are constantly agitating us. When these two properties remain unimpaired, every office must be duly performed.

It is true that the muscular or the nervous systems may be tasked, for a short period, without detriment; provided, that a corresponding degree of rest be allowed, for the weakened energies to be restored to their natural state. This is witnessed in severe bodily or mental labour; the immediate effects of which are, fatigue, lassitude, and diminished muscular and nervous energy. If this be succeeded by a due allowance of sleep, the waste of force is repaired, and the body resumes its healthy tone. If, however, this labour be continued beyond a certain point, and the requisite quantity of rest be withheld, the capillaries lose their vitality, become incapable of resisting the entrance of red blood, and *inflammation*, with *fever*, is the consequence.

Indeed, it may be laid down as a general rule, that most of those causes which are capable of producing disease, act by impairing the muscular and nervous force of the tissues to such an extent as to render them incapable of excluding the red globules. We know that these globules are charged with oxygen, and that this gas, when in contact with parts of which the elements consist of carbon and hydrogen, must effect chemical changes. It matters not whether these changes are produced within the body or in the air; the results are in both instances the same.

It has been proved by the experiments of Bichat, Buniva, and Philip, that the capillaries of a healthy living animal effectually resist the introduction of fluids, even when a powerful syringe is used; but as the energies of the animal sink, they gradually lose their power of resistance, and allow the fluid to pass into them like "passive and yielding tubes." From these experiments it is evident that the capillaries are the first to lose their vitality, since the large arteries have been observed to retain their contractile power some hours after death. Thus it is that the first manifestations of disturbing causes are upon the surface, in the condition of chills, succeeded in a short time by unnatural heat and inflammation. "Push into the aorta of a living animal, by means of a syringe, different fine fluids, and you will never see them fill the capillary system, or issue by the exhalents; but when the experiment is performed soon after the death of the animal, the fluid will pass readily into the serous capillaries, and pass out by the exhalents, excretory ducts, &c."—(*Bichat.*)

From the above facts it is evident, that whenever the integrity of the extreme parts becomes impaired, the introduction of the red globules is permitted, which, according to chemical laws, must give rise to increased evolution of heat, inflammation and thickening of the capillaries, and consequent obstruction to the passage of the excretions. The retention of the products of the combustion of the oxygen of the blood and the elements of the food, is an additional source of disturbance. These irritating substances induce accelerated respirations, in order that sufficient oxygen may be absorbed to neutralize them, and thus cause exaltation of temperature, increased activity of the organs, and the phenomena of *fever*.

In all our pathological inquiries, it is of the first importance that we have a distinct appreciation of the laws which produce and regulate the phenomena of life, and, as far as practicable, of the influence of external agents in modifying these phenomena.

First, the primary source of animal heat and motion, is the chemical action which takes place in the lungs. Secondly, when the blood arrives at the extreme vessels, other and important chemical changes occur between the oxygen of the blood and the elements of the tissues, giving rise to a great amount of caloric and motion. Now as the combustion at the lungs is the principal cause of propelling the blood through the arteries into the capillaries—so it is probable that the combustion which occurs between the oxygen of the red globules, and the elements of the changed tissues at the extreme vessels, is the principal source of the motive power which forces the blood back through the veins to the heart and lungs. There can be no chemical change without the evolution of heat, no heat without expansion, and no expansion without developing *motive power.* We are obliged to reject the doctrine that the blood is brought back through the veins to the heart, by a kind of *suction,* which this organ exercises on account of the vacuum which constantly occurs within its walls; for if this motive force is all located at the heart, there is no way of accounting for the expenditure of the large amount of motive power constantly generated at the extreme points. We see two parts of the body where combustion is constantly occurring, viz., the *lungs* and the *extreme vessels;* and when we remember that the laws which govern chemical action, whether in the body or the air, are similar, we can appreciate the probable force which must be produced at these extremities.

Since then the animal heat, motive force, &c., are generated principally at the lungs, and in the capillaries, it is evident that any cause which can disturb the healthy operation of either of these important parts must produce immediate and serious disturbance throughout the whole system.

The agents capable of inducing disease here, are numerous and dissimilar.

In hot climates, the atmosphere being highly rarefied, a less volume of oxygen is absorbed at each inspiration, and consequently a less quantity afforded to enter into combination with the carbon of the system. On this account we observe a greater prevalence of liver and bilious affections in torrid than in temperate latitudes. Unless extreme care be taken to avoid animal food, liquors, and other articles which produce a large amount of carbon, this element will so abound, that the rarefied air which is inhaled will be wholly inadequate to effect those changes which serve to retain the equilibrium between the supply and waste.

from the transformations of tissues. Here, a greater quantity of the elements of nutrition are usually assimilated than the inspired oxygen can decompose. This excess of carbon and hydrogen being retained, the nervous and muscular force of the tissues become relaxed and enfeebled, so that from slight exciting causes, diseases of a bilious or congestive character are engendered.

We have said that the same quantity of carbon and hydrogen should be supplied to the blood from the elements of the food, to reproduce the organs, which is lost by the waste or exercise of the functions. That which is not acted upon by the oxygen in the lungs and at the skin, is taken up by the veins, and carried to the liver, which separates those substances (carbon, soda, &c.,) incapable of reproducing the tissues, and finally depositing them in the gall-bladder in the form of bile. When the amount of bile exceeds the retentive capacity of the gall-bladder, the surplus must run over, and a large portion of it be conveyed into the system, thus impairing the integrity of the tissues, and laying the foundation of those diseases incident to equinoctial latitudes.

In cold climates, a state of things the reverse of this ensues. Here, the air being highly condensed, a large volume of oxygen is absorbed at each inspiration, to combine with the carbon of the system, and thus generate sufficient caloric to compensate for that which is abstracted by external cold. For this condition, all causes which can impair the normal state of the digestive organs must be avoided, in order that a sufficient amount of carbon, &c., may be assimilated, to combine with the oxygen and secure the healthy equilibrium. The greater the exposure to external cold, the larger must be the supply of food and oxygen to make up for the loss of heat.

Cold, acting unduly upon the external parts of the body, produces a train of symptoms similar to those caused by miasmata and other noxious exhalations when inhaled. The first effects in either instance, are to impair the energy of the extreme vessels, inducing constriction and chills, to be succeeded by diminished resisting power, and other phenomena which characterize inflammation.

The increased action of the circulatory vessels which usually follows the chills, has been referred by some writers to the stimulus of a greater volume of blood being thrown upon these organs than is natural, and the increased heat which accompanies this exaltation as a result of the action itself. No greater error than this could be promulgated, for the entire source of animal heat is chemical action, and all of the involuntary motions must bear a direct ratio to this evolution of heat. If the skin, lungs, brain, or any other part, becomes from any cause incapable of affording the normal resistance to the oxygen which is constantly brought into contact with it, an augmented chemical action must occur in it, with the invariable concomitants, increased heat, congestion, and fever.

"If a given part of the body is acted upon by continued and intense cold, while the other parts retain their natural temperature, there occurs, after a time, in consequence of the loss of heat, an accelerated change of matter in the cooled parts. The momentum of the force of the vitality, in the parts which are not cooled, is expended, as before, in mechanical motion; but the whole action of the inspired oxygen is exerted on the cooled part. In the cooled part of the body, the living tissues offer a less resistance to the chemical action of the inspired oxygen: the power of the oxygen to unite with the elements of the tissues, is, at this part, exalted. In the cooled part, the change of matter, and with it the disengagement of heat, increases; while in other parts of the body, the change of matter and the liberation of heat, decrease. But when the cooled part, by the union of the oxygen with the elements of the metamorphosed tissues, has recovered its original temperature, the resistance of its living parts to the oxygen conveyed to them again increases, and as the resistance of other parts is now diminished, a more rapid change of matter now occurs in them, their temperature rises, and along with this, if the cause of the change of matter continues to operate, a larger amount of vital force becomes available for mechanical purposes. If the heat is abstracted from the whole surface of the body, the whole action of the oxygen will be directed to the skin, and in a short time the change of matter must increase throughout the body."—(*Liebig.*)

From these facts we are led to conclude, that a large amount of those articles which abound in carbon and hydrogen should be consumed in cold climates, in order that sufficient materials may be constantly furnished to the tissues, to afford the requisite amount of resistance to the inspired oxygen. This is the only means by which the animal temperature can be kept up sufficiently to counteract the loss of heat which is constantly occasioned by external cold. Disease must always occur, when cold so intense and protracted as to impair the normal resisting force of the tissues, is applied to the body, in such a manner as to induce atony in the capillary vessels, chills, lassitude, pain, and other symptoms of inflammation. One of the most prolific causes of disease, in cold climates, is generally active from without, in the form of sudden changes of temperature, excessive exposure to cold when the body is enfeebled, and in going from heated rooms into the cold while perspiring. In these instances the effects produced are, debility and constriction of the extreme vessels, (chills,) lassitude, and pains in the limbs and head, followed, as soon as reaction comes on, by accelerated respiration, circulation, and other symptoms which constitute fever. In regard to the part or organ affected, much will depend upon the predispositions and constitution of the patient. As a general rule, however, the greatest impression is usually made, and the force of the disease expended, upon the most enfeebled part. If the lungs are predisposed to disease, the exciting cause will develop pneumonia. If the brain or digestive organs have been debilitated by excessive exercise, phrenitis or gastritis will ensue. The same principle holds true with regard to the other organs and structures of the economy. If the whole system be in a normal and sound state, atmospheric vicissitudes will commonly merely predispose the organs to a disordered action from whatever farther exciting cause may occur. But repeated exposure to sudden changes of temperature, even in a sound state of the organs, may produce actual disease.

The immediate effect of the above enumerated, as well as of almost all other causes of disease, is to impair the integrity of the capillaries to such an extent as to render them incapable of excluding the red globules. The intromission of these "carriers of oxygen," must of necessity give rise to an increased and unnatural change of matter, with its concomitants, augmented heat and motion. This inflammation of parts produces obstruction to the passage of the excretions, causing them to be retained within the system to serve as an additional source of disturbance. The nature and activity of the exciting cause, the part affected, and the constitution of the patient, will determine the violence and danger of the disease.

It may then be assumed with safety, that the chief influences which predispose to disease in all countries, are extremes of heat and cold, and abrupt changes of temperature.

In cold latitudes, those affections prevail which are induced by undue exposure to cold, and from the condensed state of the air respired. Hence pneumonic and other diseases of a purely inflammatory character.

In hot regions, where the respired air is highly rarefied, we observe those disorders which proceed from a deficiency of oxygen to neutralize the elements of the food, and from exposure to the burning rays of a torrid sun. Liver complaints, yellow and congestive fevers, and those diseases which an excess of carbon, circulating in the blood, would produce, are here found in abundance.

The diseases of moderate latitudes are of a more mixed character, milder, and more subservient to the power of remedies. Here frequent and sudden atmospheric changes exert the greatest influence in disturbing the healthy equilibrium, and in inducing disease.

Every living body possesses a certain definite and

limited capacity of resistance. This capacity can only be taxed to a fixed point, without deranging some of the functions and causing disease. We have seen that the first and most essential requisite to ensure health, is a due proportion between the elements of the food and the inspired oxygen. Now, if moderation and regularity be exercised in all the duties and habits of life, a sound state of the organs and a due performance of all the functions will follow.

Among the parts of which the normal action is highly essential to the well-being of the individual, and upon which disturbing causes usually act, are the digestive and respiratory organs, the skin, and nervous system. Of these, the lungs and skin are by far the most frequently affected. Exposed incessantly to noxious exhalations, impure air, extremes of heat and cold, and sudden changes of temperature, it is not a matter of surprise that most exciting causes operate primarily upon one or both of these important parts.

Almost all inflammations of important organs are ushered in with feelings of general lassitude, pains in different parts of the body, irregular respirations, and chills. It matters not whether the first impression has been made by atmospheric changes—extremes of heat or cold—or undue mental or corporeal exertion: one important phenomenon is witnessed in nearly all instances, that is, a spasmodic or constricted state of the extreme vessels. This constriction of the capillaries is always attended with more or less debility, which prevents them, when re-action comes on, from resisting the intromission of red blood. Thus result obstruction to the excretions, accelerated change of matter in these parts, and the other phenomena of inflammation and fever. Now, whatever organ or structure is most predisposed to diseased action, must receive the greatest detriment from the retained secretions, and the exalted and unnatural action which pervades the system.

According to many authors, the causes of inflammation may be either *predisposing* or *exciting*. If two individuals, one robust, and regular in his habits, and the other delicate, and irregular, be exposed to the same morbific influence, the former will escape, while the latter will receive injury; or, if the exciting cause be still more active, an impression will be made upon the first, which will predispose his system to disordered action, while in the latter, the same influence will cause actual disease. If the morbific agent be very virulent, actual disease may be induced in both instances, but in different degrees of severity.

If this is true, it may be asked why it is that in hot climates the robust are more liable to be attacked with fevers, than those of a feeble appearance? The reason is obvious. The system of the vigorous man abounds with those elements which, when properly decomposed by oxygen, generate the vital activity, and produce strength and health. Now, if he indulges his appetite as usual, while he inhales a highly rarefied atmosphere, disease must of necessity result; for unless the amount of oxygen absorbed into the system be proportionate to the elements of the food assimilated, much of the latter must remain unacted upon, and thus serve to contaminate the blood, and derange the functions of the organs. Here, a cause of disease exists, to which the feeble man is but little exposed. His system is characterized by a deficiency rather than an excess of carbon; his digestive organs being so weak that no more of the elements of nutrition are assimilated than the inspired oxygen can neutralize. Thus, in his case, the equilibrium between the supply and waste of matter is retained, and the organs remain healthy.

In the first example, a strict abstinence from animal food, liquors, and other articles abounding in carbon, with care that the healthy function of the skin be not disturbed, will secure as great freedom from disease as in the other instance. It is not that the robust man is necessarily more prone to disease than the other, but because, either from ignorance or imprudence, he often exposes himself uselessly to an exciting cause to which the latter is not liable.

We contend that the man of stout frame and vigorous constitution is better able to resist diseases in all climates than one of a more feeble organization, provided, that he adapts himself by his habits and dietetic regulations, to the climate in which he resides. The grand essential consists in keeping up a due proportion between the elements of the food and the inspired oxygen. So long as this proportion is preserved, a vast amount of exposure can be sustained in any climate, without detriment.

In northern latitudes, those who are feebly organized, or of nervous or sanguine temperaments, suffer far more than the robust and bilious. In such cases it is necessary that the amount of carbon and hydrogen assimilated to repair the waste of the tissues, be very large, in order to supply the system with sufficient material to resist the action of the absorbed oxygen. Let it be remembered, that disease ensues whenever any part of the body becomes incapable of affording a definite amount of resistance to the action of this gas. The principal source of this resistance is the carbon and hydrogen of the changed tissues; and if no unusual or deleterious causes operate to depress the system, all will be well. If, however, the digestive organs become disordered, and assimilation checked—the body being at the same time exposed to excessive cold—the oxygen will act upon the debilitated structures themselves, in order to find sufficient fuel for combustion, so that the animal temperature may be retained.

The phenomena of life depend upon the constant operation of two antagonistic elements. Their presence and activity, in suitable proportions, impart heat, strength, and life, while the absence of one makes the other an active agent in causing disorganization and death. According to Lavoisier, a quantity of oxygen is constantly being inspired by the healthy adult, equal to 32½ oz., or 46,037 cubic inches, daily, the tendency of which is to neutralize and destroy the elements of the body. To counteract this destructive agent, the elements of the food are constantly being assimilated, and are finally brought into contact with it. In this manner, so long as the proportion between these agents is equal, those chemical changes take place which generate the animal heat, corporeal vigour, and motive power, serving to keep in operation the whole machine and ensure the normal action of every organ. The immense importance, then, of fully comprehending and appreciating the mutual influence, and dependence upon each other, of the respiratory and digestive organs, will be understood by all.

Extreme cold produces disease by permitting more oxygen to be absorbed by the blood than can be decomposed by the products of the metamorphosed tissues. Those parts of the body possessing the least vitality must then be acted upon, and inflammation, and perhaps disorganization, ensue.

Extreme heat generates disease from causes directly the opposite, viz., a deficiency of oxygen, to neutralize the assimilated carbon and hydrogen. In both instances the *nervous* and *muscular* force of the capillaries is so impaired as to render them incapable of excluding from their structure the red globules. Obstruction is thus caused, a large amount of heat is evolved, and the redness, swelling, and pain, which characterize inflammation, is present.

The *primary* cause of most inflammations is a disproportion between the action of the oxygen of the blood and the elements of the changed tissues. The cause of this disproportion—acting upon those parts of the body most susceptible to its influence—gives rise immediately to an impaired state of the nerves and muscular fibres of the extreme vessels, rendering them incapable of preventing the intromission of the red blood. The *first effect* upon these vessels is *stimulant;* indicated by *contraction*, or *spasm*, and *chills*. This is soon followed by the *secondary* or *atonic stage*, which is indicated by distention or congestion of the capillaries with red blood, heat, redness, and other symptoms, which show that the small vessels have lost their power of resisting the entrance of the destructive " carriers of oxygen." The *immediate* cause of the disturbance and disorganization which results in inflamed parts, is dependent solely upon the *chemical action* of the oxygen of the red globules, upon the elements of the affected structure. If this is the case, it will be asked why, then, disturbance and inflammation do not take place from the red globules in the act of *blushing*, or from friction? Because, in these instances, the nervous and muscular force of the capillaries remains unimpaired, and they are thus enabled speedily to throw off this temporary accession of red blood, and resume their normal resistance to its further entrance. It is only by impairing the resisting force of these vessels, in such a manner that the arterial blood continues to enter them, that inflammation can occur.

Even in the act of *blushing*, a perceptible increase of *heat* is apparent, and when the emotion acts intensely, and for a considerable period, phenomena similar to those which occur in very slight superficial inflammations, are observed; as uneasy sensations, fulness, perspiration, &c.

The virulence of the morbific influence acting upon the extreme vessels, and the extent to which their resisting power is impaired, will determine the violence and danger of the inflammation.

It has been ascertained by Wilson Philip and others, "that where the inflammation of a part is greatest, the vessels are more distended, and the motion of the blood is slowest." This is owing, undoubtedly, to the *diminished contractile power* of the capillaries; and it is probable, in inflammations of a congestive character, that this contractile or resisting power is almost entirely destroyed. This fact is important, in a therapeutical point of view, inasmuch as it directs us to apply our remedies in such a manner as to restore the loss of tone of the extreme vessels, as the most direct method of cure. We shall hereafter take occasion to advert to this subject again, when we shall dilate upon it more fully.

CHAPTER III.

DOCTRINES RESPECTING A VITAL PRINCIPLE, NERVOUS FLUID, DYNAMIC INFLUENCE, &c.

All authors upon physiology and medicine, have written much about a "*vital principle*," a "*nervous force*," &c. They speak of them as immaterial and mysterious agents, which perform all of the most wonderful offices in the human economy. They are supposed to be distinct from the intelligence, or soul, and to possess a kind of subtle and mysterious power, which accomplishes all those difficult operations, in the phenomena of life, which physiologists are unable to understand or explain.

"There is not," says Paine, "in the whole range of medical literature, one author, however devoted to the physical and chemical views of life, who does not evince the necessity of admitting a governing *vital principle*, as a distinct entity, distinct from all other things in nature. I say, there cannot be produced *one* author of any consideration, who does not summon to the aid of his discussion *a vital principle*, whenever he touches upon the abstract phenomena of life."

But what proof have we that such a principle actuates the body? What good reason is there for assuming the existence of a peculiar, immaterial power, independent of the soul? "To speak of the vital forces, to give them a. definition, to interpret phenomena by their aid, and yet to be ignorant of the laws which govern them, is doing nothing, or rather is doing what is worse than nothing. It is to attempt an impossibility, it is to content the mind to no purpose, to stop the search after truth. To state that the liver separates the elements of the bile from the blood by means of the *vital force*, is merely to assert that the bile is formed in the liver. By thus varying the expression, a dangerous illusion is established."—(*Matteucci on Living Beings*, p. 29.)

We know that every part of the organism has its

own special function, the physical operation of which we can fully comprehend; but superadded to all of these parts, there is, undoubtedly, a subtle and mysterious agency, the soul. Shall we now add to the system a power which was never disclosed by the Creator—an assumed, vague, and indefinite principle, concerning which we are entirely ignorant, and which can serve no purpose but to cover up ignorance, and securely conceal absurd hypotheses? Shall we pretend that when God created man from clay, and "breathed into his nostrils the breath of life, and he became a *living soul*," he also infused *another principle*, similar to but distinct and independent of the soul?

We are of opinion that much error has arisen from the general idea, that the intelligence is established *exclusively in the brain*, and that it possesses only certain limited powers. That its highest and most important manifestations proceed from this organ, there is no doubt, because the special senses are located here. Sight, hearing, smell, &c., are all recognised and appreciated *here*, because the organs *through which* we are sensible of these phenomena, are in this vicinity; but in other parts it exercises its influence directly and often independently of the brain and spinal cord.

In regard to the nature of the intelligence, or soul, and *how* it acts upon the material parts, to aid in producing the phenomena of life, can never be known. We are able to see its results and appreciate its wonderful influences, but the mode of its operation is absolutely inexplicable. It pervades every part of the body, acting as a stimulus to each organ, giving rise to sensation in the organs of sense, motion in the organs of motion, digestion, absorption, assimilation, respiration, circulation, &c., in the organs provided for these functions.

All modifications or derangements of structure, alter the peculiar effects of this spiritual stimulus; for it acts only through the medium of the organs as they actually exist. All deviations therefore from the normal organization of parts, induces corresponding alterations in the manifestations of the intelligence.

The soul has no particular location, but pervades every portion of the nervous system, exercising a constant and direct influence over every organ and tissue. This is clearly apparent from the experiments of Philip, Stilling, Hall, and others, which prove "that the power of the heart and vessels of circulation is independent of the brain and spinal marrow," and "that the power of the muscles of voluntary motion, vessels of secretion, and peristaltic motion of the stomach and intestines, are independent of the nervous system, and that their relation to this system is of the same nature with that of the heart and vessels of circulation—the nervous power influencing them in no other way than as other stimuli and sedatives do." From these and other experiments, Dr. Philip supposes that the vessels possess "a principle of motion independent of their elasticity," and identical with galvanism.

The experiments of Majendie have shown, "that the hemispheres of the brain and cerebellum may be removed in a mammiferous animal, and it will continue to experience sensation, odours, sounds, and sapid impressions. Vision, however, is abolished."

Dr. Dowler, of New Orleans, has very recently instituted a series of experiments on the alligator, which demonstrate in the clearest manner the position which we have advanced, respecting the peculiar operation of the soul, or intelligence, upon the organism. In one experiment, Dr. D. divided the muscles of the neck, the cervical vertebræ, and the spinal cord, also the spinal cord between the shoulders and hips, destroyed the sympathetic nerve, and removed the intestinal viscera, "yet, for a period of more than two hours, the alligator exhibited *complete intelligence, volition, and voluntary motion in each and all divisions of the body. It saw, felt, and defended itself; showed anger, fear, and even friendly attentions to its keeper, a black boy.*" In another experiment, "the upper portion of the skull, including a horizontal stratum of brain, was removed. The animal performed a series of voluntary motions, intelligibly directed, to ward off injuries. *The entire brain and the medulla oblongata were now removed, without diminishing its power to direct its limbs to any part that was pained by the slightest touch of a pin or knife.* A metallic rod was passed many times within the spinal cord, completely destroying the spinal marrow beyond the hips. It was still found that both voluntary motion and sensation remained, though their manifestations were greatly impaired." Dr. D. concludes from these and numerous other experiments of a similar nature, "that voluntary motion is neither directly communicated from nor regulated by the brain, or the cerebellum; that the muscles, in connection with the spinal marrow, perform voluntary motions for hours after having been severed from the brain; that these motions are not only entirely independent of the brain, but may take place, though imperfectly, after the destruction of the cord itself; *that the trunk, as well as the brain, thinks, feels and wills, or displays psychological phenomena; that the sensorium is not restricted to a single point, but is diffused, though unequally, or in a diminished degree, in the periphery of the body; and that actions which take place after decapitation, as described above, are in absolute contrast to* REFLEX ACTIONS, *being sensational, consentaneous, voluntary, and in other respects dissimilar.*" Is it any more wonderful that the soul conduces to the phenomena of digestion, assimilation and appropriation, when the natural stimuli of these organs are presented to them, than that *sight* is appreciated when the natural stimuli of the eye, the rays of light, are applied to this organ? Is it any more singular that this spiritual stimulus should endow each structure with power to exclude all noxious substances, and *select* each its natural excitant, than that the sense of hearing should only appreciate *one* voice, in the midst of a hundred other voices and instruments, whenever the will so directs?

In order to acquire a correct idea of the functions of life, it is necessary, in the first instance, to contemplate the body as a perfect machine—adapted in every part by a definite and special organization, to receive different impressions according to the nature of the substances or excitants presented, and the offices which they are destined to perform. Without doubt *chemical* and *mechanical* forces exercise an important influence in the operations of this machine. The combustion of oxygen with the carbon at the lungs, and in other parts of the system, must develop heat, expansion and motive power, and mechanical causes may operate somewhat in adding to this force, yet all of these influences are wholly inadequate to accomplish and perpetuate the more complicated phenomena of life. It is then essential that another important agency should be every where present, in order to enable the organs to respond properly to their special stimuli. Consequently we have "superadded to the body" an intelligence which affords a specific stimulus to every part; acting solely through each particular structure as it exists, and modified in its operation according to the modifications or alterations in the organs themselves. If the structure of the eye is injured, an imperfect image will be formed upon the retina, the intelligence will manifest itself through this injured structure, and this sense altogether impaired. If the structure of other organs be altered, so that their natural stimuli cannot be brought to bear as usual, the operation of the spiritual stimulus will be modified in proportion, and disordered function result.

This stimulus acts at each particular part, specifically, and in a measure independently of other parts, causing irritability of different grades in the muscular fibres, and exercising those peculiar properties every where, which have been erroneously attributed to a different and independent principle, the vital force. The influence likewise which it exercises upon the body as a cause of disease has never yet been properly appreciated. This is due, first, to the erroneous supposition that the operations of the soul are confined to simple conception, judgment, comparison, and other intellectual phenomena; and, secondly, to the beforementioned arbitrary custom, derived from antiquity, of attributing all other phenomena connected with the organism, which cannot be explained by the known laws of matter, to the agency of *another influence*, to which Hippocrates gave the name of *phusis*, Paracelsus and Van Helmont of *archeus*, and Stahl of *anima*, but which medical men of the present day designate as the "*vital principle*," "*vital properties*," "*vis vitæ*," "*vis insita*," &c.

But what reason is there for limiting the influence of the soul to the mere intellectual operations? What good reason for supposing that the soul is located exclusively in the brain, and that the rest of the body is only acted upon indirectly and secondarily by this subtle and immaterial power?

In the ordinary waking state, the operations of the soul are manifested directly through the media of *all* the physical structures, and these manifestations are limited in extent and variety, and subject to certain fixed laws, having reference to the *structures* and the *stimuli* acting upon them. Thus, the power and extent of vision is determined by the physical condition of the eyes, and the brain (which furnishes them with bloodvessels and nerves), and the number and intensity of the rays of light which strike the retina. *Light*, in this instance, is the *material stimulus*, which passes through the structure of the eye in the same manner as it passes through an optical instrument, producing the reflection of images upon the retina in a manner analogous to images formed in a *camera obscura*. The soul takes immediate cognizance of these images upon the retina, in precisely the same manner that it recognises the images in the *camera obscura*. It is worthy of note, that these images may be formed upon the retina, and yet the soul be entirely unconscious of them: so may an absent-minded man look into a *camera obscura*, filled with reflected figures, and derive no impressions from them. Without this invisible, incomprehensible, and eternal soul, the eye would be but a mere optical instrument, perhaps taking the first rank amongst such instruments, but entirely on a par with them, and subject to similar laws. No material agent, like electricity, magnetism, galvanism, or what has been termed animal fluid, could ever enable it to appreciate impressions, or perform a single act of intelligence.

Every structure of the organism, whether situated within the cranium, chest, abdomen, or in any other part, is in a similar condition in relation to the soul.

and, without its presence and influence, is subject only to the ordinary laws of matter. Let those chemical theorists who suppose that the organism is actuated by electricity, galvanism, magnetism or caloric, instead of by an *immaterial and incomprehensible* spirit, adduce a single example in which the former agents have acted on matter in such a manner as to produce *an idea*, or anything analogous to reason, and we will then allow that such doctrines are worthy of consideration.

It is the office of the soul to preside over the necessities of the physical man—to guard against and ward off injurious influences, and to respond to all impressions made upon the textures. So long as the normal physical condition exists, and no undue influence is exerted upon the mind, a spiritual, or, (as others will have it,) a *vital* equilibrium, is maintained throughout the system; but if a part be attacked by an enemy in the form of inflammation, or if an undue impression is made upon the mind, this equilibrium is disturbed—the spiritual force is unequally distributed, and disordered action follows.

We append a few examples to illustrate the influence of mental impressions in modifying the action of the tissues: An individual in perfect health, and undisturbed by any external influence, finds himself in a gallery of paintings. At one point a devoted daughter is seen braving the horrors of a foul dungeon, to offer from her own breast sustenance to an aged and starving father, and while we look, the lachrymal glands are excited, and unbidden tears flow freely. At another point, an inhuman monster has seized an innocent child, and is in the act of dashing out its brains against the wall, and while we gaze, the blood mounts to the brain, the cheeks glow with indignation, and the heart throbs violently at the bare contemplation of the outrage. Another tableau meets the view, and we see the executioners in the act of casting a struggling criminal into a den of poisonous serpents, and, as we behold the reptiles coiled up for a deadly spring, with fiery eyes and forked tongues, the blood forsakes the surface, the stomach sickens, the heart sinks, and a cold shudder steals over the whole system. Another scene presents itself: we behold a table loaded with the most tempting viands and fruits, and an immediate change occurs in the salivary glands, the mouth fills with saliva, the stomach indicates its want, and a general perturbation of the digestive system ensues. The mere sight of an epileptic often induces a corresponding complaint in others; the indulgence of bad habits in one member of a family, like snuffling, distortion of the mouth, eyes, &c., frequently bring about the same habits in other members of the family. Violent emotions from sudden intelligence, whether good or bad, often induce *diarrhœas, syncope, catalepsy, apoplexy, mania*, &c.; fear and apprehension are most powerful *predisposing* causes of disease, and when excessive, often act as *exciting* causes, particularly during the prevalence of epidemic and contagious affections, as *cholera asphyxia, small-pox, yellow and typhus fevers*, &c. Protracted grief is a common cause of chronic diseases, like *dyspepsia, jaundice, neuralgia, hypochondria, phthisis pulmonalis*, &c. Intense and exclusive application to any given subject, eventually causes disease of the brain and nervous system, and mental derangement. The hypochondriac, who suffers under the effects of some morbid fancy, continues to feed his malady by pondering over his imaginary ailments; the monomaniac, as he dwells upon his delusion, fans the flame which is consuming him. If an individual in the most perfect health be told by several different persons that he looks pale, haggard, and sick, it is more than probable that the impression will exercise so powerful an influence, that he will actually feel sick, and take to his bed: we have witnessed more than one example of this kind. In disease, also, the manner, bearing and expression of the physician, often exert the most surprising effects upon the patient, either in ameliorating or aggravating his malady. Most diseases are attended with an exalted state of the nervous system, and with a highly sensitive and irritable condition of the mental faculties. In this condition, a doleful expression of countenance, or words of doubt, discouragement and sadness, are often capable of plunging the patient into the most profound state of mental and physical depression, and thus aggravating, to a serious extent, his malady; while on the other hand, a cheerful face, a lively and agreeable manner, and words of hope and encouragement, usually exercise an influence of the most favourable character, and conduce very materially in bringing about a curative reaction of the organism. It should never be forgotten, that courage, hope, confidence, and a cheerful state of mind, are powerful *tonics*, and often enable the healthy system to resist the influence of contagious, epidemic, and other noxious impressions, and the sick organism to combat successfully the destructive effects of disease; while fear, apprehension, grief, despair of recovery, sadness, and depression of spirits, by impairing the resisting powers of the economy, become both predisposing and exciting causes of disease. Show me a physician who has attained a high reputation in the treatment of difficult and dangerous cases of disease, and I will have confidence that he is one who carries a cheerful face; who delights in dwelling upon the bright and pleasant things of life, rather than upon those which are gloomy and dismal; and who does not fail to infuse into his patients, and all around him, confidence, hope, and comfort. The expression and bearing of such a man always act as a beacon of hope, to arouse the sinking energies of the patient, and to encourage him to strive against the depressing influence of his malady. In these, and other analogous instances, it is the intelligence alone which is operated on, and which diffuses its influence, not over any vital properties of the organism, but upon the respiratory, circulatory, digestive, and nervous systems.

We have, then, constantly operating upon the machine, first, what may be termed the *material*, or *natural stimuli*, and second, the *immaterial*, or *spiritual stimuli*, both of which are absolutely essential to the continued performance of the functions. In some parts of the organism, these material excitants must be constantly present, in order that the system may be kept in operation. The heart and blood-vessels, and the respiratory organs, must be incessantly acted upon by the blood and atmospheric air, in order to ensure life. Other parts, like the stomach, lacteals, capillaries, &c., may be deprived of their natural stimuli for a length of time without causing death, but not without inducing derangement of function, and disease. These *material stimuli* not only exercise a highly important influence in the phenomena of life, but it is upon them that morbific and other noxious impressions are often made in causing disease. According to Liebig, "the slightest action of a chemical agent upon the blood, exercises an injurious influence." Any material deviation, then, from the natural properties of the inspired air, or the other stimulants of the organism, must constitute a source of disease.

The other agency exerts a not less important influence over all parts of the body, and gives rise to its manifestations in accordance with the peculiar organization and modification of each structure. This property, which has been attributed to the "vital principle," or "nervous force," is due solely to an *immaterial*, or *spiritual* agency—the intelligence, or soul.

The operation of this intelligence upon the organs, produces that peculiar state which enables them, when supplied with their *material stimuli*, to accomplish their functions. It manifests its power in the capillary system in enabling these vessels to exclude the red globules; over the lacteals, in enabling them to exclude all but the nutritious portions of food; over the organs of involuntary motion, in enabling them to respond with uniformity and regularity to their material excitants; over the nerves of sensation and motion, in enabling them to take cognizance of injurious foreign impressions, and to exercise voluntary motions; over the organs of the special senses, in enabling them to appreciate sight, hearing, smell, taste, and touch. This spiritual influence operates only through the *medium* of these organs and tissues, developing specific and harmonious manifestations, according to the peculiar use and structure of each part. Under its guidance the molecules are appropriated, and become a part of the organism. Through the same influence the system is enabled to resist, to a certain extent, morbific and other injurious impressions. It is this stimulus which endows each tissue with its specific irritability, causing each part to recognise and respond to its own natural material excitant, and offer resistance to the application of all disturbing agencies.

The soul does not leave the body, until the structures are so much injured, that the functions *all cease operation.* Many organs may be destroyed, or rendered incapable of transmitting mental or spiritual impressions, yet the intelligence, entire and unaltered of itself, will still pervade the remaining portions of the organism. It will still manifest itself just so far as it finds normal organs and tissues to operate through or manifest an influence upon. The *material* parts alone may be impaired or obliterated, but so long as there is life, the *immaterial* part must pervade the body, unaltered, although its manifestations may be entirely changed.

The objections which we have advanced in relation to a vital principle, apply with equal force to the arbitrary and improper use of what is termed *dynamic influence.* Hahnemann, when alluding, in his Materia Medica, to the therapeutic power of the sixtieth potency of thuja, remarks in a note as follows: "The discovery that trituration and succussion develop the medicinal properties of drugs, in proportion as these processes are carried on further, until the material substance shall have been transformed, as it were, into medicinal spirit, is of inexpressible value, and so undeniable, that those who, from a want of knowledge of the resources of Nature, consider homœopathic attenuations as mere mechanical divisions of the original drug, must be struck dumb whenever they consult experience."

We regret that the great Hahnemann has fallen into the fatal and universal error of the allopaths, since the days of Hippocrates, *of calling things by their wrong names,* and of endeavouring to *explain phenomena which cannot be explained in the existing state of science.*

Experience teaches, that minute atoms of certain drugs possess more power to impress the structures of the organism, than larger quantities of the same drug in a crude state.

Hahnemann, carrying his trituration and succussion to a great extent, and still finding powerful remedial effects, hastily and quite arbitrarily concludes, that "the *material substance* has been transformed into a *medicinal spirit*." This inference, in our humble opinion, is altogether absurd and unwarrantable. Who supposes it possible, that a *material substance* can be transformed into a *spiritual* one? Who supposes that matter can be reduced, by any process, into any thing but matter, in a different state of attenuation? *Medicinal spirit*, and *dynamic properties*, are vague, and as we believe, absurd expressions, calculated to lend an air of mystery to explicable phenomena, and lead to erroneous views respecting homœopathy. We unhesitatingly assert, from positive observation in many instances, that high attenuations of drugs possess the power to impress the human organism, under certain circumstances; but what reason has Hahnemann, who made this important discovery, to assert that such drugs have been transformed, by trituration and succussion, into a *spirit*, or an *immaterial nothing?* Because the *present* knowledge of chemistry does not enable us to analyze and detect *minute atoms of matter*, has any man a right, for this reason, to declare that a *material substance* can be reduced into a *spiritual* and *immaterial one?* Because our scales are not sufficiently delicate to weigh the medicinal atoms existing in high attenuations, — or our optical instruments sufficiently powerful to see them, shall we say that they absolutely *have no weight*, or *that matter has been annihilated?*

Are there any who suppose, that the miasmatic particles which arise from vegetable decomposition and produce fevers, or the contagious effluvium which arises from smallpox, scarlet fever, or measles, or the vapours which arise from ether, chloroform, hydrocyanic acid, &c., have become obliterated, annihilated, and extinct, so that they possess no form, weight or substantial existence whatever, as soon as they escape into the air in imponderable atoms, though becoming capable of impressing the structures of the body so violently? Are there any who doubt, that in all these instances, *something material* is introduced into the blood, and conveyed to certain textures to produce an impression by contact? Let us rather acknowledge that the still imperfect state of science does not enable us to analyze and detect these minutely attenuated atoms, rather than resort to an absurdity, to cover our want of knowledge, by calling them *spiritual*, *vital*, or *dynamic*.

The great stumbling-block which has always been in the way of real advancement in medical knowledge, is the propensity which has existed to *explain* things which were difficult, or perhaps not at all susceptible, of explanation, by vague and unmeaning terms, instead of acknowledging our ignorance, and awaiting farther developments in science. Shall we say of atmospheric air, azote, oxygen, hydrogen, carbonic acid, and other gases, that they are *spiritual* and *immaterial*, and exercise their effects upon the organism *dynamically*, simply because we cannot weigh or behold the precise form and size of the minute molecules of which these gases are composed? Is it supposed, when air is introduced into the lungs, that an *immaterial* substance enters into chemical combination with the carbon of the blood, changing it from a dark to a bright red colour, and giving rise to the legitimate effects of chemical action between two *material* substances, viz., caloric and expansion? When we pour a heavier into a lighter gas, as for example, carbonic acid gas into common air, is it supposed that the former falls to the bottom and usurps the place of the latter, by some *vital*, *spiritual*, or *dynamic* influence, or simply by the force of *gravity* or *weight?* Or when the balloon, inflated with hydrogen, rises into the clouds, does the phenomenon occur through some *immaterial* agency, or because hydrogen is *lighter* than oxygen and nitrogen, and is consequently forced upwards by the pressure of these two combined gases? And yet the atômic molecules, composing these gases, are as much *attenuated* as the higher attenuations of a homœopathic medicine. Science is even progressed so far, that we can now *compress* certain gases, like the carbonic acid gas, &c., into an *actual solid body*.

Spallanzani, Prevost and Dumas have proved, that if *three grains* of the fecundating fluid of a frog be dissolved in *a pound of water*, a single drop of this solution is sufficient to vivify many thousands of eggs by *simple contact*, and yet this globule of water only contains 2,994,687,500th part of a grain! In this case an infinitesimal quantity of matter has impressed other crude substances *by contact*, in such a manner as to produce *visible changes* in these substances,—a *new action*, and one the most wonderful in nature—*life*. And the *vitalist* of the old and the *dynamist* of the new school, would attribute this phenomenon to some *mysterious vital* or *dynamic* influence: but can these minute *atoms of fluid* be *annihilated* or termed vital, dynamic, spiritual or immaterial properties of the fluid, and the effects resulting from their *contact* with the eggs, vital, dynamic or spiritual effects? Because we cannot handle, smell or taste the atoms dissolved in the globule of water, shall we assert that some mysterious change has been wrought upon this material substance, and that therefore it is not subject to the ordinary laws of matter, but must operate in a spiritual manner? Common sense forbids.

If we take the thousandth part of a grain of an organized substance and submit it to the lens of a powerful microscope, we behold all the separate parts of its organization, and containing within itself innumerable distinct nuclei, which may be again subdivided into perfectly organized molecules, until the microscope can no longer appreciate the separate particles; and yet no one supposes that the substance ever becomes annihilated or spiritualized. Even *one* part in *ten thousand* of chloroform, may be detected in the blood, by converting it at a red heat into chlorine and hydrochloric acid. How true then the axiom of Lavoisieur, *Nothing is lost, nothing is created.*

Away then with all unmeaning expressions, like *medicinal spirit, vital power, dynamization;* let us own our ignorance respecting the precise changes which drugs undergo by trituration and succussion, and their exact *methodus modendi*, and no longer imitate allopathy, by resorting to *spiritual subterfuges*, in order to give some *explanation* of the great facts which Hahnemann has discovered, but which cannot yet be fully explained or understood.

CHAPTER IV.

THERAPEUTICS.

At the present time, there exists no uniform or general system of therapeutics, because there is no theory of disease in which universal confidence is reposed. The medical world being divided into several distinct schools, each inculcating different doctrines concerning pathology and the methods of cure, and all endeavouring to sustain their favourite systems, without much regard to accuracy respecting facts, or to logic in their inductions, it is not surprising that the science of medicine is so often looked upon by the public with distrust and disrespect. We behold the vitalist, denouncing the doctrines of the chemist and mechanician, as inconsistent and highly dangerous in practical operation, while all agree in ridiculing that system which is alone founded on accurate observation of facts, homœopathia.

It is doubtless true that many new and valuable ideas may be derived from each of these conflicting schools by the medical philosopher, whose sole object is truth. Indeed, the coincidence of opinion between the father of homœopathia and many of the most prominent advocates of the vital theory, like Paine, Bichat, Philip, &c., in regard to physiology and pathology, is remarkable. These eminent authors not only agree respecting the "properties and laws of healthy beings," but they concur as to the changes and modifications which take place in diseased states of the organism. Although they entertain totally different views concerning the practical application of remedies, it will be observed that the allopath often adopts the precept "*similia similibus*," in effecting his cures.

Nor are there men wanting,—men who stand high in the ranks of allopathy,—who unhesitatingly place the pathological and therapeutical doctrines of homœopathy, far above those of either the chemical or physical schools.

Thus, Paine, in his "Institutes of Medicine," observes, "It is due to truth (*fiat justitia ruat cœlum*), that the physiologist concede to the homœopath that his hypothetical views may be directed by an enlightened understanding of the properties and laws of healthy beings. Upon this ground, indeed, his hopes can alone repose; and even his doctrines in pathology and therapeutics are a thousandfold better, more rational, more consistent, more conducive to health and to life, than any or all of the tenets of the chemical or physical schools."

We shall not be surprised at this concession, when the opinions of Hahnemann are contrasted with those of many allopathic authors who have written since his day.

The vitalists hold, "that all disease consists in a modification of the vital properties and a consequent change of function, and is, therefore, only a variation of the natural states; that the artificial cure consists in a restoration of these properties and functions by making upon the former certain impressions which enable them to obey their natural tendency to a state of health; that remedial agents of positive virtues operate like the truly morbific, but less profoundly in their therapeutical doses, and that the philosophy of their cure consists in establishing, in a direct manner, certain morbid alterations in the already diseased properties and actions of life, which are more conducive to the natural tendency that exists in the vital properties to return from a morbid to their natural states." (*Paine.*)

Hahnemann and many of his disciples also suppose that* "it is solely the morbidly affected vital principle

* Hahnemann's Organon.

which brings forth diseases; that in disease this spontaneous and immaterial vital principle, pervading the physical organism, is primarily deranged by the dynamic influence of a morbific agent, which is inimical to life. Only this principle, thus disturbed, can give to the organism its abnormal sensations and incline it to the irregular actions which we call disease."

So also of the operation of remedies, Hahnemann has it, "that the brief operation of the artificial morbific powers, which are denominated medicinal, although they are stronger than natural diseases, renders it possible that they may, nevertheless, be more easily overcome by the vital energies, than the latter, which are weaker. Natural diseases, simply because of their more tedious and burdensome operation, cannot be overcome by the unaided vital energies, until they are more strongly aroused by the physician, through the medium of a very similar, yet more powerful morbific agent—(a homœopathist medicine). Such an agent, upon its administration, urges, as it were, the instinctive vital energies, and is substituted for the natural morbid affection hitherto existing. The vital energies now become affected by the medicine alone, yet transiently; because the medicinal disease is of a short duration."

The vitalists of both schools also suppose that natural, morbific and remedial agents, possess certain peculiar and distinct properties which enable them to exercise an influence only on particular parts of the system, through the means of particular nerves; "*passing over, in the fulfilment of this law, various intermediate nerves of more direct anatomical connection.*" (*Paine*).

Although we are not advocates of the vital theory, yet it must be conceded that this principle of elective affinity is so universal, as applied to the operation of morbific and remedial agents, that the influence which any substance of either class exerts upon the organism, may, with propriety, be denominated its *specific effect.* The miasms of plague, of intermittent, yellow, and certain other fevers; the infection of contagious diseases; the virus of hydrophobia, syphilis, gonorrhœa, &c., all produce peculiar and specific effects upon the system. Each of these substances possesses the property of *selecting* that tissue for which it has an affinity, and of expending its entire primary action upon the particular part selected.

It is owing to this specific law, that medical men have been able to classify diseases; to predict with certainty, that exposure to the influence of particular morbific agents, under certain circumstances, will give rise to abnormal action in certain parts, attended with a definite and uniform train of symptoms.

It is also in virtue of this specific law, that medicines may be administered which operate with certainty upon particular tissues and organs, and effect those primary and sympathetic modifications in diseased states of the organism, which enable nature to bring about safe and speedy cures.

One of the chief objections urged against the therapeutical doctrines of homœopathia, is the supposed "fallacy of reasoning from the effects of remedial agents, upon healthy to morbid conditions." * The reason adduced for this opinion, is the fact that *diseased* parts become modified in their action, and far more susceptible to the operation of remedies, than when *healthy*. This last statement is doubtless true, and it stands, as we shall endeavour to show, at the foundation of the homœopathic method of administering medicines.

Although the axiom, "*contraria contrariis opponenda*," is almost universal among the different schools of allopathia, so far as *theory* is concerned, yet in *practice*, the principle "*similia similibus curantur*," is, as we have before observed, not unfrequently adopted.

In order that a clear understanding may be acquired of the manner in which medicines operate, as exhibited by the old and new schools, we shall attempt to demonstrate :—

1st. That most morbific and remedial agents operate *specifically* and with much uniformity, both in health and disease, as causative and curative agents.

2d. That all drugs produce upon the human body *primary* and *secondary* effects, the first of which appear speedily, and when the dose has not been exces-

* Paine's Institutes of Medicine.

sive, are of short duration, and are then succeeded by the second, which are of an opposite character, and permanent.

3d. That in *disease*, the susceptibility of the affected parts to the action of remedies, is vastly greater than of the same parts when in *health*.

4th. That medicines, when administered in a crude form and in large doses, according to the doctrines and ordinary practice of the old school, whether applied directly to the diseased organ or tissue, or to a healthy structure remote from the diseased part, are not only incompetent to eradicate disease in a safe and speedy manner, but generally serve to aggravate the already existing symptoms, and by superinducing additional medicinal disease, complicate, to a serious extent, the original natural affection.

5th. That when a curable natural disease has been excited in the organism, attended with a definite train of morbid symptoms, a medicine capable of causing (in large doses) a similar series of symptoms, in health, will become speedily curative of such natural disease, if administered in the attenuated doses of homœopathy.

CHAPTER V.

SPECIFIC EFFECTS OF MORBIFIC AND REMEDIAL AGENTS.

All are aware that the naturalpoisons of certain animals; the virus of hydrophobia, syphilis, gonorrhœa and sycosis; the miasms of plague, and of yellow, typhus and intermittent fevers; the infection of contagious diseases, &c., exercise, when introduced into the circulation, *specific effects* upon the human system, and give rise to definite and easily recognised symptoms.

There are other morbific agents, like intense and protracted heat and cold, atmospheric vicissitudes, excessive physical and mental exertion, violent emotions, &c., that operate in a more general, but not less specific manner. Their operation, when carried so far as to become morbific, induces debility of the nervous system; loss of irritability in the capillary vessels, which makes them incapable of excluding the red globules, and as a consequence, developing augmented heat, swelling, redness, and pain.

Eberle, in his Practice of Medicine, asserts that "the influence of almost every agent, whether morbific or medicinal, appears to possess a kind of elective affinity for some particular organ or structure of the organization." This fact is so apparent, in regard to *morbific* agents, that it scarcely requires notice; but there are many authors who still entertain doubts respecting the specific action of *medicines*. An attentive examination of the following facts, must, however, settle the question satisfactorily in the minds of all impartial inquirers.

Remedial agents operate in the same specific manner, both in health and in disease; but with the difference that in the latter condition, only a very minute quantity of the specific agent is requisite to produce a salutary impression, on account of the augmented susceptibility to remedial impressions, which diseased parts acquire.

1. "A medicine administered in certain doses, and during a certain period of time, can produce pathological lesions analagous to those that characterize certain diseases."

2. "This same medicine, given to a healthy individual, on the same principles, produces the characteristic symptoms of the diseases whose pathological lesions it gives rise to."

3. "This medicine is a specific of these same diseases."

4. "Specificity is not therefore an isolated fact, but the law which should guide medical treatment."—[Des Specifiques en Médecine, Paris, 1847; par L. J. J. Molin.]

The experiments of Majendie, Blake, Pereira, Rau, Liebig, Müller, Orfila, Griesselich, Molin, Matteucci, and Philip, prove conclusively, that most morbific and remedial agents produce their effects after having been absorbed into the blood. It has also been proved with equal certainty, that foreign substances, when absorbed into the circulation, are conveyed to those structures for which they have a special affinity, and there make a specific impression, which modifies the function of the part, according to the nature of the agent and predisposition of the individual. The blood serves as the conducting medium merely, and if the absorbed substances do not possess the power of exercising an influence upon any tissue, they may continue to circulate through the lungs until the inspired air gradually neutralizes them, or they may remain for an indefinite length of time,(as sometimes happens in cases of hydrophobic virus and fever miasms, without affecting the system,) and yet retain their activity. The reason of this may be, that the tissues upon which they act, are in so perfect a state of vigour, as to be able to resist the power of the noxious agent, until some cause shall enfeeble the part to be affected, and thus predispose it to receive the injurious impression.

It will not be denied, that both in healthy and diseased states of the organism, cantharides, copaibiæ, cubebs, the turpentines, juniper, squills, colchicum, digitalis, apis, mel, cajuputi, and most other diuretics, produce their effects by acting directly, or *specifically*, upon the kidneys, as topical irritants; that the preparations of mercury, nitric acid, iodine, &c., exercise a direct and *specific* action upon the glands, mucous membranes, and skin; that senega, phosphorus, ipecacuanha, tartarized antimony (whether taken into the stomach or injected into the veins), and many of the resins, exercise a specific action upon the lungs; that aloes, gamboge, colocynth, act specifically upon the stomach and rectum, while senna, rhubarb, scammony, jalap, and certain other cathartics, spend their effects upon all portions of the intestinal canal; that ergot, savin, pulsatilla, madder, tansy, &c., operate *specifically* upon the uterus; that belladonna, opium, stramonium, strychnia, hyoscyamus, conia and coffea, impress specifically some portion of the nervous system; and, in a word, that almost every drug impresses certain tissues in preference to others, and that a knowledge of the manifestations to which these different impressions give rise, can alone enable us to combat diseases. That the above enumerated substances are actually absorbed, and exert a topical effect, is apparent from the fact that they have often been detected in the blood, secretions, excretions, and even the solids of the body.

It is asserted by Flourens, "that opium acts *specifically* on the cerebral lobes; that belladonna, in a limited dose, affects the tubercula quadrigemina, and in a larger dose the cerebral lobes also; that alcohol, in a limited dose, acts exclusively on the cerebellum, but in a larger quantity, it affects also neighbouring parts; and, lastly, that nux vomica more particularly affects the medulla oblongata." He also states, "that in birds it is possible to observe, through the cranium, changes of colour (some alterations in the vascular condition of the parts) which these agents effect in the brain."

Pereira, in his Materia Medica, also declares that "the ammoniacal, empyreumatic, and phosphoric stimulants, containing ammonia and its salts, the empyreumatic oils, phosphorus, musk, and castoreum, all agree in producing a *primary* and *specific* effect on the nervous system, the energy and activity of whose functions they exalt. On account of their *specific* influence over the nervous system, they are administered in various spasmodic or convulsive diseases, especially in hysteria, and also in epilepsy and chorea. The beneficial influence of some of the vegetable tonics (as cinchona) in intermittent diseases, should probably be referred to the *specific* effects of these agents on the nervous system. The preparations of arsenic, silver, copper, bismuth, zinc, &c., are usually, but, as I think, most improperly, denominated tonics. They are agents which, in small and repeated doses, as well as in large and poisonous doses, *specifically* affect the nervous system."

We are also assured by Liebig, in his work on animal chemistry, that "we can by remedial agents exercise an influence on every part of an organ by substances possessing a well defined chemical action."

It will be observed that we have adopted, in part,

the views of Müller, in regard to the operation of morbific and remedial agents. This distinguished physiologist supposes that the blood is only the "vehicle of introduction," and that as it passes through the tissues of different organs, the medicinal particles with which it is impregnated "act on one or more parts which are endowed with a peculiar susceptibility to their influence. He also supposes "that a change is effected in the composition of the organic matter of the part acted on."

That medicinal substances induce modifications in the functions of the organs, by topical action, is proved, as we have before observed, from the fact that the medicinal particles are often found in the excretions of the affected part. The inference must follow, from a careful consideration of all the facts bearing upon the subject,* that the functions of the organism are generally morbidly altered by the direct action of noxious substances.

In regard to the mode in which these substances operate, we suppose that their primary impression is made upon the sentient extremities of the nerves, impairing their integrity, and rendering them incapable of conducting the spiritual stimulus (which is an essential condition of *irritability*) to the extreme vessels.

It must be borne in mind, that in all inflammations, the capillaries are the "instruments of disease;" that the primary impressions of all deleterious agents are made upon these delicate structures, and that all of our remedies must be directed with reference to the state of these vessels, in curing disease. "Upon these vessels all remedial agents exert their curative effects, whether by their direct action, or through the instrumentality of the nervous power."—(*Paine*).

The extreme terminations of the nerves are so highly impressible, that the very minutest quantity of a specific agent is capable of producing prompt and decided effects, while the same agent would prove powerless, if applied to the *larger* nerves. Thus it is

* For further proofs respecting the doctrine of absorption and topical action of drugs, see the experiments of Müller, Tiedemann, Gmelin, Majendie, Matteucci, Liebig, Rau, Flourens, Dutrochet, Blake, Herring, Mayer, Christison, Orfila, and Dumas.

that imponderable substances and mental emotions are so often the causes of disease. Here we have one reason, also, why medicines, when administered homœopathically, produce those happy modifications in the affected parts which dispose them so speedily to recovery. In connection with this, if we take into consideration the extreme sensibility which diseased parts acquire to the operation of medicinal agents, we shall be unable to doubt the propriety of administering medicines according to the homœopathic method.

Müller supposes that when impressions are made by specific substances, "changes are effected in the composition of the organic matter of the parts acted on." Of this, however, there is no satisfactory evidence. On the contrary, we know positively that very many cases of disease occur without giving rise to any change whatever in the organic construction of the parts affected.

One of the first indications generally observable in an abnormal state of an organ or tissue, is a loss of tone, or irritability and perverted function of the capillary vessels. In the experiments performed upon the blood, by Philip, Alston, and Gallois, it was observed that the smaller vessels were the first to succumb to foreign influences, and then, if the potency of the agent were increased, the larger vessels would become affected.

Now, when we reflect, that *irritability* is dependent, 1st, upon a normal organization of parts; 2d, a regular and uniform supply of *natural material stimuli*, the arterial blood, &c.; and 3d, a healthy action of the mind, in order that the *spiritual stimulus* shall make its due impression, we can readily conceive how slight a cause, moral or physical, morbific or remedial, may disturb or impair this irritability, and thus induce disease. "Every part of the organism depends, for the performance of its proper functions, on the receipt of arterial blood and of nervous influence; so alterations in the supply of either of these essentials may modify or even suspend the functions of a part." *

* Pereira's Mat. Med.

The nerves are simply the *conductors* of the intelligence, and so long as their integrity, tone, or conducting power, remains unimpaired, this essential condition of irritability will remain. If, however, any cause acts upon them in such a manner as to injure or destroy this important property, the stimulus of the superintending spirit, or as the vitalist would say, the nervous power, is not transmitted, and, as a consequence, disease must result from the absence of one of the important requisites of irritability or contractility.

Injurious impressions may be made upon the extreme nerves, either by deleterious matters absorbed into the blood, and brought into direct contact with them, or by certain external applications, like electricity, magnetism, heat, cold, and exercise.

Inflammation may be excited by the operation of either of these causes, by a primary effect upon the sentient extremities of the nerves, which induces loss of tone and conducting power, and as a consequence, loss of irritability and resisting power in the capillaries. This impression is not made, as some theorists would have it, upon an *immaterial principle*, but upon something material, tangible, and demonstrable, viz., the nerves themselves.

Poisons and other noxious substances, when taken into the blood, are rapidly conveyed to all parts of the body; and when they arrive at the structures, upon which they have a specific action, nature makes an effort to expel them through these particular parts. If the substance be active in its effects, the impression which is made upon the minute nerves of the part, will be in a corresponding manner severe. The length of time required for foreign substances to produce their effects, is extremely variable. Some articles, like several of the salts of potash, juniper, the turpentines, asparagus, indigo, madder, &c., are expelled through the urinary organs in a few moments, while other substances may remain in the blood for an indefinite period of time, or until some predisposing cause shall act upon the system in such a manner as to augment its susceptibility, and place it in a condition to be affected by the morbific agent. In some instances, the morbific agent remains harmless in the circulation, for months, and even years, when suddenly, some tissue becoming enfeebled and incapable of resisting the action of the specific agent, the disease, in all of its violence, bursts forth. In cases like these, it is quite evident that the injurious impressions cannot be made upon the *vital properties* of parts, for the effects must be sooner propagated and rendered apparent. Neither can we suppose, with the advocates of the chemical hypothesis, that the constituents of the blood become altered and contaminated with the peculiar miasms or virus, for such blood introduced into the circulation of a healthy individual gives rise to nothing like the original disorder. We again repeat, that the blood is simply the vehicle which conveys the poison, and that no effects are produced, until the structure for which the poison has the greatest affinity has become ready, from some predisposing cause, to receive the impression of the deleterious agent, and thus is specifically affected.

Why it is that morbific and remedial agents *select* particular organs and tissues to exert their action upon, we do not know; but that such is the fact, all medical observers will bear witness. Nor is it more surprising than that some of the natural fluids, like the urine, gastric juice, bile, &c., remain with impunity in some parts of the body, while if they gain admission to other parts, as the cellular substance, or peritoneum, they occasion inflammation, sloughing, and death.

Some writers attribute the operation of medicines to an electrical influence. "All bodies," says Bischoff, "by contact with each other, act as electrics, without, however, necessarily undergoing any chemical changes. Therefore, when a medicine is applied to the organism, its action is electrical." The instantaneous effects of very minute quantities of hydrocyanic acid, sulphureted hydrogen, and carbonic acid gases, and of strychnia, conia and morphia, certainly bear a close resemblance to the overwhelming shock of lightning, and go far to sustain this opinion.

Whether remedies act as *topical stimulants*, or as *sedatives*, *dynamically* or *electrically*, may admit of a question; but it is quite certain that their primary impressions are made upon some portion of the nervous system, and generally on the extreme nerves of the parts impressed, and those modifications of irritability produced, which exert either a salutary or injurious influence over the part acted on. Even in those instances where the primary influence has been exerted upon some portion of the cerebro-spinal or ganglionic systems, the capillaries receive an almost simultaneous impression through the sympathetic nerves, which at once gives rise to disordered function in these important vessels.

Absorption may take place in almost every structure of the body—lymphatics, lacteals, blood vessels, skin, cellular substance, &c. ; but many circumstances exert an influence in deterring the rapidity of the process, as well as the quantity absorbed.

Müller asserts that "the more the matters are soluble, divided and fitted for entering into combination with the organic juices, the more easily are they absorbed." Absorption also varies according to the quantity of liquid which exists in the organism, and is in the inverse ratio of the plethoric state of the animal." Dutrochet and Edwards have demonstrated that animals absorb water most rapidly after transpiration. Majendie and Orfila have proved that dogs having lost large quantities of blood, rapidly absorb strychnia and die ; while those into whose veins large quantities of water had been injected, remained unaffected by the same amount of the poison. These facts will enable us to understand why diseases are not easily contracted when an individual is in vigorous health, or after a *full meal.*

"Within certain limits, absorption is in proportion to the temperature of the absorbing body, and of the body absorbed." (Matteucci.) Therefore, inflammations of all kinds, fevers, &c., facilitate absorption. For this reason it is, that in acute inflammatory diseases, the higher attenuations prove efficient, which would be productive of no effect in the ordinary condition of the system.

Although, therefore, morbific or medicinal agents may be absorbed into the mass of blood, on account of protracted hunger and thirst, or other cause, it does not follow that any manifestations will be apparent;

for if the whole organism be in a sound and vigorous condition, it will resist the specific action of the substance for an indefinite period. Therefore it is that certain poisons often remain latent in the circulation for months, and even years, without being able to exercise their specific action, until some part of the system becomes disordered in such a manner as to be incapable of longer resisting the noxious influence. In many cases of absorption of morbific substances, where the organism is healthy, it is probable, from their constant circulation through the lungs, where they come in contact with that powerful decomposing agent, the inspired oxygen, that they become neutralized after a time, and their noxious qualities destroyed. On the contrary, if the following conditions are present, viz., irritation, inflammation, fever, deranged digestion, debility from loss of fluids, insufficient nutriment, &c., the morbific agent will be absorbed with facility, and speedily produce its specific impression.

CHAPTER VI.

PRIMARY AND SECONDARY ACTION OF DRUGS.

Homœopathy teaches that the impressions which drugs produce upon the organism, in health and in disease, are analogous in their character. But there is this important difference between healthy and diseased structures, that large quantities of the drug are required to produce appreciable impressions upon the former, while the susceptibility of the latter is so morbidly augmented that the most minute atoms of the medicine are instantly effective. Not only so, but even the natural material stimuli of the structures cannot be tolerated, but become immediate and additional sources of disease, and if persisted in, of fatal disorganization.

If, then, we desire to know the precise effects of drugs in disease, it is necessary to prove them by taking large doses in health—doses sufficiently large to affect the structures sensibly and decidedly. Even if *contraria contrariis opponenda* be adopted as the law of practice, this is an important discovery, for we may then administer the remedies with a full knowledge of the parts they impress, and of the exact symptoms they induce, and thus remove allopathy a single step from empiricism. Some eminent writers of the old school have distinctly recognised the importance of this subject: Thus, Dr. Paris, in his Materia Medica, remarks, that "observation and experiment upon the effects of medicine are liable to a thousand fallacies, unless they are carefully repeated under the various circumstances of *health* and *disease*, in different climates, and on different constitutions."

Professor Dunglison, on the seventh page of his New Remedies, says, "To treat disease methodically and effectively, the nature of the actions of the living tissues, in both the healthy and morbid conditions, must be correctly appreciated; the effects, which the articles of the Materia Medica are capable of exerting under both those conditions, must be known from accurate observation, and not until then can the practitioner prescribe with any well-founded prospect of success."

Pereira assures us, "that in order to ascertain the action of remedial agents on the living body, it is necessary that we examine their influence both in *healthy* and *diseased* conditions. For, by the first we learn the positive or actual power of a medicine over the body; while, by the second, we see how that power is modified by the presence of disease."—(Pereira's Mat. Med. and Ther. Vol. 1, p. 126.)

Other equally distinguished allopathic writers now entertain the same views upon this point, but without taking into consideration some very important circumstances connected with the provings. We have reference to the great fact inculcated by Hahnemann, that all drugs exercise upon the organism *two effects*, a *primary* and a *secondary*, and that these secondary effects are always the *reverse* of the primary. A knowledge of this truth will enable us to classify both the primary and the curative results of medicines, and thus more clearly to appreciate the phenomena which should guide us in their application. The primary symptoms make their appearance soon after the medicine has been taken into the stomach, and continue for a longer or shorter period, according to the magnitude of the dose, and the condition of the health, after which they disappear, and the secondary or opposite series of phenomena manifest themselves, and remain until the organism recovers its equilibrium. But in a few instances the power of drugs is displayed in such a manner that these primary and secondary effects appear in alternation for a considerable time, when the primary symptoms yield to the secondary, or serious organic derangements ensue. The mode of operation in these instances, is probably analogous to that of the miasm of intermittent fever, in producing alternate chills and heat. Medicines of this description are termed *polycrests*.

No one who has candidly tested the operation of drugs with reference to this law, can for an instant deny its truth and importance; and the law applies not only to large doses of drugs, but to every other cause which unduly impresses the structures; that is, in such a manner as to disturb that healthy balance in the operations of the organs which constitutes health. Let us examine the ordinary effects of *cathartics* in health: first, the mucous membrane of the intestinal canal is irritated or inflamed, and the natural consequence of inflammation follows in the form of increased mucous and serous secretion, increased peristaltic action, and a painful and loose state of the bowels: this is the *primary effect*. After several thin discharges from the bowels, a *debility* and a *depression* of the parts occur (bearing an *inverse* ratio to the amount of *primary inflammation*); the peristaltic action becomes impaired or suspended, and *constipation* results as the *secondary* effect of the drug.

There is no exception to this rule, unless the cathartic operates so violently as to produce a permanent inflammation and disorganization of the mucous membrane, in which case the primary symptoms may be continuous and constitute a permanent affection. Even in cases of this kind, however, partial reactions sometimes occur during the course of the malady, and secondary symptoms are manifested, in the form of constipation alternating with diarrhœa. These violent primary symptoms rarely continue beyond a few days without resulting in serious structural lesion, or a healthy and permanent reaction.

The *primary* effects of *opium*, in large doses, are to induce sleep, lessen nervous and muscular sensibility, cause agreeable dreams, and diminish or suspend all of the secretions, with the exception of perspiration, which is augmented. If the quantity taken has been moderately large, a pleasurable excitement for a short time precedes the soporific influence, as a primary symptom. These first results continue from twelve to forty-eight hours, according to the magnitude of the dose, when the organism reacts; the exhilaration is succeeded by depression, the sopor by constant and prolonged wakefulness, morbid irritation of the whole system, a return, in preternatural quantities, of all the secretions which had been suspended, and a suppression of the cutaneous secretion, which had been morbidly augmented; and the *secondary* effects of the drug are thus manifested.

So long as *diuretics* continue to irritate the kidneys, they are forcibly stimulated to pour out an unusual quantity of urine; but as soon as the specific is omitted, the organism reacts against the temporary irritation set up by the medicine, and a corresponding diminution of the urinary secretion follows, until the organ recruits from the previous overaction, and the disturbed equilibrium is restored.

The *primary* operation of *stimulants* gives rise to an exaltation of the mental and physical powers, while a corresponding depression and abasement invariably result as *secondary* consequences.

The *primary* operation of *digitalis*, in large doses, is to *retard* the action of the heart and arteries. The reaction of the system against the drug, or the *secondary* effect, is an augmentation of this action.

The *primary* symptoms caused by *aconite*, are intenser action of the circulatory vessels; the *secondary* consequence consists of a reduction of the pulsations, in some instances as low as thirty-five in the minute.

The *primary* effect of intense cold, is to stimulate and invigorate the whole system; and the *secondary* results are loss of muscular and mental energy, stupor, and death.

This law of *primary* and *secondary* action applies not only to *medicinal*, but to a large proportion of *morbific* agents. On this supposition we may readily account for the remissions and exacerbations which are observed in most fevers. It is only when the morbific influence has been very active, and the resulting inflammation violent, that no reactions or remissions occur. It may nevertheless be set down as a general law, that no structure of the human body can be called into preternatural action, or stimulated *beyond a given point*, without a speedy tendency to reaction on the part of the organism. In severe forms of disease, this reaction may not be apparent for weeks, and perhaps until organic lesion occurs; yet, sooner or later, some reaction, with secondary symptoms, manifests itself. There is a healthy point in the functional actions of the organs—an equilibrium, if we may be allowed the expression, of the respiratory, circulatory, digestive, absorbent, assimilative, secretory, and excretory functions—which cannot be disturbed with impunity. Stimulate one of these beyond its natural point, and a corresponding depression must necessarily ensue before the normal balance is restored. Each tissue possesses only a definite amount of resisting power, and therefore every undue expenditure of this power entails future debility. Nature is constantly striving to maintain the functions in their natural condition, and this she accomplishes by inducing in the different parts *a reaction the reverse of the disturbing cause,* and bearing an *inverse ratio to this cause.* The amount of strength and resisting power which is acquired from the food, &c., is fixed and definite; and this force is expended in limited and definite quantities throughout the economy, and thus secures the healthy performance of the functions.

The practical deductions which legitimately arise from these views of this subject, are of the most interesting character, as regards the application of remedies; for if the ideas which have here been adduced are correct, it is plain that the antipathic doctrine of cure is erroneous, while the truth of the homœopathic becomes equally apparent.

CHAPTER VII.

SUSCEPTIBILITIES OF ORGANS AND TISSUES TO THE INFLUENCE OF REMEDIAL AGENTS, VASTLY GREATER IN DISEASE THAN IN HEALTH.

ONE of the principal arguments which has been adduced against Hahnemann's system of therapeutics, is the supposed fallacy of judging of the effects of medicines in *disease*, from their operation in *health*. It is considered that the modifications which occur in what are termed the "vital properties" of parts, in a state of disease, also alter the action of remedial agents in a corresponding manner.

The fact is incontrovertible, that tissues in a state of inflammation, do acquire properties very different from what they possess in the normal state; but respecting the nature of these acquired properties, numerous facts go to prove, firstly, that the parts actually inflamed, become extremely sensitive to the impressions of specific remedies; and, secondly, that the facility of absorption is promoted throughout the whole system. The recent experiments of Müller and Matteucci have demonstrated the fact, that in proportion as the tone of the nervous and muscular systems becomes impaired, or inflammation obtains, up to a certain point, just in the same ratio will absorption be promoted and foreign agents exercise their influence.

We have seen that inflammation consists in a "congestion of the capillaries," induced by debility, and the want of resisting power in these structures, to exclude the arterial blood, and that the effects of inflammation of a particular organ upon the general system, are lassitude, pains, and other symptoms which indicate diminished nervous and muscular energy. That condition, therefore, which is termed *erethism*, is not, as is sometimes supposed, indicative of increased nervous energy, but results directly from loss of strength.

In health, the capillary vessels possess the power of

excluding all of those constituents of the blood except the colourless fluid which is their natural stimulant. Although the capacity of these minute tubes is sufficiently large to admit the red globules with ease, yet they are endowed with a peculiar property which enables them to resist their entrance.

Any cause, therefore, capable of impairing this *natural irritability*, becomes a source of debility and inflammation.

It has been proved that, in health, most medicinal substances may become absorbed into the blood; but unless they possess some peculiarly noxious qualities, they will act upon those parts for which they have a specific affinity, and be thrown off in the form of excretions, causing in their passage through the structure on which they act, only a slight and perhaps unappreciable irritation.

When taken in disease, these same substances are absorbed with far greater facility, and exercise the same specific affinity for particular parts as in health; but with the difference, that they make impressions upon the inflamed tissues, far more energetic and strongly pronounced, than when taken in a healthy state of the organism. Nor is this augmented susceptibility to the influence of remedies, confined to the tissues primarily affected, but the whole system becomes far more impressible than during health. It is a well established law, that no one structure can be inflamed, without giving rise secondarily to sympathetic symptoms in other parts of the economy. It matters not whether the part *primarily* affected, be the lungs, stomach, skin, or any other structure, the whole system may be ultimately disordered, through remote, contiguous or continuous sympathy. The connection between the different parts of the human body, through the media of the sympathetic nerves, is so close and direct, that no organ can be acted on by a morbific agent, without developing secondarily sympathetic symptoms more or less violent, according to the nature of the agent, the severity of the primary impression, and the constitution of the individual. All of the organs are so designed and constructed by the Supreme Architect, that, in health, a certain harmony of action prevails throughout every part of the machine, causing every function to be executed with uniformity, so that no disturbance can accrue to any single part, without impairing this healthy equilibrium.

Paine advances the following sentiments, which have a powerful bearing upon this subject. Probably no allopath has ever written whose theoretical views coincide so nearly with the doctrines of Hahnemann, as those of this distinguished author ; and we only wonder that their practical deductions should differ so materially.

"It appears therefore to be a most important law, that *morbid states* call into operation the function of sympathy among organs, which, in their *natural state*, manifest but feeble, and perhaps no direct relations whatever; and that in consequence of morbid changes, remedial agents will operate sympathetically through the stomach, &c., upon remote parts, when they would have no such effect in the healthy state of the organs. New vital relations being developed by disease, our remedies continue to operate through those acquired relations so long as they exist."

Again, "In proportion, therefore, as the susceptibility of the system at large is increased by morbid changes, or predisposed by morbific influences, so, in a general sense, will the alterative action of remedial agents be felt in a corresponding manner."

Again, "It is one of the most important laws in medicine, that the susceptibility of tissues and organs to the action of remedial agents, is more or less affected by disease. Many agents which operate powerfully in certain *morbid* states, and in certain doses, both locally and sympathetically, may be perfectly inert in the *natural* states of the same organs."

Finally, "It is worthy of repetition, that such is the analogy between morbific and remedial impressions, that the organs which sustain the former are thus rendered susceptible of the latter, when they might otherwise be insensible to the same remedial agents, in their appropriate remedial doses. Take many of the most powerful agents, *arsenic, tartarized antimony, iodine*, &c., and when administered in certain small and repeated alterative doses, they bring about the cure of the most obstinate and formidable conditions of disease; while the same doses may not manifest any action upon the system, or on any part of it, under circumstances of health. This manifestly depends upon an increased susceptibility of the organic properties, in their diseased conditions, to the action of foreign agents, and upon an increased disposition to undergo changes. This law, which unfolds a principle *latent in health*, and by which morbid organic properties acquire susceptibilities to salutary influences from agents which in health, would either produce no effects, or lead to untoward results, and its ally, the great recuperative principle, impose the highest obligation upon physicians to become medical philosophers."*

Most of the positions laid down by Dr. Paine, in the above quotations, are doubtless correct; but in all his inductions, he is labouring under an important error in supposing that morbific and remedial agents exercise their influence only upon certain *immaterial principles* or *vital properties.*

Can it be supposed that when *tartarized antimony* or *Ipecacuanha* are taken into the stomach, in emetic or diaphoretic doses, they act upon an immaterial property of this viscus, in causing emesis or diaphoresis? Can it be believed that the diuretics, *copaibæ, cubebs, turpentine,* &c., operate upon the vital properties of the urinary apparatus, in producing diuresis, or that *belladonna, stramonium, strychnia, conia, alcohol,* and the vapours of *ether*, or *chloroform*, expend their force upon the spiritual properties of the brain and nervous system; or that the preparations of *mercury, iodine,* &c., exercise their powerful influence upon the organism, by impressing immaterial, imponderable, or vital properties?

We think it is more consistent with known facts and sound logic, to suppose that all such agents exert their influence primarily upon the sentient extremities of the nerves, modifying the functions of those parts which they supply, increasing their susceptibility to the influence of foreign agents, and thus establishing inflammation or a new action.

* Paine's Institutes of Medicine.

It has been remarked by Paine and others, that *arsenic, antimony, iodine, mercury*, etc., given in certain small and repeated doses, in disease, are productive of decisive effects, while the same doses in health, would exert no appreciable influence. For this reason, they assert and would have us believe, that the conditions and properties of diseased parts are so modified and altered *in all respects*, as to be incapable of responding to the action of those medicines which operate specifically in health.

It is quite certain that most medicinal substances may be taken in *very small doses* during health, without any apparent effect, on account of the power which the system then possesses of resisting the aggressions of slight foreign agents; but if the same substances be taken *in large doses*, most decided, powerful, and specific results will follow *in all states of the system.* If taken in still smaller quantities, the effects are yet perceptible, but less strongly marked. These results will be unequal in point of intensity in normal and abnormal states of the organism, according to the amount of disease present; but in all instances, *their specific operations* will be uniform.

Tartarized antimony and *ipecacuanha*, in large doses, both in health and disease, exercise a specific influence upon the stomach, lungs, and skin, as is indicated by vomiting and augmented secretions from the respiratory organs and skin. In doses of one-sixth or one-eighth of a grain, no effect is produced upon the respiratory muscles or stomach, but the influence is yet *visible* upon the skin. If the quantity be diminished still farther, even to an attenuation of Hahnemann, the impression may not be *perceptible*, either upon the stomach, lungs, or skin, yet we find them capable of influencing the extreme nerves in a decided manner. It does not follow, because a patient does not vomit, purge, or sweat, that a medicine has no effect. On the contrary, we know that morbific agents give rise to the most virulent diseases without creating the slightest sensation in the system at the period when the noxious impression is made. The direct and sympathetic effects of such causes are, however, severe and dangerous.

The experiences of a host of honourable and scientific men have proved, beyond a doubt, that minute quantities of medicinal agents may produce salutary influences in the same manner; and the law obtains with regard to all specific medicines. The effects in these instances may not indeed be sufficient to induce emesis, catharsis, or other *violent* effects in any part of the body; yet from the great sensibility of the minute nervous ramifications, they must receive impressions and be modified in their action, when the trunks, or larger branches of nerves, would remain unaffected. Who shall decide *when* the quantity has become too small to produce an effect upon the most sensitive parts of the body? Shall the allopath, because he does not witness vomiting, purging, or sweating; or the homœopath, who from accurate observation in numerous instances, notes from infinitesimal doses, prompt and decisive curative effects?

To illustrate our meaning more fully, we will suppose a certain medicine possesses the power, when given in large doses, during health, of affecting a particular tissue. The same substance, administered in very small doses under the same circumstances, has no apparent influence. If, now, the tissue for which it has a specific affinity, *becomes inflamed*, its susceptibility is so acute, that an extremely minute quantity of the specific agent is capable of making potent and salutary impressions.

The other parts of the organism which become disordered through the media of the sympathetic nerves, also acquire an exalted sensibility which renders them highly impressible, and capable of being acted upon by infinitesimal quantities of specific medicinal agents. Homœopathic remedies, as Paine has well observed of medicines generally, act only through these "acquired relations," and their power ceases as soon as these acquired relations have been removed and health re-established.

We shall appreciate, then, the importance of selecting a remedy which shall cover, not only the symptoms resulting directly from the tissue primarily affected, but which shall embrace all of the remote sympathetic effects. In other words, we must prescribe for the "totality of the symptoms."

"It will now be apparent, from what has been said in the preceding section, how it is that remedial agents will call into salutary reacting, sympathies in various parts of the body not affected by disease, but whose susceptibilities are increased by morbific sympathies reflected from the seat of absolute disease, and upon which parts the remedial agents might otherwise be inoperative. Whatever, too, may be the complexities of disease, the right remedy will be at least compatible with the whole condition." *

"A particular state of one organ, such as inflammation, or a secreting action in it, often causes the production of a similar state in other parts." And, "the principle of the balance of sympathy teaches us how we must avoid aggravating the morbid condition of one organ by the means which we apply to another."†

An adherence in all cases to Hahnemann's axiom, "similia similibus," in our remedial measures, is the only means by which this last objection can be obviated with any certainty or success.

It is proper to remark, before concluding this chapter, that there are a few apparent, though not real exceptions to the principles which we have advanced. A most remarkable one is observed in the case of *tetanus*, where enormous quantities of *opium*, both in a crude form and in tincture, may be administered by the stomach or rectum, without producing any marked effect. This fact, however, by no means proves that the susceptibility of the parts for which *opium* is a specific, is diminished; but it proves only that *absorption is prevented.* If *opium* is injected into the veins, under these circumstances, it has been found by Majendie, Orfila, and Müller, that it exerts its influence in the same manner and degree as when taken during health.

We suppose, therefore, that in *tetanus*, the lacteals and other absorbents, are *in a state of spasm*, and thus mechanically exclude the entrance of all substances

* Paine's Institutes of Medicine.

† Müller's Physiology

from their structure. In this manner, opiates and other drugs are shut out of the circulation, and consequently, cannot be brought into *contact* with those parts of the nervous system upon which they exert their specific force, and where alone they possess the power of producing their legitimate effects.

All cases of this description, are simply apparent exceptions to the general rule, and do not in the slightest degree invalidate the general principles which we have advanced.

CHAPTER VIII.

ALLOPATHY.

It would be very difficult at the present time, to give an accurate definition of the above term. The axiom which is adopted by a portion of the disciples of the allopathic school, and upon which their hypothetical doctrines are founded, is "*contraria contrariis opponenda.*" Although distinctions are recognised between the *antipathic* or *palliative*, the *allopathic* or *heteropathic*, and the *chemical*, methods of practice, yet in point of fact, they may all, with propriety, be resolved into one and the same school. All employ venesection, emetics, purgatives, diaphoretics, and alteratives, to reduce inflammations; opium to allay pain and suppress unnatural discharges; bark, iron, brandy, &c., as tonics; blisters, setons, moxas, issues and escharotics to produce counter-irritation; revulsives, derivatives, and indeed all of those means which are termed allopathic.

Allopathists do not, however, uniformly adhere to any of the above doctrines, but often unconsciously encroach upon homœopathic ground, and by *practising* according to the law of "*similia similibus,*" effect their speediest and safest cures.

Thus, rhubarb and calomel, when administered in large doses during health, cause irritation or inflammation of the membranous tissue of the bowels, as is indicated by griping pains, and discharges of watery or mucous fluids; yet these are favourite allopathic remedies for diarrhœa and dysentery: copaibæ, cubebs, turpentine, and cantharides, when given in large and repeated doses in health, induce inflammation of the mucous membranes of the urino-genital apparatus; yet these specific medicines are almost invariably prescribed in the acute and chronic affections of these parts: ipecacuanha in doses of twenty to thirty grains, is the most common emetic of the old school; yet this same school are constantly in the habit of administering this drug in doses of one-twelfth or one-sixteenth of a grain, in cases of obstinate nausea and vomiting, with the most happy results: inhalations also of the particles of ipecacuanha, cause asthma, cough, dyspnœa, &c.; yet it is a common remedy in small quantities for the cure of these complaints: excessive use of alcoholic liquors or opiates, often induces *mania a potu;* yet opium and brandy, which exercise the same specific effect upon the brain, are the principal allopathic cures of this dangerous malady: the preparations of mercury, when given in considerable quantities, cause ulceration and sometimes gangrene and sloughing of the mouth and throat, pains in the muscles and bones, eruptions upon the skin, and inflammation of the bowels, attended with tenesmus, and mucous and bloody stools; yet for syphilitic and other ulcerations of the throat, pains in the limbs, eruptions, and bowel affections, the use of small doses of this mineral, in some form, is deemed indispensable by the allopath. Sir Astley Cooper, in his Lectures, observes,* "Children often contract syphilis *in utero*, and within twenty-four hours after their entrance into the world, have the palms of their hands, the soles of their feet, and the nates, covered with copper-coloured eruptions; and the nails begin to peel off, and if care be not taken, the little patient will sink under the effects of the disease. In these cases, you give the *mother* a quantity of mercury, the influence of which is communicated to the child,

* Cooper's Manual of Surgery, by Castle.

through the medium of the milk, and it becomes cured of the syphilitic disease." This is excellent homœopathic treatment: the mercury in this instance is attenuated in the mother's milk to a very great extent—probably to such a degree that no analysis can detect it, or any scales *weigh* it, and yet Sir Astley Cooper assures us that the infinitesimal quantity of mercury which finds its way to the milk of the mother, is sufficient to effect a speedy cure upon the child. In this instance nature, instead of art, attenuates the drug. Tartarized antimony exercises a specific effect upon the lungs, stomach, and secretory organs, causing, according to Majendie, an inflammation or engorgement of the two first named organs, whether taken into the stomach or injected into the veins; yet this is the sheet-anchor of allopathy in pneumonia, pleurisy, and in the first stages of gastric or bilious fevers. Arsenic has a specific influence when taken in large doses, in health, upon the nervous system, heart, skin, and alimentary canal; and this is an important old-school remedy in neuralgia, epilepsy, chorea, angina-pectoris, cutaneous affections, and intermittent fevers. When nitrate of silver is absorbed in health, it makes a specific impression upon the nervous system and the corium; allopathists employ it in epilepsy, chorea, and in morbid sensibility of the gastric and intestinal nerves. Large and repeated doses of nux vomica or strychnia, taken in health, produce "rigidity and convulsive contractions" of the muscles; yet in cases of traumatic tetanus, strychnia has effected cures in the hands of allopathic physicians, in doses of $\frac{1}{14}$ to $\frac{1}{20}$ of a grain:* its specific action under all circumstances, is upon the cerebro-spinal system, and thus its efficacy when properly exhibited in tetanus, epilepsy, chorea and hysteria. Belladonna, taken in health, gives rise to inflammation of the throat and a scarlet eruption upon the skin; and yet this remedy is highly extolled and extensively used by many leading men opposed to homœopathy, as a prophylactic against scarlatina. An

* See report of tetanus cured with strychnia, by Dr. Fell. 8th number of N. Y. Med. and Surg. Reporter.

eruption resembling psora is often produced by an excessive use of sulphur and iodine; still these are the grand remedies in cutaneous affections of this kind. Pereira prescribed prussic acid to a lady who had been suffering for months from gastrodynia; in a few hours, to the astonishment of every one, she was quite well. "It can hardly be imagined," says Pereira, "that irritation of the stomach can be rapidly removed by a substance which is *itself an irritant.*" The direct application of blisters to surfaces affected with rheumatic, erysipelatous, and other natural cutaneous inflammations, is constantly recommended at the present time by the Hippocratics. "Erysipelas and other cutaneous inflammations may be removed by the direct action of cantharides upon the part inflamed. The remedial agent, in these cases, varies the mode of inflammation, and thus introduces a modification in which the properties of life are brought into recuperative action" (*Paine's Institutes of Medicine*); yet they affect a superlative contempt for the law of "similia similibus curantur!"

It is from experience alone that the old school physicians have learned that ipecac., in doses of $\frac{1}{12}$ to $\frac{1}{16}$ of a grain, arrests nausea and vomiting, and imparts tone and vigour to the stomach; that calomel, in doses of $\frac{1}{20}$ of a grain, is invaluable for the cure of inflammation of the mucous membranes of the bowels: "in cases of inflammation of the mucous tissue of the intestines attended with frequent watery discharges, there is nothing comparable with calomel, in doses varying from the twentieth to the eighth of a grain, once in four to twelve hours:"—(*Paine's Institutes of Medicine.*) That quinia, in doses of $\frac{1}{16}$ or $\frac{1}{20}$ of a grain, is more efficient in removing remittent and intermittent fevers, and as a general tonic in diseased states of the system, than when exhibited in quantities of from one to ten grains at a dose: "quinia in the dose of 5 or 10 grains, may speedily arrest an intermittent fever by its *febrifuge* virtue; but this is bad practice, since, by its associate *tonic* virtue, it is likely to increase or to induce local congestions; thus leaving the patient imperfectly cured, and subject to relapses: I have seen, in my own family, the most formidable grade of remittent fever, of long duration and attended with the foregoing complications, ardent heat, thread-like pulse, loss of mind, &c., and where hope of recovery had been abandoned, *yield to less than a grain of quinine, divided into sixteen doses*"—(*Paine's Institutes of Medicine*); that strychnia, in very minute quantities, will cure tetanus; that the class of remedies denominated *alteratives*, are capable of producing powerful effects upon the organism, and that too, in a manner altogether unknown and imperceptible.

But how do these physicians know that the virtues of these medicines cease at these points? Have they ever made honest trials of them in a *pure form*, and in doses of $\frac{1}{50}$, $\frac{1}{100}$, or a still smaller proportion of a grain, and learned from *actual observation* that they have then lost their power of impressing diseased structures? We venture to affirm, never, or they would long since have deserted the standard of allopathy.

This leaning towards the modern theory is not altogether confined to the few practical cases which we have cited, but some of their most eminent writers have approached so near to the views of Hahnemann, that we are at a loss whether to rank their theoretical doctrines as homœopathic or allopathic.

The distinguished Pereira, in his Materia Medica and Therapeutics, writes as follows: "Unguents and lotions are used in cutaneous diseases, ulcers, &c.; gargles in affections of the mouth and throat; collyria in opthalmic diseases; and injections into the vagina and uterus in affections of the urino-genital organs. *In all such cases, we can explain the therapeutical effect in no other way than by assuming that the medicine sets up a new kind of action in the part affected, and that the new action subsides when the use of the medicine is suspended or desisted from.*"

This explanation is the true one. The medicines in these cases, as well as in all other instances where appropriate specific remedies are used, do "*set up a new kind of action in the part affected*," creating a *medicinal disease* which supersedes the *natural one*.

The only fault we have to urge against allopathists

in the treatment of these and analogous cases, is, that they give much too large doses, and thus create a far more violent medicinal disease than is necessary to bring about their cures. Notwithstanding, however, their errors in exhibiting medicines in a crude and impure form, and in unnecessarily large doses, we must give them the credit, (*fiat justitia ruat coelum*,) of occasionally curing disease (although unwittingly) in a "rational and consistent" manner.

Paine, in his Institutes of Medicine, remarks, "that when the intestinal mucous tissue is affected with that condition of disease which results in a preternatural watery secretion, and consequent evacuations, which is called diarrhœa, and rhubarb is administered in a certain dose, this substance first impresses the membrane in such a way as to determine an increase of the peristaltic movement; *but it simultaneously alters the morbid state of the intestinal mucous tissue in such a way that the natural secretion is arrested.* Whether, therefore, the rhubarb purge, or prove astringent, or tonic, a common principle, and common laws are concerned throughout; *and all the sensible results depend upon certain alterations which the agent effects in the vital properties and actions of the vessels or tissues which are the seat of the morbid conditions, or in which the various phenomena may take place.*"

The same principle directs the practitioners of the old school in the treatment of many other diseases, and yet they sneer at homœopathy, and hold up their own inconsistent and uncertain doctrines as philosophical and correct! Gentlemen of the old school, your practice too often belies your profession: you pretend to be allopathists and antipathists, while constantly administering medicines after the manner of the homœopathist. Instead of abiding by the theoretical doctrines which have come to you from rude and dark ages—doctrines which have received seals of approbation from the alchemist, the astrologer, and the sorcerer—you have stealthily, and, doubtless, in many instances, unwittingly, abandoned your legitimate ground, and *practised* upon the principles of our modern heresy! Where is your pride, where your consistency? You have the boast of antiquity, you have received your "*bundle of ideas*" from Hippocrates and Galen, to whom you pay reverence and allegiance; you disdain innovations, and despise discoveries and improvements; you have withstood the changes of more than two thousand years, and, by your powerful dicta, have continually discouraged all original induction, and endeavoured to crush in the bud every advancement in medical knowledge. Where is now your former pride, that you so often *practically* abandon your time-sacred axiom, "*contraria contrariis*," and adopt the new heresy, "*similia similibus?*" Perhaps the light of modern science and discovery breaks, against your will, through the crevices of your unjointed and heterogeneous theories, or you are startled from your propriety by the whelming accumulations of fact which Hahnemann and his disciples have displayed so bravely before the world; or, possibly, the disrespect and abuse of some of the most eminent and able of your caste, has impaired all confidence in, and respect for, your own dogmas and their applications, and you are at sea in search of a system. Are we wrong? If so, we have excuse in the following, from the distinguished editor of the British and Foreign Medical Review, Dr. Forbes, who asserts:

"1. That in a large proportion of the cases treated by allopathic physicians, the disease is cured by nature, and not by them.

"2. That in a less, but still not in a small proportion, the disease is cured by nature in spite of them; in other words, their interference opposing instead of assisting the cure.

"3. That, consequently, in a considerable proportion of diseases, it would fare as well or better with patients, in the actual condition of the medical art, as more generally practised, if all remedies, at least all active remedies, especially drugs, were abandoned. We repeat our readiness to admit these inferences as just, and to abide the consequences of their adoption."

Beware, then, most ancient goddess, survivor of all thine earlier contemporaries—of alchemy, and astrology—lest thou fall, and thy doctrines, handed down through the dark ages, through the juggling temples of idolatrous priests, be swallowed up in the deluge of new facts and discoveries which the nineteenth century is pouring upon the world. But, seriously, it is a matter of no little surprise, that while *anatomy* has made most rapid strides, unfolding the secrets pertaining to the most minute structures of the animal organism; while *botany* and *mineralogy* have displayed before our eyes the wonders of the vegetable and mineral kingdoms, and pointed out the laws of their formation, development, and even of their very existence; while *chemistry* has grasped some of the most subtle agents in nature, and developed improvements in the arts and sciences which have continually startled and astonished the world, as well for useful as for purely scientific results,—*medicine*, until the time of Hahnemann, has been crushed under the weight of antiquated doctrines, and the legalized power and oppression of the schools.

We have thus far made allusion to that part only of the allopathic *practice* which bears some approximation to the correct method. In most of the instances enumerated, *specific medicines* are employed—medicines that produce a similar state when given in health, to that which they are to cure. Although large quantities of crude and impure drugs are used in these instances, and the medicinal diseases are thus rendered violent and complicated, still it must be admitted that occasional cures are accomplished.

But we come now to a more interesting and momentous part of our subject. It becomes our duty to lay before our readers the doctrines and practice of allopathy, as they actually exist; to note their many inconsistencies, and to point out some of the innumerable evils which they entail upon mankind.

We have seen that in the treatment of disease, the old school physicians make an indiscriminate use of the *palliative*, *heteropathic*, and in a few instances, the homœopathic methods of practice.

A general idea prevails, that all diseases consist in "local determinations of blood," and that no two affections of any consequence, can exist in different parts of the same organism, at once. On this account it is, that new diseases are created in healthy parts, for the purpose of removing the primary natural one.

Physicians have been led to adopt this mode of reasoning from observing that the spontaneous appearance of cutaneous eruptions, discharges of blood, profuse perspirations, &c., occasionally afford relief to morbidly affected internal organs. Without reflecting that these results are *merely symptoms* of the internal disorders, and that the causes upon which these signs depend are located in the blood, they attempt to annihilate diseases, by imitating artificially *these symptoms.*

In regard to the first position, we affirm that their premises are untrue. There are no facts which warrant the statement, that "no two excessive determinations of blood can exist in the same individual at the same time." Neither is it true, that the appearance of cutaneous eruptions, spontaneous sweats, diarrhœa, and discharges of blood, are invariably, or even generally, indications that the affected organ is in process of restoration, or that the system at large is recovering its lost energy and vigour ; since it often occurs that the symptoms of the complaint are all aggravated, upon the supervention of either of the above occurrences.

Dr. Wilson observes, that "there is often a remarkable tendency to the worst species of hæmorrhages from the bowels, towards the termination of fatal cases of phrenitis."

Dr. Eberle, in his Practice of Physic, remarks, "On the day preceding the fatal termination of a case of phrenitis which came under my own observation, an exceedingly copious discharge of dissolved blood took place from the bowels, and on the following morning the hæmorrhage occurred also from the mouth and gums."

Let us suppose a case of phrenitis. We have here an inflammation, or a congested state of the capillaries of the brain. To relieve this inflammation, and withdraw a portion of the fluid which is concerned in the congestion, blood-letting, both general and local, is resorted to as a primary and indispensable process of cure. By this means, the general strength is reduced, the pulse increased or diminished in frequency, and the temperature of the skin altered, but the congestion still continues, and the morbid and debilitated state of the extreme vessels (in which the disorder alone resides) remains the same as before.

A resort is then made to *revulsives* and counter-irritants, in order that new inflammations may be created in healthy structures, which shall supersede that already existing in the brain. To effect this object, purgatives of the drastic kind are exhibited, and blisters applied to the head, neck, and lower extremities, in order that the intestinal canal, and portions of the skin, shall be placed in a state of artificial inflammation.

Let us understand the case clearly. We have a disease consisting solely in a loss of tone and irritability of the serous vessels of the brain, which prevents them from excluding the red blood, and of performing properly their functions. To obviate this condition, a quantity of blood is abstracted, and artificial or medicinal inflammations are caused in the intestinal canal, and upon different parts of the surface of the body.

We now inquire in what manner these violent means can, by any possibility, reach the *seat* of the malady, and impart tone and vigour to the weakened capillaries, so as to enable them to exclude from their structure the red globules, and resume their healthy function?

All will concede that inflammation consists in loss of tone and irritability in these vessels, and that no cure can take place, until this impaired irritability is restored. In inflammation, according to Philip, Hastings, Eberle, Wilson, and Allan, the capillaries of the part are in a state of *debility*, and *passive relaxation.* The immediate exciting cause of inflammation may be either *stimulant* or *sedative.* In both instances the impression is made upon the nervous filaments of the capillaries, and if the cause acts as a *stimulant*, the reaction which must follow this augmented action, will leave these delicate nerves in a state of debility proportionate to the amount of the previous excitement.

If the primary cause is directly *sedative*, no reaction will occur, but a similar state of relaxation will obtain as in the former instance.

How, then, we repeat, can venesection, cathartics and blisters affect the necessary object? They do not certainly prevent the red blood from still entering the relaxed capillary tubes, for the whole *remaining* mass must continue to circulate through the brain, as well as other parts of the organism, every few minutes.

By lessening the quantity of blood, we also abstract a portion of that natural stimulus of the organism, which is one of the essential conditions of *irritability.* "Every part of the organism depends, for the performance of its proper functions, *on the receipt of arterial blood and of nervous influence; so alterations in the supply of either of these essentials, may modify or even suspend the functions of a part.*"*

How absurd and pernicious then, in inflammations, the very essence of which is debility and loss of tone, to detract from one of those conditions upon which this very tone and vigour depends! As well might you remedy the breach through which the waters of a raging torrent are madly rushing, by turning off from its course a small quantity of this element. As well attempt to suppress the leak of a storm-tossed vessel, by diverting a portion of the stream on which she floats, from its natural channel.

It is not the blood which is at fault; but a portion of the organism. Correct therefore the *cause* of the disturbance by direct and appropriate specifics, and you may then, and not until then, effect cures, safely and philosophically. Seek not to deprive the system of that fluid which is so essential to the organism, and on whose integrity its functions depend; for by so doing, the *cause* of the malady will remain untouched.

It is very true, that when a large quantity of blood is abstracted, during inflammation, there will seem to be in some instances an apparent amelioration of all the symptoms, but this effect is only temporary; for as soon as reaction comes on, the enfeebled capillaries again admit the destructive "carriers of oxygen" as before; the state of congestion and inflammation remains, while the system at large has lost a portion of that stimulus which conduces so materially, not only

* Pereira's Mat. Med.

to sustain the normal integrity of the functions in health, but to aid in the restoration of enfeebled and diseased parts.

The remedies which stand next in importance in the old school method of treating phrenitis, are *revulsives* and *counter-irritants*. It is supposed that by exciting the intestinal exhalents, inflaming the membrane of the bowels, and portions of the skin, the circulation is diverted from the brain and directed especially to these parts.

But by this means is the brain in reality relieved? Is the whole mass of blood thus prevented from circulating as usual through this organ once in three or four minutes, or the character of its red globules changed? By exhausting the energies and resisting force of distant healthy structures, and creating sympathetic symptoms throughout the body—thus complicating the already existing disease, and impairing the entire nervous and muscular energies—are the inflamed capillaries of the brain placed in a more favourable condition to recover their impaired tone and irritability? Every man who has a correct idea of the laws which govern the organism in health and disease, and who is willing to banish prejudice and be guided by common sense and true philosophy, must answer in the negative.

We object to these remedies, however, not only because they are incompetent to produce salutary impressions upon inflamed parts, but because of the evils of a positive character to which they give rise.

The chief remedies of the old school, are the preparations of mercury, opium, antimony, and bark. In a vast majority of all the cases treated by the practitioners of this school, one or more of these articles is made use of. Indeed, scarcely a single malady of any moment can be named, in which one of these medicines is not considered indispensable.

Let us then examine some of their effects, in allopathic doses, upon the healthy and diseased organism.

1. MERCURY.

This mineral is more uncertain in its action, in all states of the system, than any other article in use. It possesses the power in different constitutions, and under certain circumstances, of affecting nearly every organ and tissue of the body; and it is not in the power of the most judicious physician to say beforehand, *where* or *in what manner*, it will exert its force.

Some of the more common deleterious effects of the use of mercury, are, *excessive salivation, ulceration, gangrene and sloughing of the gums, mouth, and throat, gastro-enteritis, mercurial erethism, dysentery, cutaneous eruptions, inflammation of the periosteum and bones, nodes, excessive derangement of the nervous system, paralysis, tremors, necroses of the maxillary and other bones, rheumatism and opthalmia.*

When mercury is administered, even in a moderate quantity, no human being can be at all certain that one or more of these evil consequences will not result. Indeed, it is the direct object, oftentimes, to produce some of them, to operate as *counter-irritants.*

Whether it is employed in large or small quantities, solid, or in the form of vapour, is of little importance, so far as its power of affecting the system is concerned. The following, from the Ed. Med. and Surg. Journal, illustrates the baneful influence of the vapour when inhaled: "In 1810, the Triumph man-of-war, and Phipps schooner, received on board several tons of quicksilver, saved from the wreck of a vessel near Cadiz. In consequence of the rotting of the bags the mercury escaped, *and the whole of the crews became more or less affected.* In the space of three weeks 200 men were salivated, *two died*, and all the animals, cats, dogs, sheep, fowls, a canary bird,—nay, even the rats, mice and cockroaches, *were destroyed.*"

The following cases resulting from the employment of calomel, have come under my own observation, viz., three cases of necrosis of the inferior maxillary bones, requiring the removal of portions of the jaw; several cases of gangrene and sloughing of the mouth and throat, which have terminated fatally; a number of cases of mercurial palsy; numerous instances of ulceration of the nose, throat, &c.; skin diseases, affections of the bones, nodes, rheumatic affections, &c., &c.

Professor Chapman, after descanting upon the woful effects which have so often been produced by calomel, and referring to many disgusting cases of mercurial disease which have come under his own observation, thus concludes: "*Who is it that can stop the career of mercury, at will, after it has taken the reins in its own destructive and ungovernable hands?* He who, for an ordinary cause, resigns the fate of his patient to mercury, is a vile enemy to the sick; and if he is tolerably popular, will, in one successful season, have paved the way for the business of life; for he has enough to do ever afterwards to stop the mercurial breach of the constitutions of his dilapidated patients. He has thrown himself in fearful proximity to death, and has now to fight him at arm's length as long as the patient maintains a miserable existence."

And this dreadful poison is the most common,—yes, the daily remedy of allopathy, for almost every disorder, whether mild or severe, acute or chronic. This is the agent with which artificial diseases are created in healthy parts, to cure primary or natural ones! This is the substance with which unfortunate mortals are drugged, from the time they come into the world, until their wretched and too often premature departure, with its well-known and generally admitted evils and dangers,—from the contemplation of which the well-instructed and experienced allopath shrinks with instinctive dread,—and its questionable value in most instances of its prescription, it may justly detain our attention. Calomel and opium are the common remedies in the traditional practice. We shall see to what degree they may be used in a practice that is philosophical.

By glancing at the standard works on the practice of medicine, it will be observed that there is scarcely a single malady, either acute or chronic, in which one or both of these articles is not recommended as an important if not indispensable means of cure. Taking Eberle's Practice of Medicine — an approved allopathic work—as a fair illustration of their views and practice, it will be seen that of the *one hundred and thirty-nine diseases*, upon which these two volumes treat, there are *only ten*, in which *calomel* or *opium* in some form is not recommended. The following are the names of these exempt diseases, viz: mumps, ring-worm, nettle-rash, scurvy, chronic cystitis, hysteritis, asphyxia, roseola, hæmatemesis, and nose-bleeding. Nor are these remedies advised simply as auxiliaries in the treatment, but in a large majority of cases, they constitute the principal means of cure.

The allopath is taught to believe that mercury excites the functions of all the organs—acts specifically upon the liver, salivary glands, heart, lungs, and nervous system—and therefore that it may be administered almost universally. Regardless of the secondary sympathetic affections to which it usually gives rise, he attributes all of these symptoms to the natural disorder, and if the patient succumbs before the combined attacks of the primary disease and the medicinal one, he consoles himself with the reflection that he has followed his authorities and prescribed as his predecessors have done for centuries before him.

Ask him what are his views concerning inflammation, and he answers that it consists in a debilitated and congested state of the capillaries of the part affected. Ask him what is the *modus medendi* of mercury in the cure of inflammation,—how any of its effects can reach the seat of the malady, the congested capillaries, and restore to them their impaired tone and healthy functions,—and he either avows his ignorance or offers an unsatisfactory explanation.

2. OPIUM.

If we except calomel, this drug and its preparations are more frequently used by the medical men of the old school, than any other article in the Materia Medica. Possessing the power, as it does in an eminent degree, when exhibited in large doses, of *covering* (not curing) symptoms, and of *shutting* the mouths of clamorous and inquiring patients, it is used constantly and indiscriminately in nearly all protracted maladies.

Let us then briefly examine the effects of opium in health and disease, and see if it possesses the wonderful property of reaching every structure, and of counteracting so many diverse and contradictory symptoms.

Its effects upon the human system, in medium doses, are in the first instance *stimulating*, succeeded in a short time by diminished sensibility and desire to sleep.

"This continues from eight to twelve hours, and is followed by *nausea, headache, tremors, and other symptoms of diminished and irregular nervous energy. All of the secretions, with the exception of that from the skin, are either suspended or diminished.*"* These effects, with a very few exceptions, are uniform under all circumstances, so far as we can judge.

How, then, is this substance applicable to the treatment of so many diseases?

We have remarked that in all maladies, there exists an inflammation of an acute or sub-acute character, in some part of the organism, and it is the presence of this inflammation which maintains and perpetuates them.

We have also observed that all inflammations consist in a congested state of the capillaries of the part affected, caused and kept up by a loss of tone, resisting power, or irritability, which disables them from resisting the intromission of red blood.

It is apparent, then, that in order to prove efficient, such remedies should be exhibited as are capable of acting upon the seat of the complaint, and of restoring the delicate capillary nerves to their normal state of integrity. Opium cannot accomplish this, for its operation tends to impair the nervous energy, instead of adding vigour, to dry up most of the secretions, instead of aiding nature to give vent to the poisonous and pent up fluids, it induces *nausea, headache, tremors,* and many other medicinal symptoms of sufficient severity to make a healthy man sick, or to complicate to a serious extent any existing natural affection.

If it be urged that opiates have the power of allaying pain, while other more efficient measures are pursued to effect the cures, we reply, that by covering up the pain, the *real* state of the case is concealed; other new symptoms set in, which will be unnoticed by the benumbed patient, while secondary sympathetic affections will be propagated to every part of the body, aggravating and complicating the original disorder.

Opium is also highly extolled in low forms of fever,

* Wood and Bache, U.S. Dispen.

and other complaints, where the powers of the system are in an exhausted condition. But let it be remembered, that the *stimulating* effect of this drug is of short duration, and that the corresponding *reaction* or *depression* will bear an exact ratio to the previous exaltation. This law is fundamental; for the system possesses but a definite and limited amount of vital power, and is capable of resisting only a limited degree of unnatural action or disease, so that we can readily perceive how opiates, and other stimulants, must ultimately prove deleterious.

It is true that perspiration is promoted by the use of this narcotic, but this does not cure. Sweating is merely a symptom, and it may be favourable or otherwise. When excited artificially by medicine, it is not productive of benefit, because this adds nothing towards invigorating the weakened capillaries.

"Perspiration induced by medicine is of little moment, unless the remedy simultaneously impresses, directly or indirectly, *the parts diseased*; and then the salutary results, so far as the surface is concerned, depend upon special vital influences exerted by the remedy upon the skin and reacting sympathies. This is exemplified by the profound effects of tartarized antimony and ipecacuanha, the uselessness of hot water, *and the frequent pernicious results of the compound powder of ipecacuanha*, when free perspiration may follow the administration of either. The effect, therefore, depends but very little upon the evacuation from the skin, as produced by what are called sudorifics."*

It is proper to observe that opium may, and sometimes does, effect cures in the hands of allopathists, when given as a *specific*. Its curative virtues in *mania a potu* and intoxication, even in large doses, are well known. In these instances, the remedy *impresses directly the part diseased*, and cures *homœopathically*. It is quite true that an infinitesimal quantity of the drug, properly prepared, will always prove more efficient, speedy, and safe, in accomplishing the object, and will not give rise to the unpleasant medicinal

* Paine's Inst. of Med.

symptoms which necessarily attend the employment of large doses; yet the fact must be conceded, that clumsy and unscientific cures are occasionally effected by the course alluded to.

An interesting case is related by Pereira, illustrative of this. "Opium is sometimes employed by drunkards to relieve *intoxication.* I knew a medical man addicted to drinking, and who for many years was accustomed to take a large dose of laudanum whenever he was intoxicated, and was called to see a patient." The *specific effects* of the alcoholic stimulants and opium, given during health, are exerted as remarked at page 43, upon the same organ; and we should therefore expect that a malady *caused* by the excessive use of the one, might be *cured* by the specific action of the other.

TARTARIZED ANTIMONY.

This salt has been several times formally banished from the Materia Medica, on account of its dangerous qualities, and as often revived again.

The Faculty of Medicine, at Paris, in 1566 and 1615, passed solemn decrees against it, as a virulent poison, and these decrees were even sanctioned by parliament, though afterwards formally reversed.*

Since this period, some have loudly extolled its virtues in the treatment of a great variety of diseases, while others have as earnestly condemned its use, as deleterious in all cases.

The celebrated Professor Nathan Smith, in his Essay on Typhus Fever, remarks, "I have seen many cases in which persons in the early stages of this disease were moping about, not very sick, but far from being well, and who, upon taking a dose of tartarate of antimony, with the intention of breaking up the disease, *have been immediately confined to their beds.*" He arrives at the conclusion, after much experience, that "tartar emetic should not be used in this affection, even at its commencement; and in the latter stages of the disease, that it is sometimes followed by fatal consequences."

* Vale.

In emetic doses, tartarized antimony irritates the stomach, causes congestion, and sometimes inflammation of the lungs, attended with more or less constitutional disturbance. When it fails to produce emesis speedily, it often acts violently upon the bowels, giving rise to severe griping pains and watery evacuations. The tenderness of the stomach and intestines, and the constitutional disturbance which succeeds its emetic and cathartic operation, indicates the injury which these delicate structures have sustained.

The primary impression of antimony is not the only objection against its employment; for, like calomel and opium, it gives rise to numerous secondary symptoms in remote parts, which tend to aggravate in a serious manner any natural affection which may be present. One of the most important of these secondary evils, is dilatation of the ventricles of the heart. Having witnessed this result in several instances, one of which occurred in my own family, my attention has been particularly directed to the subject, and I am fully of opinion that cases of this description, from the use of antimony, are by no means unfrequent.

CINCHONA.

In intermittent fevers, general debility, and in certain stages of most other affections, Peruvian bark and its preparations are usually employed by the old school. For the cure of the former, especially, quinine is the remedy upon which universal reliance is placed; possessing the property, when used in large and repeated doses, of speedily arresting the chills and fever, it is constantly prescribed for this malady, without the slightest knowledge of its processes, and without any regard to the dangerous medicinal disorders which it superinduces.

All allopathists who have had much experience in the treatment of fever and ague, are aware that the mere suppression of the paroxysms by no means restores the patient to health; for in a great majority of instances, he lingers for months or even years in a diseased and miserable condition. In these cases it is probable that a medicinal affection is induced by the remedy, so serious in its character, as to supersede temporarily the primary one. This is evident, from the fact that after the effects of the medicine have somewhat subsided, the original disorder again generally makes its appearance. In some instances, however, the medicinal affection is so severe as to constitute a permanent disease, and thus entirely usurp the place of the fever.

"Experience shows that, though bark, and its alkaloids, in large doses, will often arrest intermittent fever suddenly, such doses are liable either to induce some congestion, especially of the liver or of the mucous tissue of the stomach, or will aggravate and establish some co-existing congestion; and thus while the patient is for the present relieved of the fever, *he is dismissed with an insidious local complaint that not only renders him a permanent invalid,* (resulting often in indurated enlargements,) *but which local malady may, and often does become, in process of time, the exciting cause of another attack of fever.* In respect to relapses, it is not unfrequent that, when intermittents are suddenly stopped by a large dose of quinine, the paroxysms return as soon as the patient begins to exercise much, or to take his ordinary food."*

We should naturally suppose that these untoward results would deter practitioners from using so frequently these dangerous remedies; or at all events, as rarely and in as small quantities as possible.

On the contrary, it seems to be peculiar to allopathy, that her advocates take credit to themselves, when they succeed in administering this, as well as other medicines, *in larger doses than any of their contemporaries*, without *destroying* their patients. Indeed, so far has this destructive system been carried, of experimenting upon disease, that the enormous quantity of a scruple and even half a dram of quinine has been exhibited at a dose, and repeated several times a day. These monstrous quantities create † gastro-enteritic irritation, nausea, griping, purging, head-ache, giddi-

* Paine's Inst. of Medicine. † Wood and Bache.

ness, fever, somnolency, in some cases delirium, in others stupor," &c. Paine asserts that he has witnessed many of these effects "from five grains only;" yet, as patients sometimes *live* in spite of this treatment, many persist in adopting these desperate innovations.

There are many other medicines employed by allopathy in the treatment of disease, besides those to which we have alluded, but in general they serve only as *auxiliaries*. In this list may be ranked diaphoretics, diuretics, expectorants, refrigerants, emmenagogues, emollients, errhines, &c., but the articles belonging to each of these classes, in a crude state and in large doses, are liable to important objections.

The fault of those medicines which operate specifically, like diuretics, emmenagogues, &c., in the hands of allopathists, is the aggravation which they must necessarily cause, if the part acted upon be irritated or inflamed. This objection will be clearly appreciated, when it is remembered how extremely sensitive to specific remedial impressions, organs and tissues become during inflammation.

The evils resulting from the use of those medicines which are not specifics, are, first, their inability to reach the seat of the complaint, and secondly, the sympathetic derangements to which they give rise in various parts of the body, the direct tendency of which, is to retard and counteract the recuperative efforts of nature.

As an example of the first class, let us take the diuretic copaibæ, as a remedy for gonorrhœa. In this example, the remedy doubtless impresses directly the inflamed membrane of the urethra, but the impression is so violent that either a decided increase of the inflammation ensues, or the discharge is suddenly suppressed, and some other organ, as the bladder, kidneys, testicles, or lungs, takes on diseased action. Indeed we are decidedly of opinion, that not one *genuine* case of virulent gonorrhœa can be adduced where a safe and permanent cure has been effected by large doses of this balsam.

A not unfrequent effect of copiabæ in moderate quantities, is to excite serious disorder of the lungs. This consequence I have often witnessed, and I have a patient at this time, who assures me that he is unable to take a single dose of it, without being afflicted with a pain in his chest, and cough.

Gastric and intestinal disturbance, also, usually result from its use. In some instances, a troublesome eruption makes its appearance, rendering it necessary to discontinue its employment for a time. And yet with all of these artificial consequences, the disease is very rarely, if ever, cured by this nauseous substance.

Diaphoretics were introduced into practice by the advocates of the humoral pathology, under the supposition that their sweating qualities would aid nature in throwing off the morbid humours. When the hypothesis universally obtained that fevers were caused by an excess of one of the four humours, blood, phlegm, and yellow and black bile, and that this superabundance must be expelled through the pores of the skin, kidneys, &c., it was a rational deduction that the employment of diaphoretics and diuretics should conduce essentially to aid nature in the cure.

But when more correct ideas in regard to the nature and seat of diseases were introduced, and medical men had learned that spontaneous sweating, diuresis, discharges of blood, diarrhœa, &c., in the latter stages of diseases, occurred *in consequence* of a natural *amendment* or a sudden *prostration* in the powers of the affected parts, and not as an effect of the medicines, it is a matter of surprise that these uncertain remedies should have been retained.

The late Professor Nathan Smith, makes use of the following language, replete with good sense: "As there is more or less sweating in the decline of most febrile diseases, and as a general perspiration is often accompanied with other symptoms of amendment, it has been looked upon as the natural cure of the disease. Under this impression, it has been a pretty universal practice to encourage sweating; but with respect to the grounds upon which this practice is founded, it is a question whether the effect has not, in this case, been mistaken for the cause; that is, whether the sweating is not the effect of the amendment, rather than the cause of it; and if so, it is still more questionable, whether sweating, produced by art in the beginning of the disease, would be attended with good effects. *In all cases, where I have seen this sweating regimen adopted, the practice has been obviously injurious.*"

Many other eminent professors, as may be readily proved, entertain similar views in regard to this subject.

Physiology teaches us that no unusual disturbance, no inflammation, and no functional derangement, can accrue to any part of the body, whether by a moral, physical, morbific, or medicinal agent, without being followed by secondary sympathetic symptoms in remote parts, more or less severe according to the violence of the exciting cause. The stomach and bowels, more especially, being the grand centre of junction of the ganglionic system of nerves, are so intimately connected with all parts of the economy, that disturbances at either of these points are reflected through the sympathetic nerves upon remote healthy structures, thus complicating to a serious and often fatal extent, any disorder which may already be present.

There is scarcely any part of the machine which is not called into morbid sympathetic action, by derangements of the stomach and intestines. Even the presence of bile, or acid, in unusual quantities, causes pains in the head and limbs, nausea, and other affections of a distressing nature, until the offending substances are removed.

All of the organs and tissues are so closely connected by the nervous system, that it may be laid down as a general rule, that no disorder can happen to one part without implicating, more or less, other parts, whether diseased or healthy.* "A particular state of one organ, such as inflammation, or a secreting action in it, often causes the production of a similar state in other parts. The principle of the balance of sympathy teaches us *how we must avoid aggravating the morbid condition of one organ by the means which we apply to another.*"

* Müller's Physiology.

How reasonable, then, to expect that artificial medicinal inflammations of the sensitive structures of the economy, should give rise to secondary affections of a grave and permanent character.

In conclusion, the theoretical and practical doctrines of allopathy may be briefly summed up as follows:

1. In the rude ages of the world, when the arts and sciences were in their infancy,—when vague, indefinite and absurd notions were entertained respecting diseases,—when anatomy, chemistry, physiology, pathology, botany, and even correct methods of induction, were entirely unknown,—when the imaginations of men, instead of ascertained facts, were appealed to in establishing theories,—and when systems of practice were founded upon merely fanciful conjectures; then it was that blood-letting, cathartics, diaphoretics, diuretics, refrigerants, revulsives, derivatives, counter-irritants, and most of the other remedies of allopathy, made their first appearance. As the *pathological* doctrines of this period were all entirely erroneous, it is but fair to conclude that their *therapeutical* inferences must have been equally incorrect.

2. Whatever may have been the changes in respect to the *theory* of disease, from age to age, long established customs, the force of habit, education, prejudice, &c., have served to retain until our own period, most of the violent, unnatural and pernicious methods of *treatment*, invented and adopted by the founders of medicine.

3. At the present time, everything pertaining to the theory and practice of the old school is indefinite, obscure, and uncertain. Scarcely two different allopathists entertain the same views in regard to pathology, and not one can determine beforehand, with any kind of certainty, precisely what effects his medicine will produce; yet, in the treatment of nearly all cases, *venesection, calomel, opium and antimony* are empyrically, and, we might almost say, universally employed. In those cases where refrigerants, diuretics, expectorants, &c., are used, they can only be looked upon as auxiliaries, and are usually administered without any

accurate knowledge as to whether they promote or retard the designs of nature.

4. Owing to the absence of any generally received or consistent theory of disease, allopathists are obliged to prescribe at random. They strike at the *name*, and not at the *seat* of maladies, where alone remedies can prove efficient. Thus it is that patients are so often reduced to the lowest point, by medicines, while the disease continues its progress, unchecked.

5. Lastly, there is every reason to believe, that the production of violent artificial diseases in healthy structures, for the suppression of natural maladies, is, upon the whole, far more productive of deleterious than of beneficial consequences.

In view, therefore, of the present condition of the medical art, we most earnestly request the allopath to pause, and reflect deeply and seriously, before persisting in the use of *venesection, revulsives, derivatives, alteratives*, and *counter-irritants*. Let him remember that a high responsibility attaches to his position,—that the welfare, happiness, and lives of his patients hang upon his judgment and decision,—and that an improper exhibition of remedies may so complicate and aggravate the natural disease, as to consign his patient to a premature grave. Let him look about, candidly and impartially, and see if there are really no improvements in the practice of the healing art, since the times of Hippocrates and Galen. Let him submit new discoveries and new doctrines to a *rigid practical test*, and decide from the results—from the cures effected—what system is most correct and best calculated to promote the welfare of the human race. Let him no longer reverence ancient doctrines and ancient names, simply on account of their *antiquity*, but seek after *truth alone*, whether of ancient or modern discovery, and found his practice only upon this certain basis.

CHAPTER IX.

HOMŒOPATHY.

When Hahnemann first promulgated to the world his pathological and therapeutical views, their novelty, their entire variance from all preconceived opinions, and their alleged superiority over all other systems, when applied to the practice of the healing art, induced physicians to suppose the man mad, and his ideas the offspring of a disordered imagination.

It was difficult to conceive that acute maladies could be cured without venesection, emetics, cathartics, sudorifics, refrigerants, alteratives, and counter-irritants, and on this account the great discoveries of the father of homœopathy were for many years coldly received, and his arguments answered only by impudent sneers, or senseless ridicule.

Like the illustrious Fulton, who—when he announced to his countrymen the powers of steam, and first applied this agent to the propulsion of a vessel—was declared, even by his nearest friends, insane, and his projects visionary; like Harvey, the discoverer of the circulation of the blood, who was bitterly attacked "by the bigoted abettors of old established systems, with whispers, inuendoes, and controversial writings," and himself pronounced a reckless innovator, and unworthy of public confidence as a practitioner; like Galileo, who, after demonstrating the truth of the Copernican system, was persecuted by his rivals, and twice compelled by the inquisition to abjure a system which he knew to be correct; like Columbus, Newton, Locke, Jenner, and many other benefactors of the human race, Hahnemann has been aspersed, and his doctrines, like theirs, have been ridiculed, misrepresented, and contemned; but time has cast all the calumniators of Columbus, of Galileo, of Newton, of Locke, of Harvey, of Jenner, of Fulton, into a deserved oblivion, while the names of these eminent persons stand high on the roll of fame, and their discoveries remain to benefit the world.

The public of Europe and America are fast rendering the same justice to Hahnemann and his doctrines, and the time will ere long arrive, when the united world will rank him by the side of those great men to whom we have just alluded. It is even now conceded by many eminent allopathic writers, that the hypothetical doctrines of homœopathy are correct. By referring to page 65, it will be observed that the pathological views of Hahnemann, and some of the professors of the old school, coincide in a very striking manner. Indeed, it is a matter of doubt whether there can be found in the medical ranks, two more staunch advocates of the " vital theory," than Samuel Hahnemann, the homœopathist, and Martyn Paine, the allopathist.

But when we come to the therapeutical inferences deduced from these opinions, we find a wide and essential difference. The latter, in summing up his method of treatment, has retained all of the violent and barbarous remedies of antiquity, with very little knowledge of their mode of operation upon the human system, and with as little certainty as to whether they will ameliorate or aggravate disease.

The former has pursued a different course. In consideration of the facts, that the action of no two medicines upon the economy is the same,—that almost every agent exercises a peculiar and specific influence upon certain structures only, and that this specific effect obtains both in health and disease, he instituted a series of accurate experiments during health, in order to arrive at the pure effects of different medicinal substances. The illustrious founder of homœopathy not only tested the operation of medicines upon his own person, but he induced others—men of science and undoubted integrity in different parts of Europe—to make trials of the same substances, without informing them of the results of his own experiments; and when their observations were completed, he instituted comparisons, and found that the effects of the medicines upon the different individuals were almost uniformly the same. Having now ascertained with certainty the pure effects of a number of articles during health, he commenced exhibiting them for the cure of diseases, in accordance with the principle which he had conceived to be philosophical and true, *similia similibus curantur.* We need not repeat, that the results of these experiments were in the highest degree satisfactory.

In the early part of his career, Hahnemann made use of the pure mother tinctures, in ordinary doses, but he observed that the primary effects were too active,—there usually occurring a temporary augmentation of the symptoms. This induced him to reduce his doses until he came to make use of attenuations and dilutions ; and he found, that when the medicines were properly prepared, they still had their specific action, and that disease was more speedily removed than when stronger preparations were employed.

But the principal objection which was formerly, and which still, to a considerable extent, is raised against the system of homœopathy, is the supposed inefficiency of *infinitesimal* quantities of medicines when administered as curative agents. Nor is this at all surprising, for it has been customary for three thousand years, when disturbance prevails in the human citadel, to storm it with agents of destruction. Blood is made to flow, the delicate membranes of the stomach and intestines are raked with broadsides of emetics and drastics, the nervous system is shattered by narcotics and stimulants, and the functions of every organ deranged by the showers of destructive allopathic missiles with which the enfeebled body is constantly assailed. By these summary means the disturbance is smothered, but the citadel is in decay, its resources exhausted, its foundations impaired, and its strength forever diminished.

Homoeopathy, however, resorts to a different mode of procedure. In her remedial measures, she uses no unnatural violence, nor seriously disturbs the function of any organ; but her remedies are exhibited with a definite object ; the affected organ or tissue is acted upon with almost mathematical certainty, and that too without creating disease in healthy parts, or in any way complicating the natural affection. But she usually administers her medicaments in *infinitesimal doses,* and we now come to the question whether such minute quantities of matter are capable of producing salutary impressions upon the organism when labouring under disease?

No one will deny that the human body during health is constantly being acted upon and disturbed by influences or agents so subtle, that neither the chemist nor physiologist can analyze or even detect them. The simple application of substances to the surface of the body is sufficient to produce decided and permanent effects. Turnbull says, that "so small a portion as the *one hundredth part of a grain* of aconite, made into an ointment, and rubbed upon the skin, has produced a sensation of heat, pricking, and numbness, that has continued a whole day."

A leaf of tobacco applied to the wrist or sole of the foot, will excite the action of the respiratory muscles, blood-vessels, glands, and skin, causing nausea, vomiting, &c.

If the leaves of hyoscyamus or belladonna be applied to the eye, *an effect will be produced which will remain for several weeks.* It is asserted by Pereira and Sigmond, that "a dilatation of the pupils may be produced by *only approximating* the leaves of hyoscyamus or belladonna to the eyes."

It is also well known,* that "violent erysipelatous inflammation over the whole surface of the body, is often induced from *approaching within a few yards of several species of rhus.*"

The wild buffalo scents the hunter for a distance of more than a mile, and hastens from the vicinity of danger.

The carnivorous bird recognises the odoriferous particles arising from a dead carcass, miles distant in the air, and with hasty wing, pounces upon the prey.

The medicinal quality of *cod liver oil* (*ol. jec. aselli*) consists of *iodine* distributed in infinitesimal quantities throughout the oil. According to an analysis made by Falker, the *iodine* forms only the one-forty-thousandth part of the oil, being about equal to a third or fourth homœopathic attenuation of iodine. The value of this *naturally* attenuated medicine in the treatment of scrofula and consumption, is at the pres-

* Paine's Inst. of Med.

ent time generally conceded. The analyses of Stein, De Jongh, and Balard, fully confirm that of Falker.

The very minutest quantity of the natural poison of certain animals, the virus of hydrophobia, small-pox, kine-pox, syphilis, and gonorrhœa, is sufficient, when placed in contact with an abraded or delicate surface, or otherwise introduced into the system, to give rise to all of their corresponding maladies. Other diseases, like scabies, leprosy, &c., may be communicated by the mere *touch*, or from inhaling the breath of an infected person.

Miasmata, animal exhalations, electricity, magnetism, heat, light, and even mental emotions, are all, under certain circumstances, capable of disturbing the organism and causing dangerous maladies, and yet, as Liebig, in his Animal Chemistry, truly observes, "with all our discoveries, we shall never know what light, electricity, and magnetism are in their essence. We can ascertain, however, the laws which regulate their motion and rest, because these are manifested in phenomena. In like manner the laws of vitality, and of all that disturbs, promotes, or alters it, may certainly be discovered, although we shall never learn what life is."

Let it be ever borne in mind, *that most substances, both in the organic and inorganic kingdoms, possess certain active principles which are latent and unappreciable in the natural state, and are only called forth and developed by the influence of some agent or process, which effects a transformation or metamorphosis of the crude material.*

Heat, electricity, and magnetism, become apparent when certain physical substances operate upon each other in such a manner as to disturb or change the original state of cohesion of particles.

Caloric is a property common to all material substances. In the natural state of these substances, this active principle is latent, and cannot be appreciated by the senses; but if *friction* be used, this agent is set free, and its power becomes manifest.

Electricity also, pervades all material bodies, and only becomes sensible when the natural state of these bodies is disturbed by *friction*.

It is probable, likewise, that iron and other substances contain magnetism in a *latent* state, and only require the operation of certain influences, to develop in them the phenomena of magnetism. This is evident from the fact, that "the same magnet may successively magnetize any number of steel bars, without losing any portion of its original virtue; from which it follows, that the magnet communicates nothing to the bars, but only develops, by its influence, *some hidden principle*."*

Large quantities of vegetable, animal, or mineral substances, may be taken into the stomach in a crude state, with impunity; but if their elementary particles become separated by decomposition, or otherwise, and then introduced into the system, they give rise to the most baneful results. It is a matter of little consequence, whether this minute subdivision of particles is effected by the action of solar heat and moisture, by trituration, or succussion; the ultimate effects are the same: The elements of the substance are separated, the essence or medicinal part is set free from the crude, material, and non-medicinal portions, and reduced to such a state of attenuation as to become readily absorbed, and yet retain all the specific qualities pertaining to the original agent.

Indeed, so minute and subtle are the miasms from vegetable and animal decomposition, the exhalations arising from contagious disorders, &c., that no one has yet been able to appreciate their physical or chemical properties, by the most accurate tests of chemistry or optics. Who, however, for this reason, will presume to deny or doubt their tremendous, although mysterious, power upon the human system?

When ether or chloroform evaporates, the cohesion between the particles of the liquid is destroyed; its elements float in the air, and are capable of impressing the organism in a much more powerful, and in a totally different manner, from any impression which could be produced by these constituents in a less attenuated state—as, for example, that of the original

* Beck's Chemistry.

liquid. If a large quantity of ether be swallowed, but slight effects will result; but if an imponderable quantity be introduced into the blood through the lungs, in the form of vapour, it is immediately brought into contact with the brain and nervous system, and the most astonishing effects speedily ensue.

"If the 10,240th of a grain of tartrate of mercury be diffused through the substance of a mere hard sweet-pea, the beautiful germ of a graceful flowering herb, which lies folded up in its horny pericarp, shall never come out and be expanded, though you imbed it in the softest mould, and solicit it by every art." (*Leuchs.*)

Professor Dôppler, of the Royal Institute of Prague, in speaking of the modus operandi of infinitesimal particles, writes thus: "From the moment in which the substance of the atoms succumbs to the influence of their surfaces, and apparently independent of the law of gravitation, they move with the greatest facility in every direction, and, as it were, become alive; from that moment only, in my opinion, drugs acquire the capacity of penetrating the organism, and of exciting there a curative effect. For if drugs, prepared in this manner, be brought in contact with the invisible extremities of nerves, their hyper-microscopical atoms will enter the organism at the same time with their *superficial electricity*, and will, if the nerves be in a perfectly natural state, be thrown out of the system without impediment, *after having penetrated it in every direction.* But if a body in a state of health be accompanied by an activity of the nervous system, perfectly unimpeded and equally free in every direction, we cannot, on the other side, but presume, that in a state of imperfect health the power of conduction, proper to the nervous substance, will be materially diminished, partially and in individual organs, either in consequence of a chemical change, or for some other reasons. But to use rather a material, but, nevertheless, by no means unfit comparison, as streams deposit the sand and pebbles they carry along, on those spots only where their currents meet with an impediment, and their rapidity seems broken by obstructions, so in a similar manner, in the diseased organism, may the electric currents, however feeble, *leave the atoms of drugs at the diseased spots*, where they, according to their individual properties, exert either a curative or detrimental influence."

If, then, *imponderable* substances possess powers so unequivocal and potent upon the healthy subject, when the organs are in a high state of vigour, and consequently in a good condition to resist the influence of foreign impressions, why may we not infer, with perfect propriety, that medicinal substances, equally *imponderable*, are capable of impressing the organism during disease, when the affected structures are unusually susceptible to extraneous influences?

Homœopathists suppose that the mode in which their tenuations operate is analogous to that of infection by miasms; that the inert matter of the substance is destroyed, and the active principle set free; and that the smallest quantity of this active principle, triturated with sugar of milk, or diffused in water or alcohol, is capable of communicating to the vehicles its properties, and thus to the organism its peculiar action.

The essential principles of all vegetable substances constitute but a very small proportion of the original crude article, and the more perfectly we separate these *active* from the *inactive* portions, the more pure and powerful will the remedy become. Like caloric, electricity, and magnetism, the strength remains latent in the crude state of the substance, and can only be developed by the important agency of heat, friction, or trituration.

Peach-blossoms, the bark of mountain-ash, the kernels of peaches, cherries, and plums, bitter almonds, &c., contain, in a latent condition, the active poison known as prussic acid, which may readily be obtained from either of these articles by a chemical process.

Ipecacuanha is indebted for its virtues, to a principle called *emetia*. Pelletier found, upon analysis, that the brown ipecacuanha bark contains only sixteen per cent. of *impure* emetia; and the red bark fourteen per cent. According to Bergelius, the impure emetia possesses only one-third the strength of the pure. We therefore find, that of one hundred parts of crude ipecacuanha, only five parts possess the medicinal virtues of the drug. Nor is it at all improbable, that farther researches will enable the chemist to free this principle from other impurities, and thus develop a still more potent medicine.

Opium contains but a very small per cent. of its narcotic principle, morphia. The crude substance contains, in addition to morphia, at least fourteen other ingredients, all of which are destitute of any particular virtues. Only about eight or nine per cent. of morphia is obtained from Turkey opium, and this is quite impure and unfit for use, containing narcotina, &c.

Cinchona is composed of ten or twelve ingredients of which, all but quinia and cinchonia, are inert. Even these last, as usually obtained, are highly adulterated, and do not by any means represent the active principle of bark in its purity.

The same rule obtains in relation to most other substances. The essential properties are distributed but sparingly throughout ligneous, resinous, and other matters, and it is only by the utmost care and nicety, that we can separate and develop these properties.

Indeed, there are many instances where the skill of the chemist is unable, not only to develop artificially certain principles of vegetable and animal substances, but even to analyze them when they become spontaneously disclosed by the action of heat and moisture. Miasmata and other noxious exhalations are examples of this kind.

It is a fundamental law of therapeutics, that the *active properties* of all medicinal substances can only be manifested from their *surfaces;* and it follows as a consequence, if we would develop the full powers of drugs, that they must be made to occupy *as great a surface as possible.*

If a compact piece of wood be ignited, but a small blaze can be produced; while if the same wood be cut into small portions, so as to expose a *large surface*, and then ignited, a large and powerful flame will appear.

Only a limited amount of electricity can be drawn from a given surface of glass; but if the same glass be made to occupy double the space, an additional amount of the fluid may be set free.

If a hole be rapidly bored through an ordinary piece of iron, the surface of each chip so detached will be found to possess magnetic properties; and a singular circumstance connected with this, is the fact, that when the boring is accomplished in a *perpendicular* direction, the chips are more highly magnetized than when it is effected *horizontally*. Here, again, is an instance where *friction* has developed properties entirely unappreciable in the natural state.

A single grain of matter may be made by trituration to pervade every part of one hundred grains of sugar of milk, and each molecule thus separated may be still farther subdivided into corpuscules, which in their turn may be diffused intimately through additional quantities of the medium. In this manner only, can we call forth all of the latent properties of drugs, and reduce them to that state of attenuation which is compatible with absorption, and which enables them to exert those salutary specific influences which the homœopathic practitioner so uniformly observes.

Each atom thus minutely separated, retains the power of exercising its *specific influence* upon the organism. *Quantity* is of but little consequence, provided that the substance is properly prepared; for an imponderable quantity in its highest state of development, is quite as capable of producing its peculiar effects in certain conditions of the body, as a much larger amount.

It is undoubtedly true that an atom, either morbific or medicinal, which possesses an affinity for a particular structure, is capable of communicating to such structure its peculiar action, the influence being propagated from one molecule to another, and each acquiring the properties of the original atom, until the influence is expended.

Examples of this kind of action are constantly presented to the physician in the form of *continuous sympathy*.

One inhalation of a noxious miasm, under favourable circumstances, is as capable of causing its specific contagion, as a thousand, or more. One thousandth part of a grain of a natural or morbid virus, is as capable of imparting the peculiar action of the poison to all parts of the organism susceptible to its influence, as a larger quantity.

So also, when an atom of a medicine is absorbed into the system and comes *in contact* with an organ or tissue already diseased, upon which it exercises a specific influence, it communicates to the surrounding atoms its peculiar action until the whole tissue is involved, and thus, if the remedy be homœopathic to the malady, it will supersede the primary affection.

La Place and Berthollet have advanced the opinion, that "a molecule, being put in motion, can communicate its motion to others, if in contact with them."

This law is applicable to both animate and inanimate matter, under certain circumstances. Thus, the smallest point of decayed vegetable or animal matter, if placed *in contact* with healthy vegetable or animal substances for which it has an affinity, will communicate to the latter its own morbid action.

The smallest point of decay in a tooth, continually propagates its peculiar action to the surrounding parts until the whole tooth is destroyed, or the diseased portion is removed.

The slightest spark of fire, put *in contact* with a combustible material, communicates its action to all parts susceptible of combustion.

A minute nucleus being once formed in the mineral kingdom, possesses the power of attracting to itself in a regular and uniform arrangement, all of those particles near it, for which it has an affinity, and the different varieties of minerals communicate to these particles their own peculiar action and arrangement.

It is asserted by the supporters of the chemical hypothesis, "that substances in a state of putrefaction, by entering the blood, impart their peculiar action to the constituents of that fluid, and all the substances of the body are induced to undergo a modified putrefaction."* Liebig affirms that "a body, the atoms

* Paris Pharmacologia.

of which are in a state of transformation, may impart its peculiar condition to compounds with which it may happen to communicate."

These assertions, however, are not sustained by facts. There is no proof that the blood becomes contaminated by the atoms which enter it in a state of transformation; nor is there any proof that such atoms are capable of "imparting their peculiar conditions," indifferently to other "compounds with which they may happen to communicate."

Every substance in nature, whether morbific or medicinal, possesses its own characteristic and distinct mode of action, and is only able to exercise or communicate this action, in a specific manner, to particular structures. Thus, the contagion of scarlatina imparts its peculiar action to the throat and skin. The contagion of scabies acts exclusively upon the skin. The miasms which occasion many kinds of fever, appear to expend their effects upon the nervous system. The virus of gonorrhœa is specific and uniform in its results upon the mucous membrane of the urethra. The virus of syphilis, although more general in its operation, affects only a certain class of structures. All of these poisonous matters are incapable of imparting their peculiar influence, unless they are brought *into contact* with those tissues for which they possess a "*kind of elective affinity.*" There is no reason to suppose, that in any instance we have named, the blood itself is contaminated, but it serves merely as the vehicle which conveys the morbid particles to the different parts of the body.

What we have advanced in regard to the *modus operandi* of morbific, is equally true of medicinal agents. We have before shown that most drugs possess well-defined specific actions, which can only be manifested after having been conveyed by the blood to their destined structures.

It will be perceived that the views here advanced in regard to the mode of operation of morbific and medicinal agents, differ essentially, not only from those of the chemical school, but also from those of most writers who have hitherto appeared as advocates of homœopathy. From quotations made at page 22, it will be observed that Hahnemann himself is a firm advocate of the "vital theory." In common with many distinguished writers of the old school, he supposes all diseases to consist of certain alterations of the "vital properties" of parts, and that medicines cure these diseases by acting upon these (supposed) immaterial properties in such a manner as to restore them to a normal state. In advocating these doctrines, Hahnemann has virtually rejected the theory of absorption, the truth of which has been so amply verified by Müller, Pereira, Blake, &c., and thus has marred a portion of his beautiful system.

It may seem impossible, at a first view, that *attenuated* drugs can be *absorbed* into the system, and exert their influence *topically* on the different structures; but in support of this opinion we beg leave to submit the following ideas.

Medicines, as has been previously remarked, are often detected in those structures on which they have exerted their effects. Mercury, iodine, sulphur, nitrate of silver, the salts of lead, iron, bismuth, copper, &c., have all been found in different tissues of the economy; and even Liebig himself advises us that many of these substances often form "permanent compounds with the different tissues." The same author also remarks, "if by the introduction of a substance certain abnormal conditions are rendered normal, it will be impossible to reject the opinion, that this phenomena depends on a change in the composition of the constituents of the diseased organism, *a change in which the elements of the remedy take a share.*"

The elements of the remedy do most certainly take a share in this change, but only so far as the disordered organ or tissue is concerned. It matters not whether the specific agent be imponderable in quantity, administered through the lungs, stomach, or skin, or injected into the veins; it seeks that part for which it has an affinity, and there manifests its force.

I have known persons to become salivated by the use of less than one-half of a grain of the first trituration of corrosive sublimate, given in divided doses. This can be explained in no other way than by supposing that the remedy is rendered innoxious to the absorbent vessels by the peculiar mode of preparation; for so small a quantity of the crude article has never, to our knowledge, been known to produce this result. By trituration, the crude particles of the mineral are so minutely separated and diffused through the vehicle, that the delicate absorbents admit them into the circulation with facility, while in an unprepared state the remedy would be recognised as an *irritant*, and consequently excluded.

When salivation is produced by large doses of calomel, or blue-mass, it is highly probable that *evaporation* occurs from the heat of the stomach and intestines, and that this vapour, impregnating the chyle, is absorbed. It has been said by the opponents of absorption, that the preparations of mercury cannot be absorbed on account of their *insoluble nature*, and therefore that salivation is caused by an impression which is made upon the "vital properties" of the stomach, and that this impression is reflected to the salivary glands, through the sympathetic nerves. But if the advocates of this doctrine will reflect that mercury evaporates at a *common temperature*, and that this vapour, when inhaled, exerts all the specific effects of the mineral, they must admit that when submitted to the higher temperature of the stomach and bowels, this evaporation and absorption will be augmented. "I believe," says Pereira, "with Buchan, Orfila, and others, that metallic mercury, in the finely divided state in which it must exist as vapour, *is itself poisonous.*"

An argument which we deem conclusive upon this point, is from the fact that traces of *mercury itself* have often been detected in the secretions, excretions, and solids of the body; and if any "vital properties" have reflected the influence, they must have conveyed the *solid substance* along bodily to the affected glands, etc.

In considering the subject of absorption and the topical action of attenuated drugs, it must be remembered that the absorbing structures are very delicate and sensitive, so that they are enabled to exclude all crude and irritating substances; and also that the extreme terminations of the nerves, in all parts of the body, are exquisitely susceptible to the influence of specific foreign agents; and a cause capable of affecting powerfully these minute filaments, would be entirely without energy and unappreciated, if brought to bear upon the trunk or larger branches of the same nerve.

Another fact illustrative of the truth of absorption and topical action is, that substances always exercise their specific effects more promptly and potently when introduced directly into the mass of the blood, than when taken by the stomach. "Medicinal or poisonous agents, injected into the blood-vessels, exert the same kind of specific influence over the functions of certain organs, as when they are administered in the usual way, but that their influence is more potent."*

Liebig also assures us, that "we can by remedial agents exercise an influence on every part of an organ by substances possessing a well-defined chemical action."

Here is a distinct recognition of the principle of the *topical* or *specific* action of remedial agents, although the character of this action is supposed to be chemical. Without entering into any discussion upon this point, or attempting to explain *how* morbific or remedial agents produce their peculiar effects, we shall remain satisfied with the positions we have before laid down, and simply refer our readers to the numerous instances, within their own knowledge, of the *topical* action of substances, both ponderable and imponderable, with the addition of a few examples of the latter, which can be understood and appreciated by all.

1st. *Odours.* When odoriferous particles are brought *into contact* with a certain nasal structure, (the schneiderian membrane,) the minute and sensitive nerves of the part take cognizance of the stimulus, a decided impression is made upon the whole membrane, and an odour, agreeable or otherwise, according to the nature of the exciting cause, is the result. In this instance, *physical*, but *imponderable* particles, operate

* Pereira, Mat. Med. and Ther.

upon the nasal tissue *by absolute contact*, and impart that peculiar action which enables us to appreciate odours.

2d, *Light.* According to Sir Isaac Newton, light is a *physical*, but *imponderable compound*, and can only manifest its power when its atoms are in contact with the organ of sight. These particles of light are the natural stimulus of the eye,—*material, imponderable, specific.* When this compound is separated into the different primary rays, each particular ray, when brought into contact with the eye, exercises a special and distinct influence, giving rise to the perfect appreciation of the different colours of the prism. Here again we are presented with an example of the specific influence of imponderable atoms upon a certain part of the system.

3d, *Caloric.* Newton also maintained that caloric is "a *distinct material substance*, the particles of which repel one another, and are attracted by all other substances."

When caloric is given off by a heated body, its atoms impart to all other atoms with which it comes *in contact*, its own peculiar action, and the sensation of heat, with its attendant phenomena, expansion, &c., is the consequence. Here we are afforded with a still more striking instance of the power of an imponderable substance in altering and modifying the character and properties of all substances upon which it exercises its action. This active principle, present in all bodies, hidden and unappreciable except when set free by *friction, percussion, mixture, electricity*, or *combustion*, possesses properties when thus liberated, surpassing in power and influence every other substance in nature ; yet it is more subtle and imponderable than the most attenuated medicines of homœopathy.

4th. Electricity, galvanism, magnetism, and the various gases, are all *material* substances, and manifest their influence *physically* by contact with the body.

It must not be supposed that light, heat, electricity, magnetism, etc., are immaterial nothings—mere properties of matter—because they cannot be weighed handled, and made subservient to all of those which govern more crude substances. Nor must it be supposed of drugs, that they possess no qualities except those which are apparent in the crude state, and can be fully appreciated by their nauseousness of taste, rankness of smell, or power of raking the stomach and intestines.

Modern science has demonstrated, that by *friction, percussion, mixture*, &c., some of the most powerful principles known may be liberated from substances, which, in a crude state, are entirely harmless. It has shown, that the more perfectly we can disencumber these principles from their inactive envelopes, the more potent they become. It has shown that the mass of ligneous, resinous, starchy, fatty, extractive, and colouring matters, which surround and enclose the active portions of vegetable substances, instead of possessing medicinal properties, serve only to nauseate and oppress the stomach and bowels, and thus complicate any existing malady.

Pereira, and other authors opposed to our system, have endeavoured to cover it with ridicule by entering into a computation respecting the *weight* and *strength* of the different attenuations. They have displayed before us tabular views showing the strength of each attenuation, and then assured us, without the trouble of testing the question practically, that such exceedingly small doses of medicines can produce no effect upon the system, but "that the supposed homœopathic cures are referable to a natural and spontaneous cure, aided, in many cases, by a strict attention to diet and regimen."* This is the principal argument urged against the therapeutical doctrines of Hahnemann.

We beg leave, however, to request those gentlemen who judge of the potency of substances by their *weight* and *dimensions*, to enter into a still further calculation, and inform us which possesses the greatest *weight*, the medicinal particles pertaining to a drop of a thirtieth attenuation of homœopathy, or the charge of electricity, which lays prostrate and senseless the strongest man—or the quantity of sulphuretted hydrogen, or carbonic acid gas, requisite to cause immediate

* Pereira's Mat. Med. and Ther.

death when inhaled? Which can be most readily detected and appreciated by *analysis*, the atoms of a high attenuation of Hahnemann, or the deleterious miasms which arise from vegetable or animal decomposition?

Which present the greatest difficulties in examination and description, the *physical structure* of the particles of a homœopathic medicament, or that of caloric, or light?

Will the respectable Hippocratic, who cannot recognise *power* in any material substance, unless it can be *weighed* or *handled*, enter into a computation, and inform us *how much* a poisonous dose of the vapour of hydrocyanic acid, mercury, or lead, *weighs?*

Let it be remembered, that not one atom of matter in the whole universe can be *annihilated:* transformations may be effected—the cohesion of particles may be changed*—atoms in their ultimate state of chemical combination may be *physically* divided into molecules, and again subdivided into lesser atoms to such an extent as to baffle detection from the most perfect tests of chemistry or optics—new powers may be developed in these atoms, the exact operation of which we may not at present be able to understand, but in no instance can we destroy one single particle of matter. We may effect an entire metamorphosis of almost any solid substance, and diffuse its elements in such a manner as to occupy and affect a very large amount of space. The elements of a few grains of gunpowder may be made with the aid of a few imponderable particles of caloric, to change their form, and impregnate every portion of the atmosphere of a large room. In like manner, a single grain of a vegetable or mineral substance may be transformed, and its atoms diffused throughout large quantities of inert materials, in such a manner as to impregnate them in every part with medicinal properties, but in no instance can a single atom be *annihilated.* Until we arrive at more accurate knowledge in relation to the laws which govern the chemical and physical action of the minute atoms of substances than we at present

* See Atomic Theories.

possess, let us not deny that they may be endowed with properties and powers, (although their modus medendi is a mystery to us,) capable of exercising an important influence upon the human organism.

In regard to the preparation of medicines, there are several points of difference worthy of particular notice, between the old and new schools.

1. Allopathy employs her drugs in a crude and consequently inactive form; while homœopathy makes use only of their pure essential principles, unencumbered by foreign matters.

2. Allopathy employs so great an amount of artificial heat in her pharmaceutical operations, that a large proportion of the active properties of her drugs is expended in evaporation; while homœopathy makes use only of expression, trituration, and succussion, and thus not only retains all of the virtues inherent in the drug, but actually develops powers which would have remained latent under other circumstances.

3. On account of the peculiar mode of preparation, the remedies of allopathy are offensive to the taste, nauseous to the stomach, and by their indigestible and irritating qualities, serve directly to induce gastric and intestinal derangements, and other serious medicinal symptoms. The medicines of homœopathy are liable to none of these objections.

4. For the reasons above enumerated, many of the remedies of the old school are excluded by the sensitive absorbents, on account of their irritating qualities, and are thrown off with the fæcal matters as foreign substances; having failed, in their passage through the intestinal canal, of producing any other effect than an irritation of the gastro-intestinal membrane. The attenuated remedies of homœopathy, being innocuous to the lacteals and absorbents, are readily admitted into the circulation and conveyed to those parts upon which they exert a specific action, thus impressing *directly* the organs or tissues actually diseased. "No substances," says Martyn Paine, in his Institutes of Medicine, "but such as exist in a fluid or *very attenuated state*, are taken up by the lacteals and absorbents."

So, also, in the therapeutical application of remedies, we claim, as far as accurate scientific principles and sound philosophy are concerned, that homœopathy is vastly superior to allopathy. We shall briefly reiterate some of the more prominent points of difference in the practice of the two schools.

The system of homœopathy is founded upon rational and scientific principles, inasmuch as its remedies are exhibited with a definite object, and the results can in most cases be predicted with mathematical certainty.

The practice of allopathy must always be indirect, uncertain, and empirical. The violence of the remedies employed, necessarily induces medicinal and sympathetic affections, which, mingling with the symptoms of the natural disease. render it impossible to distinguish between the two classes of symptoms, or to judge whether the malady, or the medicine, or both combined, are killing the patient. The fact, that so few allopathic practitioners coincide precisely in regard to the treatment of very many diseases, proves conclusively that their system is one of *guessing*, rather than one founded on scientific knowledge and ascertained facts.

Homœopathic remedies being *specific* and *certain* in their effects, operate only upon those parts which are actually diseased. Without inflaming healthy structures, debilitating the system, or disturbing the function of any organ, they induce, when judiciously exhibited, a new or alterative action in the part affected, of just sufficient severity to banish the natural malady, while the new or medicinal action subsides speedily and spontaneously.

According to the doctrines of homœopathy, no two diseases or kinds of inflammation can exist in the *same structure* at the *same time;* for whenever two exciting causes act upon the same part, the one possessing the most powerful action, must necessarily banish and supersede the weaker. Therefore, in accordance with the rules of our system, remedial impressions are always made *directly* upon the *organ* or *tissue affected,* and a new kind of action set up which abolishes the disease and usurps temporarily its place.

According to the strict tenets of the old school, remedies should be exhibited in such a manner as to impress structures which are *healthy* and *remote* from the *organ or tissue diseased*, in order that *revulsive*, *derivative*, or *counter-irritating* effects may be produced, and thus serve to attract the fluids from the *natural* affection to the *artificial* one. This plan of treatment originated, as we have seen, from the supposition that no two maladies of consequence could exist in *different parts* of the same organism at the *same time*. As this idea is at present universally conceded to be erroneous, we assert that a mode of practice deduced from such false data, must of necessity be unscientific and empirical.

By operating on *healthy structures*, the allopath accomplishes little or nothing towards restoring the impaired capillaries of the affected part to their original condition of strength and resistance, and consequently his system must be entirely inadequate to effect cures. We are, for this reason, forced to the conclusion that the modern Celsus, Dr. Forbes, is correct when he asserts, that "in a large proportion of the cases treated by allopathic physicians, the disease is cured by nature, and not by them."

It is a fundamental law of medicine, that no inflammation can be created in any part of the body, without giving rise to secondary sympathetic affections in *other and distant parts*. It is evident, therefore, that the greater the number of structures affected with inflammation, whether natural or artificial, the greater will be the number of sympathetic symptoms, and consequently the more serious and complicated the malady. Thus we perceive the force of Dr. Forbes' remark, "that in not a small proportion of the cases treated by the physicians of the old school, the disease is cured by nature, in spite of them; in other words, their interference opposing, instead of assisting, the cure."

We have before shown that organs and tissues become morbidly susceptible to the impressions of specific remedial agents *during inflammation;* therefore it is that extremely minute quantities of specific medicaments are capable of exercising powerful influences *during disease*, which, under circumstances of health, would be productive of no effects whatsoever. This is a truth of vast importance in the administration of medicines, and should be thoroughly appreciated by the practitioner who regards the welfare of his patients. Let him remember that these acquired susceptibilities are so great, that even the natural stimuli, food, gastric juice, bile, light, &c., cannot be tolerated; and from this fact, take warning lest he inflicts injury and counteracts the efforts of nature, by too active medicines.

But as we have so frequently observed, it is not so much our *principle of cure*, at which the shafts of the old school are directed, as to the doctrine of *small doses*. It is not because the adherents of allopathy *cannot* make themselves acquainted with the powers of attenuated drugs, but it is because their inveterate prejudices will not allow them to investigate the facts which are involved. They prefer *to die* of vomiting, purging, and sweating, as their predecessors have done for two thousand years, rather than to *be cured* quietly under a *new system*. These individuals are not satisfied unless they *feel and see* the poor body writhe and suffer for the sin of being sick. What care they for any interior or invisible action of a medicine, when they can be cut, racked, and tortured, by the lancet, emetics, cathartics, blisters and moxas, and that too, *secundem artem?* To be sure, they were not aware of any *visible effects when* the *morbid agent* operated upon their systems to *produce* the disease, but the *curative* part is in their own hands, and they are determined to exercise their privilege of a full and continual appreciation of the whole modus operandi of the remedial process. This part, *nature* has no power to cheat them of, but Hippocrates now reigns, and they are resolved to exercise their ancient reserved rights, and bleed, puke, purge, sweat and blister, *ad libitum*.

But why have our opponents dwelt so much upon our doses? Does not every homœopath aim and intend to give a sufficient quantity of the medicine at a time, to effect a speedy cure; and is not this quantity determined by experience of simple facts? We have different *strengths* or *attenuations* of each medicine, from the strongest tincture up to the most minute attenuations, and every homœopath selects that *strength* or *attenuation* of the drug which most speedily and safely *cures his patient.* The great point with him is, to select such a medicine as shall be homœopathic to the symptoms of the disease, and then to administer just enough of it to effect his object in the most safe and speedy manner. He finds by experience—by a mass of facts—that the tinctures and alkaloids, although often capable of subduing disease, are less prompt, less efficient, and less safe than weaker preparations of the drug. This easily demonstrated truth, was not the result of theory or hypothesis, but originated with Hahnemann, as we have already seen, through necessity, on discovering that the tinctures which were first employed by him, in accordance with his principle, often produced too violent impressions upon the affected structures. What cared Hahnemann—what care his disciples—whether they use *one* or *twenty* drops of a tincture, or *one* grain of a twentieth attenuation? Were twenty drops of a tincture, or twenty grains of a crude substance, more efficient in curing sickness than one drop or one grain of an attenuation, is there any man who supposes that Hahnemann or his followers would not have administered them in this form, in preference to any other? The chief glory of the founder of homœopathy does not consist in the discovery of the efficacy of small doses, but in the demonstration and practical introduction of the great doctrine of curing maladies by impressing diseased tissues with medicines which operate specifically upon these tissues themselves, rather than on distant parts.

It matters not, therefore, in regard to the homœopathic law of cure, whether we use this or that strength, provided the remedy is homœopathic to the disease, and exactly the requisite impression is produced upon the affected parts. The man who cures a belladonna headache with ten drops of the tincture, adheres to *similia similibus* as much as he who cures with the thirtieth attenuation of the medicine. The only question to be decided is, which strength cures most safely and quickly; and if facts prove, as all homœopaths believe, that a preparation weaker than the tincture is by far the most safe and efficient, then it is our duty to give these preparations the preference. It is found, for example, when repeated doses of tincture of belladonna are given in acute inflammation of the brain, that the primary symptoms from the drug manifest themselves too violently—that it causes dangerous and protracted medicinal aggravation, and a tardy re-action of the organism; while a dilution of the remedy impresses mildly the diseased structure, causing scarcely perceptible *primary* symptoms, and is speedily followed by its *secondary* or *curative* effects.

We shall conclude this chapter by quoting a few observations of the distinguished modern chemist (an allopathist) *Kane*, respecting the divisibility of matter, and some of the phenomena witnessed when a very high state of attenuation has been arrived at. We make these extracts for the benefit of those whose "bundles of ideas" are not already made up, trusting at least, that they may have the effect of demonstrating to such persons, that, not only morbific and medicinal power may exist in infinitesimal atoms of matter, but even *life itself.*

"It has been proved that gold may be divided into particles of at least $\frac{1}{1,400,000,000}$ of a square inch, and yet possess the colour and all other characters of the largest mass. If a grain of copper be dissolved in nitric acid, and then in water of ammonia, it will give a decided violet colour to 392 cubic inches of water. Even supposing that each portion of the liquor of the size of a grain of sand, and of which there are a million in a cubic inch, contains only one particle of copper, the grain must have divided itself into 392 million parts. A single drop of a strong solution of indigo, wherein at least 500,000 distinctly visible portions can be shown, colours 1,000 cubic inches of water; and as this mass of water contains certainly 500,000 times the bulk of the drop of the indigo solution, the particles of indigo must be smaller than $\frac{1}{2500,000,000,000}$ the twenty-five hundred millionth of a cubic inch. A rather more distinct experiment is the following: if we dissolve a fragment of silver, of 0.01 of a cubic line in size, in nitric acid, it will render distinctly milky, 500 cubic inches of a clear solution of common salt. Hence the magnitude of each particle of silver cannot exceed, but must rather fall far short of a billionth of a cubic line. To render the idea of this degree of division more distinct than the mere mention of so imperfectly conceivable a number as a billion could affect, it may be added, that a man, to reckon with a watch, counting day and night, a single billion of seconds, would require 31,675 years."

According to Dôppler, a cubic inch of brimstone, broken into a million equal pieces, a sand grain each in size, is magnified in sensible surface from six square inches to more than six square feet. It is calculable in this way, that, if each trituration of the homœopathist diminishes his drug a hundred times (an extremely moderate allowance), the *sensible surface* of a single inch of sulphur, or any other drug, shall be two square miles at the third trituration.

"In the organized kingdoms of nature, even this excessive tenuity of matter is far surpassed. An Irish girl has spun linen yarn of which a pound was 1,432 English miles in length, and of which, consequently, 17 lbs. 13 ounces would have girt the globe; a distinctly *visible* portion of such thread could not have *weighed* more than $\frac{1}{127,080,000}$ of a grain. Cotton has been spun so that a pound of thread was 203,000 yards in length, and wool 168 yards. And yet these, so far from being ultimate particles of matter, must have contained more than one vegetable or animal fibre; that fibre being of itself of complex organization, and built up of an indefinitely great number of more simple forms of matter.

"The microscope has, however, revealed to us still greater wonders as to the degree of minuteness which even complex bodies are capable of possessing. Each new improvement in our instruments displays to us new *races of animals*, too minute to be observed before, and of which it would require the heaping together of *millions upon millions to be visible to the naked eye*. And yet these animals *live* and *feed*, and have their organs for locomotion and prehension, their appetites to gratify, their dangers to avoid. They possess circulating systems often highly complex, and blood, with globules bearing to them, by analogy, the same proportion in size, that our blood globules do to us; and yet these globules, themselves organized, possessed of definite structure, lead us merely to a point where all power of distinct conception ceases; where we discover that nothing is great or small but by comparison; and that presented by nature on the one hand with magnitudes infinitely great, and on the other with as inconceivable minuteness, it only remains to bow down before the omnipotence of Nature's Lord, and own our inability to understand him." (*Kane's Chemistry, by Draper*, p. 19.)

CHAPTER X.

ATTENUATIONS OF DRUGS AND REPETITIONS OF DOSES.

In selecting our attenuations for the cure of disease, the following circumstances are to be taken into consideration: 1, the age, sex, temperament, constitution, and habits of life; 2, the condition of the disordered textures; 3, the character of the drug to be employed.

(*a*) *Age.* Infants and children of tender years, whose organisms have not become blunted by exposure to the ordinary stimuli of life, by improper food and drinks, and by abuse of cathartics and opiates, are in the most eminent degree impressible, and require the highest attenuations. It is at this period that the circulation is most active, the nervous system most delicate, and the tissues most sensitive to the influence of external agencies.

At the middle period of life, when the body has arrived at maturity, and all of the organs have acquired their full strength and vigour, the resisting power against both medicinal and morbific agencies is at its maximum. The action of the circulatory vessels is now moderate and stable, the nerves are strong, the structures have become accustomed to all kinds of stimuli, and the mind, which exercises so powerful an influence over the body, acts calmly and judiciously. At this period, our lower attenuations will often serve us more efficiently than the higher.

During the decline of life, many circumstances which have a tendency to modify the operation of medicines, are to be considered. Individuals who have passed their lives in intemperance, who have been afflicted with frequent attacks of disease, and whose systems are loaded with the cumulative poisons of drugs, usually acquire a remarkable obtuseness and inactivity of the whole organism, so that the very lowest attenuations are requisite to effect suitable impressions. On the other hand, many old people, upon the verge of second childhood, become sensitive, irritable, and so intensely impressible, that the higher preparations respond promptly and effectively.

(*b*) *Sex.* Females are more easily acted upon by medicines than males, for several reasons. Perhaps the most prominent one consists in their superior delicacy of organization: their circulation is more active, their nervous systems more irritable, and their mental powers more acute and quick, although less strong, logical and independent than those of men. J. J. Rousseau asserts, that a woman will leap to a conclusion which would require a man hours of severe thought to arrive at. It is this susceptibility and delicacy of organization which render the female more impressible than the male sex, and which should always have no inconsiderable weight in the selection of attenuations.

(*c*) *Temperament.* The temperament also has an important influence in the operation of medicines. As most morbific and remedial agents produce their effects upon the sentient extremities of the nerves, it follows that a highly susceptible condition of the nervous system is most favourable to the prompt operation of these causes. We therefore infer, that the higher attenuations are better adapted to the *nervous*, than to either of the other temperaments.

Next to the nervous temperament, in point of susceptibility, may be ranked the *sanguine*. Individuals of this temperament are characterized by great activity and energy, and by prominent development and vigour of the vascular system.

The temperaments which are the least susceptible to remedial impressions, are the *bilious* and *lymphatic*. The former is characterized by large muscular developments, tendency to biliary derangements, frequent turns of melancholy, and great powers of endurance. The latter is distinguished by a predominant activity of the glandular system, by a flabby and relaxed condition of the muscles, and by a feeble and rather obtuse state of the nervous system. These temperaments sometimes require our lowest attenuations, especially in chronic diseases.

Two or more of these temperaments often unite in the same person, when we have what is termed a *mixed* temperament. This variety may be considered, upon the whole, the most favourable to health and longevity, since no quality predominates, and the functions of the organism are more equalized.

(*d*) *Constitution.* Attenuations must also be selected with a due regard to the constitutional peculiarities of each particular case. We know of several persons who cannot take a blue pill, or a pill in which calomel is a constituent, without being violently salivated. There are others in whom opium produces furious and protracted delirium, and catharsis, as primary effects; others cannot carry ipecacuanha about their persons, or inhale the smallest quantity of it, without attacks of asthma; others cannot approach the rhus plant without being poisoned; others cannot use shell fish, and certain other sorts of food, without being afflicted with urticaria; the smell of hay causes asthma in some, and the delicate fragrance of the rose, syncope, in others. On the other hand, there are some organisms which can scarcely be impressed with even large and continued doses of medicines. Constitutions which have been impaired by abuse of stimulants, drugs, tobacco, and licentiousness, and in which there is an abasement of the nervous and physical power, demand low attenuations. In a word, it will be found on rigid examination, that each individual possesses some peculiarities which it will be necessary to take into consideration, when we decide respecting the strength or repetition of a remedy.

(e) *Habits of life.* We have read of persons who were "*music* mad," but we have often seen those who were *medicine* mad. The world is full of this class of monomaniacs, who "pass away their time in descanting on their own" diseases, and in filling their bodies with all sorts of injurious and nauseous drugs. After pursuing this course a long time, the system, by habit, tolerates enormous quantities of the poisons swallowed, and the structures lose, in a measure, their susceptibility to medicinal impressions. It is for this reason that the homœopathist experiences so much difficulty in the management of cases of dyspepsia, hypochondria, and constipation, which have been induced by long continued abuse of cathartics; also in the affections of confirmed opium eaters, habitual drunkards, and gourmands. Individuals of these classes, require low attenuations. In the same category may be ranked those operatives who make a free use of *mercury*, the salts of *lead*, the strong acids, and other poisonous substances which evaporate at the ordinary temperature.

Robust persons, who pass much time in active exercise in the open air, will require stronger doses than those of delicate organization and of studious and sedentary habits.

2. *The condition of the disordered textures.* Those parts of the system which are most amply supplied with nerves, are, all other things being equal, most susceptible to the operation of medicines. Thus the eye is more readily impressed than the arm; the lungs, stomach and intestines, than the limbs and joints, &c. Much, also, depends upon whether the specific employed, is positive and decided in its operation.

But there is another circumstance of vast moment to be taken into consideration in the choice of our attenuations, and to which we have elsewhere called particular attention. We refer to the *augmented susceptibility to medicinal impressions which inflamed structures acquire.* We have shown that the condition of inflamed tissues becomes entirely changed, and that their acquired susceptibilities become so morbidly increased, that even their natural stimuli cannot be tolerated, but when allowed to operate, become additional and powerful sources of disease. The natural and healthy material stimuli of the eye, the ear, the lungs, the stomach, the bladder, &c., are grateful during the normal state of these organs; but let inflammation occur, and the smallest pencil of light becomes intensely painful to the eye, as noises to the ear, air to the lungs, food and drinks to the stomach, and urine to the bladder.

Nor is this augmented susceptibility confined to the operation of the natural stimuli, but it applies with still greater force to the action of *specific* medicines, up to that point of inflammatory action when the sensitive extremities of the nerves succumb from intensity of excitement, and a condition bordering on paralysis or gangrene obtains. It is sometimes difficult to decide when this morbid erethism has arrived at its maximum, and the atonic state commences; but the gradual subsidence of pain, appearances of effusion or ulceration, and diminished sensibility of the affected part, will afford us the best indications upon this point. This fundamental law of homœopathy, not only serves to explain in the clearest possible manner the astonishing effects of infinitesimal doses, but it teaches an important practical fact, at present unappreciated, but incontrovertible, and which stands at the foundation of our therapeutical applications, viz., *to ascend in our scale of attenuations in proportion to the violence of the inflammation, until we arrive at that point where the nerves of the diseased part have attained their maximum of erethism, after which we must again descend the scale in the same ratio.*

This same law applies with equal force to all irritations of the nervous system, even when entirely unattended with the usual phenomena of inflammation, redness, swelling, heat, and pain. We have often seen this nervous erethism so strongly pronounced—and where there were no signs of vascular excitement—that a single grain of ipecacuanha, or the twentieth part of a grain of tartarized antimony, would produce copious vomiting and purging; or a drop of the first dilution of nux vomica, induce involuntary contractions of the muscles, especially of those parts which were unusually irritable; or a single grain of jalap, rheum, calomel, or even a mental emotion, immediately cause diarrhœa; or a cup of tea or coffee taken in the evening, prevent sleep for a whole night; or the inhalation of a few imponderable particles of ipecacuanha, give rise to both its primary and secondary specific effects upon the pulmonary organs.

There may be a few *apparent* exceptions to this rule, as in the example already referred to respecting the inefficiency of large quantities of opium and laudanum in *tetanus;* but these exceptions are susceptible of ready explanation. In this disease there exists a peculiar preternatural excitement of the nerves, which preside over the voluntary motions, and the contractility of the tissues, which induces a *spasmodic occlusion* of those textures of the digestive canal which, in the normal state, permit the absorption of opiates. This is evident from the fact, that if laudanum be *injected into the veins during tetanus,* the usual effects are manifested. In this exception, therefore, the drug is not *absorbed,* and of course cannot exercise its specific effects upon the economy.

It is evident, then, that in the selection of attenuations for chronic diseases, the precise condition of the nerves of the affected parts must always be taken into consideration, since some chronic maladies are characterized by a highly exalted nervous susceptibility, and call for the use of high attenuations; while in other cases, this susceptibility or impressibility remains at a low grade, and consequently will only respond to low attenuations.

Dr. Lobethal, in alluding to this subject, makes use of the following language:—"God be praised, the times are passed when we adhere without examination to the prescriptions of Hahnemann, and when we administered the thirtieth dilution in every case, without any regard either to the species of the medicine, or the individuality of the patient. The idea of greatness or littleness is but relative; we cannot say in a general manner, that some drops of the mother tincture of a certain medicine will be a strong dose; nor yet, perhaps, that the twenty-fourth or thirtieth dynamization of every medicine shall be regarded as a feeble dose. *The dose of each medicine should be strong enough to provoke the necessary reaction of the organism,* and, provided we are careful not to administer a too heavy one, agreeable to take, and without danger, we should always give a sufficient one.

"I am decidedly convinced, that in order to apply the homœopathic treatment with success, the physician should take cognizance of the whole scale at his disposal, from the actual dose of the old school, up to the highest dilutions of which any medicine is susceptible.

"We may establish it as a principle, that the administration of large or small doses is in inverse proportion to the richness in nerves of the individual organism, and the species of diseased organ; that is to say, the more the sentient sphere of the organism, in a given case, shows itself predominant, the more the dose of the indicated specific medicine should be feeble, and that the more the individual organism, or, in a local affection, the diseased organ, is poor in nerves, the more the doses should be large."—(*Revue Critique et Retrospective de la Matière Medicale Specifique.* Vol. iii., 1841).

Dr. G. H. Gross, of Germany, also observes, that "homœopathia, as now accepted, has determined the point, *that the physician must exercise his judgment as to the dose, varying it from the* HIGHEST DILUTION *down to* ONE OR MORE DROPS OF THE UNDILUTED TINCTURE, *as individual cases may demand.*" *

"In the Vienna Homœopathic Hospital, where a chronic case is rarely seen, the dilutions usually given by Dr. Fleischmann, range from the first to the sixth of the decimal scale. At the Linz Hospital, Dr. Reiss, though convinced of the efficacy of the highest dilutions, and occasionally prescribing them, treats the majority of his patients with the same dilutions as those employed by Fleischmann. In looking over the

* Dr. Gross wrote this in 1840; but during several years preceding his death, he was a most decided advocate of the highest dilutions.

records of homœopathic practice, we cannot help perceiving that of late years there has been a constant downward tendency with respect to the dilutions (the high potency novelty being left out of view). Not only is this true with respect to the generality of cases recorded, but also with respect to the practice of individuals. The majority of those statistics to which we so triumphantly appeal, are undoubtedly derived from the employment of the lower dilutions." (*British Jour. of Hom.* No. xxiii, p. 25.)

Dr. E. F. Ruckert, of Germany, also writes as follows: "I am satisfied that the system (homœopathia) is still progressive, and has by no means attained its perfection. In respect to *doses*, most generally, I make use of the *first dilutions*, and never exceed the twelfth, giving them in increased volume and repeating them frequently. I have been more successful in this course of treatment than formerly in the use of the smaller doses."

Similar views have recently been promulgated upon this subject, by *G. Schmid, Trinks, Griesselich, Watzke, Madden, Bigel, Drysdale, Russell,* and indeed by a majority of our school, both in Europe and America.

We have not unfrequently been able to cure disease with a high attenuation, after having failed with the first and second dilutions of the same remedy; but it has been a much more common occurrence with us, to effect cures with the first attenuation after having been unsuccessful with the higher preparations. No definite rules, therefore, can be given which will apply in all cases, but every circumstance connected with each particular case must be duly investigated, and the physician then exercise his own best judgment.

3. *The character of the medicine to be employed.*—Certain substances which are very feeble or even inert, in their natural crude state, appear to acquire new and potent qualities on trituration. Whether these new properties are communicated to the minutely divided particles by a chemical combination with the oxygen of the air, for which several, like carbon, graphite, sulphur, lime, &c., possess a very strong affinity, or whether they arise from the simple subdivision of the atoms of the drug, we are unable to determine. But these are the medicines which have been found

especially serviceable when employed in high attenuations.

On the other hand, there is a class of medicines so volatile in their nature, that trituration and exposure to the air and moisture, deprive them of their active principles. Amongst these articles may be ranked camphor, ammonia, bromine, nit. argenti, the ethers, the volatile salts, &c. Medicines of this kind should always be exhibited in the lower attenuations.

We must also be governed somewhat by the positive or negative character of the specific employed. Some medicines are very marked and prompt in their specific operation,like tartarized antimony, phosphorus, ipecacuanha, belladonna, aconite, hyoscyamus, stramonium, opium, &c., and may ordinarily be used at rather higher attenuations than those whose primary effects are less prompt and strongly pronounced.

The advantages which we obtain from a minute subdivision of crude substances, are as follows:

1st. We develop every part of the active principle pertaining to the substance, by breaking up all natural organization or arrangement between its molecules, and thus exposing a large amount of *active* surface which would otherwise have remained latent.

2d. By distributing these molecules intimately throughout an inert vehicle, (sugar or water,) they are far more readily absorbed by the delicate lacteals and absorbents, than coarse and irritating particles of matter.

3d. When these minute atoms have been conveyed by the blood to those parts with which they have an affinity, they penetrate the smallest vessels, impress the minutest sentient nerves, and become productive of results entirely unattainable by drugs in a crude form.

4th. During the act of subdivision, it is not improbable that the atoms of drugs sometimes become oxydized, and thus acquire new and increased powers.

Finally, we infer, that no new properties are developed by the homœopathic method of preparing drugs, except such as arise from the mere subdivision of their particles; and that all ideas respecting *spiritualization*, *dynamization*, and *magnetism*, in the preparation of medicines, are erroneous and untenable.

In regard to the repetition of doses, we are to be guided by the *acute* or *chronic* nature of the malady, the urgency and danger of the symptoms, and the effects produced by the medicine.

In violent and dangerous acute diseases, like cholera-asphyxia, convulsions, phrenitis, pleuritis, gastritis, &c., the remedies should be repeated as often as every fifteen, twenty, or thirty minutes—until an aggravation of the symptoms, (that is, some *primary* effect of the drug), appears, or a perceptible amelioration of the symptoms is apparent, when the medicine should be omitted, in the first case, until the *secondary* or *curative* symptoms have come on, and expended themselves; and in the latter, so long as amendment continues. If the case demands it, recourse may again be had to the same medicine; or if new symptoms have made their appearance, another appropriate remedy may be selected.

In less urgent cases of acute disease, it will be sufficient to repeat the remedy every four, six, or eight hours, until *primary* symptoms (aggravation) occur, or amelioration of the symptoms evinces the *secondary* or curative effects, when we may rest tranquil until the amendment ceases, and the medicine has expended its curative effect.

In chronic maladies, the remedy may be repeated once in twelve or twenty-four hours, until an impression is perceptible, either in the form of primary drug symptoms, or of amelioration of the morbid condition. When this result obtains, we may with great propriety wait until the full effects of the medicine have subsided, before we repeat the dose. In these cases it is far better to make use of doses sufficiently strong, and repeat them sufficiently often to induce decided primary medicinal symptoms—even if we are obliged now and then to give antidotes—rather than to remain for weeks in doubt as to whether a suitable impression has been produced by a *single* dose. It is very rare that moderate drug symptoms are productive of unpleasant consequences in chronic diseases, while the reaction thus induced in the diseased tissue, usually has the effect to bring about a much more speedy cure. Indeed, we believe it may be set down as a general rule, that the sooner we can produce a moderate, but decided medicinal action in a structure suffering from *chronic* inflammation, the sooner will a *curative reaction* follow, and health result.

"It would therefore appear that experience has confirmed the opinion of Hahnemann, that a certain amount of aggravation is essential to the therapeutic process; in the vast majority of cases this does not make itself known in any perceptible degree, but it does occur in a certain, though small amount of cases, sufficient to confirm its existence as an essential phenomenon. The cases in which it occurs with infinitesimal doses are probably only those of excessive or even idiosyncratic susceptibility, and even with these it is a phenomenon of no danger, and only slight inconvenience. Hence we may conclude, that a normal dose of homœopathic medicines, sufficiently small to avoid the liability to aggravation in a certain amount of cases, and yet sufficient to cure best and quickest in the majority of cases, is a mere chimera, and ought not to be sought for; but in seeking for doses the best for the majority of cases, we must lay our account for meeting with a certain number of aggravations, but practically these latter are of no importance.

Likewise in the case of collateral symptoms, it is affirmed by Hahnemann, that "we cannot arrange our doses so as to escape the liability to them in a small and practically unimportant degree."—(*Dr. Drysdale*: *British Jour. of Hom.*, No. xxiii., p. 22.)

In all cases of urgent acute disease, in which we can find no single remedy which corresponds to the prominent symptoms, it is necessary to select a second remedy which shall cover the remaining symptoms, and administer it in alternation with the first. *Pneumonia* is often accompanied by *cerebral* inflammation; *typhus fever*, with serious disorder of the intestinal canal, the lungs, the brain and nervous system; *intermittent fever*, with enlargement of the liver, jaundice, cough, &c.; and other maladies with affections in other parts of the body, which are not strictly connected with the original complaint. In examples of this kind, the alternation of remedies is both proper and necessary; at the same time it must be remembered, that it is far more desirable that a single medicine should be chosen which covers all the symptoms of the disease.

The same rule holds good with respect to giving medicines in *succession*. Whenever the first remedy fails in producing the required impression, or whenever important *new* symptoms arise to which the original drug does not correspond, we may resort to another which accords with the totality of the symptoms.

A large proportion of homœopathic physicians, both of Europe and America, now advocate a frequent repetition of doses in acute diseases, and in many instances give alternations of the remedies. Some of those who have expressed themselves decidedly upon this point, are, Drs. Gross, Schmid, Rau, Fleischmann, Reiss, Ruckert, Lobethal, Hartmann, Russel, Hull, Neidhard, Gray, Currie, Trinks, Griesselich, Madden, Dudgeon, and Quin.

The erroneous ideas which were formerly entertained respecting the alternate employment of remedies, are at present nearly abandoned. So long as the absurdity prevailed that our medicines operated in a kind of spiritual manner, upon certain mysterious appendages of the organism, termed "*vital properties*," it was deemed unsafe to administer two remedies in alternation, for fear of creating confusion among these dynamic influences; but since the laws of absorption, and the specific topical action of drugs, have become so fully established, there is no longer hesitation in alternating medicines whenever symptoms appear to require it.

CHAPTER XI.

GENERAL DIAGNOSIS.

It is a matter of the highest importance that the homœopath should be perfectly familiar with the most approved methods of diagnosis, in order that he may take advantage of every possible circumstance which may facilitate his investigations of disease. Although a patient may be competent in general to indicate the exact seat of his pain, and thus enable the physician to determine what organ or tissue is affected, this is by no means true in all cases.

There are many maladies which are entirely unattended with *pain*, or any other *local sign*, by which the physician can detect the suffering organ. In cases of infants and young children, who are unable to indicate the locality of their sufferings, and in some chronic affections, a knowledge of the external signs is of vast importance. In all such cases a proper skill in diagnosis will prepare the medical man to penetrate the innnermost recesses of the organism, and to understand its most profound secrets.

It is a singular and highly interesting fact, that the *pains* of the different parts of the body impart to the countenance certain characteristic and easily understood expressions. As these signs are involuntary, and almost uniformly present, all will recognise their importance as diagnostic phenomena.

In forming our diagnosis, it is essential in the first instance to notice accurately every circumstance connected with the patient which is at all peculiar or unnatural. The general expression of countenance, the tone of voice and manner of speaking, the figure, attitude, movements, etc., should be attentively marked. At the same time, age, sex, temperament, hereditary predisposition, occupation, habits of life, whether labouring under the effects of any previous malady or of mercury, and whether accustomed to the constant use of opium, should all be duly considered.

The patient should then be permitted to detail his symptoms after the manner pointed out by Hahnemann, in his Organon, (pages 126-7). In cases of inability on the part of the patient to enter into a description of the case, the friends should be called upon to give all of the information in their power, in regard to the rise and progress of the disorder. An attentive perusal of Hahnemann's advice upon this subject, is of the utmost importance to the acquisition of a perfect portraiture of every complaint.

Since, however, there are some instances in which neither the patient nor friends are able to afford any information respecting the nature or seat of the affection, it is indispensable to acquire a knowledge of all external and involuntary signs which can in any way illustrate the character of the malady.

Allopathic writers have divided diagnostic signs into those exhibited by the *countenance;* the *attitude;* the *nervous system;* the *digestive organs;* the *circulatory system;* the *respiratory organs;* the *skin;* the *lymphatic system;* the *secretions.*

As the countenance is an excellent index of what is occurring in distant parts of the organism, we should note attentively the expression of the *eyes, nose, mouth,* and *forehead,* and also whether sadness, moroseness, peevishness, despair, fear, grief, or joy, is evinced. By heeding carefully these indications, we shall be greatly assisted toward accurate opinions in obscure and complicated cases.

Thus, contraction of the features, rapid dilatation and contraction of the nostrils, dyspnœa, with expression of anxiety, indicate *acute inflammation of the respiratory organs.*

Sharp features, and expression of anguish, "forehead wrinkled, brows knit," eyes sunken, countenance pale, hollow cheeks, lips dry and bluish, indicate *pain and severe inflammation of the abdominal viscera.*

General expression of countenance flushed and excited, or dull and stupid; eyes red and brilliant, or dull and heavy; pupils contracted or dilated; protrusion of the eyes, with a wild expression; mouth drawn to one side; twitchings of the eyelids and muscles of the face, indicate *inflammation of the cerebral organs.*

Expression anxious; respiration difficult and rapid during inspiration, while expiration is comparatively easy; symptoms worse after assuming the recumbent posture; face swollen and livid; indicate *hydrothorax.*

Face flushed and swollen; lips blue; eyes prominent and unnatural; face cold; sudden startings in sleep; anxious expression; indicate *organic disease of the heart.*

Cheeks pale and blanched; lips white, and puffy; a

dark circle around the eye-lids; expression of languor and debility, indicate *chlorosis.*

Paleness and puffiness of the upper lip indicate *scrofula and verminous affections.*

"Eyes and face red; rapid respiration; motions of the nostrils rapid;" indicate ***simple acute fevers.***

FIGURE AND ATTITUDE.

Before alluding to the different attitudes assumed by the body during disease, as diagnostic signs, we shall take the liberty of digressing for a moment, in order to touch upon the importance of a proper cultivation of the physical powers, as a means for securing the most perfect corporeal development and symmetry.

In order that the organs may perform their functions in a proper manner, it is absolutely indispensable that the body should retain its normal structure and shape, and remain unincumbered by any artificial appliances which tend to impede the circulation or check the free action of the muscles. Unfortunately for mankind, it has been customary both in barbarous and civilized countries, to *distort artificially* certain parts of the body, under the absurd notion that they were improving upon nature, and enhancing the beauty of the figure which the Supreme Architect had formed in his own image.

Amongst the savage tribes of the Rocky Mountains, it is customary, and we suppose fashionable, for the natives to flatten the forehead by long-continued artificial pressure. This constitutes the ideal of savage beauty, and is the common method of improving upon the works of the Creator.

In other barbarous countries it is customary to slit the ears and nose, and hang from them large quantities of tin, brass, and other cheap ornaments. This, with the requisite amount of tattooing and painting, illustrates their notions of what the human figure should be.

In China, the semi-barbarous inhabitants compress the feet of their females, from birth, in such a manner as to prevent their growth and development; and in this abominable distortion consists their idea of female beauty. This is the Chinese improvement upon nature.

The Turks cram their women with "*pillau*," after the manner of stuffing geese, to cause enlargement of the liver, for "*pate de foi gras*,"—that they may become enormously fleshy, and thus present to the admiring eyes of their lords, figures of uniform dimensions in all directions. This is the Moslem's style of female beauty.

In the highly civilized countries of Europe and America, it is not customary to make use of artificial contrivances to flatten the head, prevent the growth and development of the feet, to slit the ears and nose, or cram their women; but, through the instrumentality of those "infernal machines," corsets and stays, the sex deem it indispensable, in order to be *genteel*, to compress entirely from its natural shape the most important and vital part of the organism. These unnatural efforts at distortion are usually commenced at an early period, and continued with perseverance, until the figure has lost its natural symmetry, the lungs are forced upwards, out of their just position, and the abdominal viscera made to accommodate themselves in the *new* situation to which they have been reduced by art.

The civilized females of the present day, affect to contemn the symmetrical figures which the Creator originally formed, and which the ancient sculptors delighted to represent in marble, and have chosen to "improve" on these old-fashioned notions, by partially cutting off the connection between the upper and lower parts of the body; thus reducing it from the shape of those models of perfection, the Venus di Medici, and the Venus of Milo, to that of a wasp or an hour-glass. We have not only the authority of the ancients in all those master-pieces of art in which they have illustrated their ideas of beauty, but the greatest of modern sculptors, our illustrious countryman, Powers, in a MS. letter before us, declines a suggestion that his exquisite statue of Eve should be exhibited, because *his* sense of harmonious proportion, as well as of physical necessity, compelled him to present the mother of mankind in the shape which the Creator approved as the ultimate product and most perfect fruit of divine intelligence and energy. "Eve," the sculptor says, with satirical humour, "is an old-fashioned body, and not so well formed and attractive as are her grand-daughters,—at least some of them. She wears her hair in a natural and most primitive manner, drawn back from the temples, and hanging loose behind, thus exposing those very ugly features in women. *Her waist is quite too large for our modern notions of beauty*, and her feet, they are so very broad and large! And did ever one see such long toes! they have never been wedged into form by the nice and pretty little shoes worn by her lovely descendants. But Eve is very stiff and unyielding in her disposition: *she will not allow her waist to be reduced by bandaging, because she is far more comfortable as she is*, and besides, she has *some regard for her health, which might suffer from such restraints upon her lungs, heart, liver, &c., &c., &c.* I could never prevail upon her to wear modern shoes, for she dreads corns, which, she says, are neither convenient nor ornamental. But some allowance ought to be made for these crude notions of hers,—founded as they are in the prejudices and absurdities of *primitive* days. Taking all these things into consideration, I think it best that she should not be exhibited, as it might subject me to censure, and severe criticisms, and these, too, without pecuniary reward."

Singular perversion of taste! wonderful and all-powerful influence of *fashion*, which can induce so many intelligent beings to suffer torture like savages, for the purpose of distorting their bodies, and bringing them into those artificial shapes which civilized nations denominate genteel and graceful!

Suppose a fashionable woman should apply corsets and stays to a favourite monkey, or a pet lap-dog, and so compress its body out of shape, would not the attempt be pronounced heartless, and its author, perhaps, be indicted for cruelty to animals? but when the same barbarity is perpetrated upon a human being, it is tolerated, because it is *genteel* and *fashionable!*

Were females the only sufferers from these cruel practices, the sin would not be so great; but their posterity participates deeply in the consequences which result from their criminal perversity. The flat and narrow chests, the stooping gaits, and the pale or sallow faces which greet us at every step, demonstrate the extent of our physical degeneration.

But the female sex are not alone censurable. Too great a proportion of the men,—of this country especially,—become round-shouldered, crooked, and deformed, from a want of free muscular exercise, and too close an application to business, in constrained, bent, and unnatural positions.

Physical education in latter times, has been quite overlooked. Parents have commenced sending their children to school in infancy, and their embryo minds have been tasked with all kinds of *mental* exercise, while their physical powers have been suffered to languish in heated and ill-ventilated rooms. Thus they have grown up with improved *minds*, but feeble, undeveloped, and perhaps crooked, or mis-shaped *bodies*.

Let it ever be remembered, that the mind and body exercise an influence upon each other, and if we would secure to the former its highest development, we must cultivate and perfect the latter. In this respect we may with advantage go back to antiquity, and copy after Herodicus, in advancing physical education.

But to return to our subject: As in health the attitude is erect, and those positions are assumed by the body and limbs which indicate muscular strength, so departures from the normal standard, induce corresponding alterations in the position and appearance of the body.

Thus, tremors; position upon the back, with a constant disposition to sink down towards the foot of the bed, indicate extreme *muscular debility*.

Distressing dyspnœa, and sense of suffocation when lying down; constant desire to assume the erect posture; general agitation, cough, and appearance of anxiety, indicate *hydrothorax*.

Common position upon the back; rigidity and morbid involuntary contractions of the flexor muscles, usually of the upper extremities, indicate *softening of the brain*.

Position upon the back, " with the knees drawn up;

head and shoulders a little elevated ; dread of motion, indicate *abdominal inflammation with acute pain.*

Position upon the belly ; pressure of the abdomen affording relief ; and very restless, indicate *spasmodic abdominal pains.*

Rigidity, and involuntary contraction of the muscles of the neck, back, and limbs, indicate *inflammation or irritation of the spinal cord.*

In the advanced stages of acute diseases, position upon the back, with the legs drawn up, indicate *retention of urine.*

THE TONGUE.

Much information may be gained, in many instances, from an examination of the tongue. The following are a few of the diagnostic signs presented by this organ:

A clean, smooth, and bright red tongue, indicate *inflammation of the gastric or intestinal mucous membrane.*

A clean and red tongue, with papilla prominent ; or a furred tongue, with red papilla appearing through the fur, indicate *scarlatina.*

A reddish, and tremulous tongue, indicates *mania á potu.*

A thick and yellow fur covering the tongue, with bitter taste, indicate *biliary derangement.*

A white fur upon the tongue, indicates slight *simple fever.*

Acute symptomatic fevers, effect but little change in the appearance of the tongue.

A relaxed, dilated, and tremulous tongue, indicates *congestive* or *nervous fevers.*

A pale and flabby tongue, " with large papilla," indicate *gastric debility*—met with in *chlorosis.*

A sharp and pointed tongue, is often observed in *irritation and inflammation of the brain.*

THE NERVOUS SYSTEM.

Tearing, throbbing, and aching pains—aggravated by contact, pressure, or movement, indicate *inflammatory action.*

Twitchings of the limbs ; jerkings and shocks of the

tendons; cramps; convulsive movements; violent contortion of the body; pains relieved by pressure; unattended with fever, indicate *spasmodic pains.*

Sharp and darting pains, unaccompanied by swelling, heat, or redness, indicate *neuralgic pains.*

Vague and wandering pains about the ancle often indicate *inflammation of the knee.*

Pains also in other healthy parts, sometimes indicate *inflammations in remote structures.*

Wakefulness, indicates *irritation of the nervous system.*

Irresistible inclination to sleep, with stertorous breathing, indicates *compression, or serious disturbance of the brain.*

Twitching of the muscles during sleep, and frequent waking from frightful dreams, indicate *organic disease of the heart;* also characteristic of *verminous irritation.*

Sudden, rapid, and jerking movements of the head and limbs, indicate *cerebral irritation, mania à potu, and some forms of insanity.*

THE ALIMENTARY CANAL.

The alvine discharges will afford many useful hints to the observing physician.

Thus, light or clay-coloured evacuations denote a *lack of bile.*

Mucous and bloody stools indicate *intestinal inflammation:* if accompanied with tenesmus, and redness or protrusion of the rectum, we may conclude that the lower part of the canal is affected.

Watery stools, with slight pain, indicate *irritation of the bowels.*

"Glairy, dark green evacuations, like chopped spinage, are characteristic of *hydrocephalus.*"

Very dry and hard fæces indicate a *relaxed and torpid state of the mucous membrane of the bowels.*

THE RESPIRATORY ORGANS.

Using the abdominal muscles principally in respiration, indicates *inflammation of the lungs.*

Using the intercostal muscles alone, indicates *abdominal inflammation.*

Irregular respiration, with stertorous breathing, indicates *compression of the brain.*

Inspiration difficult, anxious and rapid, while expiration is comparatively easy, is peculiar to *hydrothorax.*

Wheezing, short, panting and anxious respiration, with contraction of the larynx, indicate *asthma.*

Paroxysms of rapid, short, suffocating and spasmodic cough, indicate *pertussis.*

White, tenacious sputa, indicate *chronic bronchitis.*

Very thick, yellow, or greenish sputa, which sinks in water, indicative of *disorganization of the lungs.*

THE SKIN.

A yellow skin indicates *disordered liver.*

A sallow skin occurs in *chlorosis, and a few chronic ills.*

A pale and waxen skin denotes a *deficiency of blood.*

A blue or livid skin, in infants, indicates a *pervious foramen ovale.*

A hot and dry skin denote *inflammation.*

A cold skin, with internal heat, indicate *internal congestion.*

THE URINE.

Urine red and scanty denotes *inflammation.*

Urine clear, limpid, and abundant, in *nervous affections.*

Urine depositing a sediment indicates *biliary derangement.*

The above are only a few of the more common and well known diagnostic signs. Our only object is to direct the attention of physicians to this subject, for there are often many things about the general appearance of a patient which are slight and indescribable in themselves, but which will aid him materially in forming his opinions.

In order, then, to arrive at a correct diagnosis, it is necessary—

1. To note all external signs.

2. To ascertain the age, occupation, previous habits, predispositions, and peculiarities of the patient.

3. To procure from the patient a spontaneous and minute detail of his sufferings in his own language. When the patient is unable or incompetent to afford this information, get as accurate a description as possible from those best acquainted with the history of the case.

4. Ask such questions, and make such examinations by the touch, pressure, sight, hearing, percussion, auscultation, &c., as may be necessary to perfect the diagnosis.

CHAPTER XII.

FEVERS.

Much has been written, and many hypotheses have been advanced, from time to time, concerning the pathology of this important class of diseases. Within the two past centuries, the changes of opinion in regard to the nature and seat of fevers, have been almost innumerable ; and yet, with all that has been written, and the numerous bitter controversies which have taken place, we are at the present moment but little farther advanced as to any definite knowledge upon the subject, than we were centuries ago. Indeed, the opinions of the medical world at the present time, are so much at variance, that it would not be difficult to find men of distinction who advocate almost every doctrine which has ever been promulgated.

The old dogma that fevers arise from a *concoction* of something injurious to the system, has even its advocates ; thus, "substances in a state of putrefaction, by entering the blood, impart their peculiar action to the constituents of that fluid, *and all the substances of the body are induced to undergo a modified putrefaction.*"* Again, Dr. Burne says, "that the adynamic or typhoid fever has no local seat ; that its nature is a *morbid condition of the blood*, produced by the

* Paris Pharmacologia.

operation of a primary cause, the respiration of a contaminated or tainted atmosphere."

Dr. Clancy and other authors believe the proximate cause of fevers to be " a want of power in the system to form blood."

Others still, like Clutterbuck and Broussais, have contended that fevers of every denomination and degree, are the result of *inflammation.* They are supposed by these gentlemen to be *topical affections,* " the general disorder of the system being only *secondary* and *sympathetic.*" The former located the seat of fevers in the *brain,* the latter in the gastro-intestinal mucous membrane.

The vitalists suppose that fevers, in common with many other diseases, are owing to a morbid alteration of what are termed the vital properties of the textures affected.

Professor Mackintosh, of Edinburg, has advanced the opinion, " that the effects of outward causes, and inward irritations, in producing irregular determinations of blood, are the great agents in exciting diseases, and especially fevers." He supposes " that the functions of almost all organs are embarrassed in fever from the very beginning ; that internal determinations of blood take place, which rouses the system to reaction, and thus causes fevers ; that inflammations of all parts of the body will give rise to fever ; that inflammation may supervene during fever, without being the primary cause of the febrile commotion ; that the *nervous* system is involved as well as the *vascular ;* and that the blood itself must be in a diseased condition."

A majority of the profession at the present day, however, suppose with Cullen, that the prime causes which produce them, act directly upon the *nervous system,* and thus produce their pernicious results.

Our own opinion is, that fever is a *combination of symptoms* that may arise from a disturbance of any one or more parts of the body ; that the primary impression is made upon the extreme nerves of the part acted on ; and that the whole system is affected to a greater or less extent, secondarily, thus giving rise to that congeries of symptoms which constitute fever.

The skin, the nervous system, the circulation, the respiration, the secretions, and indeed the whole body partakes more or less in the general disturbance.

We suppose that the causes which produce fevers, are *specific agents* which operate by being absorbed into the circulation, and conveyed to those structures for which they have an affinity or attraction, there imparting those peculiar and specific actions which induce fevers.

The miasm which causes intermittent fever evidently impresses a different part of the organism from that which induces typhus. So also the miasms of yellow fever, the contagion of plague, smallpox, scarlet fever, &c., are all peculiar and specific morbific agents, which exercise their influences upon the system in different ways and in a manner analogous to medicinal agents. Whether this morbific influence is exerted upon the brain, the nervous system, the blood, the stomach, or the arterial coats, of one thing we are quite certain, that the miasm of intermittent fever can never cause plague, yellow, scarlet, or typhus fevers, nor can the poison of either of these maladies give rise to any disease except that of its own peculiar type.

It is probable that the contagion arising from human effluvia—of ship, jail, and hospital fevers, scarlatina, smallpox, plague, and the different kinds of malaria—are all distinct substances, composed of minute particles of matter, each possessing its own peculiar properties, and each exercising its own specific influence when introduced into the human organism. Unless this were true, we should see either of these affections constantly giving rise to any of the others indiscriminately.

In a perfectly healthy and vigorous state of the system, neither miasms nor contagious matters are capable of producing their peculiar effects, and they may continue to circulate harmlessly in the blood for months, until the system is debilitated from some cause and thus predisposed to their influence, or until their noxious qualities shall have been neutralized by frequent contact with the air respired at the lungs. The fact that physicians and other healthy persons so often expose themselves with impunity to all of the noxious agents, proves conclusively that a certain state of preparation is an essential condition to their operation.

At present the pathology of fever is so little understood, that all opinions respecting its nature and seat must be, to a considerable extent, vague and conjectural. In treating upon the different forms of fever, therefore, we shall adopt the classification of Mackintosh, on account of its simplicity and the superior facilities it affords for diagnosis. The following is the arrangement:

1st. Intermittent fever.

2d. Remittent or yellow fever: infantile remittent.

3d. Continued fever, subdivided into four orders, viz.:—

Fever from functional derangement.
" from inflammation.
" from congestion.

A mixed form of fever between these three last, but in which congestion predominates, commonly denominated typhus or synochus.

4th. Hectic fever.

5th. Fevers attended with eruptions, subdivided as follows:
Scarlet fever.
Measles.
Smallpox.
" " modified.
Chickenpox.
Miliary fever.
Roseola.
Urticaria.
Erysipelas.

6th. The plague.

In all of these fevers there are certain peculiar characteristics which serve to distinguish them from each other, and from all other maladies. Notwithstanding this, however, we scarcely ever find two cases of the same type running precisely the same course, or presenting precisely the same symptoms. So many circumstances connected with the exciting cause, as climate, age, sex, temperament, predispositions, habits, &c., tend to modify the character of each particular case, that all instances of the same malady must necessarily present different trains of symptoms. It will readily be perceived, therefore, how impossible it is to prescribe for the *name* of a disease instead of *symptoms*. We also take this occasion to express our opinion, that any classification of diseases whatever, is valuable as an aid in diagnosis rather than in the exhibition of remedies.

The course of a fever sometimes varies during its progress from its commencement to its termination, and on this account divisions are made into—

1. The forming stage.
2. The cold stage.
3. The hot stage.
4. The sweating stage.
5. Collapse.

This is a mere arbitrary division, which can by no means be relied upon, for many fevers run their course without the supervention of these stages. Let it ever be impressed upon the mind, then, that these classifications and divisions are entirely arbitrary and artificial, and can only be used for the purpose of facilitating our diagnostic examinations.

CHAPTER XIII.

CAUSES OF FEVER.

The causes of fever are either *predisposing* or exciting. Anything which debilitates the organism, or impairs the tone and resisting power of the nervous or muscular system, may be denominated a *predisposing* cause of disease. Under this head may be ranked, excessive physical or mental exertion, protracted grief, anxiety, fear, chagrin and disappointment, deprivation of well ventilated dwellings, proper food, clothing and exercise, over-indulgence in the pleasures of the table, stimulating drinks, licentiousness, want of cleanliness, and, finally, congenital causes, and those connected with some hereditary predisposition.

Those causes which induce fever by a direct impression, are termed *exciting* causes. Miasmata, contagious and epidemic effluvia, noxious gases, extreme and protracted heat or cold, and sudden changes of temperature, are examples of this class.

All of the causes, however, which we have ranked under the head of *predisposing*, may, and often do become, under favourable circumstances, actual *exciting* causes of fever.

It is equally true, also, as we have before observed, that what are called *exciting* causes, do not usually operate so as to produce fever, unless the system is prepared or rendered susceptible to their influence by debility, or some other predisposing cause.

The powers of the body may be taxed up to a certain point, by moral or physical, morbific or remedial agencies, without exciting actual disease ; but if the influence be carried beyond this point, an impaired condition of the capillaries acted on will ensue. with the usual concomitants, inflammation and fever. Even the natural maladies, scarlet fever, measles, smallpox, chickenpox, and hooping cough, seldom make their attacks unless the system is predisposed to receive their impressions. Therefore, these disorders will often attack one member of a family, while all of the rest, who are equally exposed to the contagion, will escape.

The same rule holds good in regard to the operation of morbific, as of remedial agents, viz.: in proportion to the departure of the organs and tissues from their healthy standard, so will be the acquired susceptibilities of these structures to the influence of morbific agents.

The importance, then, of a constant and regular system of physical culture, and a rigid avoidance of all those things which can in any way impair the normal integrity of the organism, will be recognised. Indeed, we believe that such a course *might* be pursued, as would secure an individual against disease until his system should succumb from old age. Such a course would involve a herculean task in our present state of physical degeneracy, yet it is not beyond the bounds of possibility.

A few of the means which we should recommend to accomplish this object would be,

1st. A proper system of physical education.

The first and most essential condition for the enjoyment of perfect health, consists in a symmetrical and well developed organization. In looking around upon the world, how few do we behold who can boast of unexceptionable physical conformations—how few who have not some imperfection which might have been avoided by an early and proper attention to physical culture!

But how shall this bodily perfection be attained?

We reply, by the universal establishment of free public gymnasiums, where those athletic exercises can be pursued which shall systematically develop and strengthen every part of the body. We repeat, let there be established, athletic sports, games, &c., suitable for all ages and conditions; where the man of mature years may occupy agreeably an occasional leisure hour with physical and mental benefit; where the growing youth can correct all incipient bodily defects, and acquire that development and expansion in every part, which will enable all of the organs to act in a free and healthy manner. Let us abolish "infant schools" for the education of infant *intellects*, and establish in their place infant gymnasiums for the culture of their infant *bodies*. Let us see no more *intellectual* "infant prodigies," with their pale, sickly faces, and their feeble and half-developed forms, but show us in their stead, *physical* prodigies with their rosy cheeks, their plump, firm, and well-grown muscles, and with elasticity and buoyancy reminding us constantly of perfect health. Show us your children of six, eight, or ten years of age, wild, bouncing, and overflowing with animal spirits, rather than your prim, well-mannered, delicate sickly, hot-house, and band-box specimens.

All physiologists agree as to the vast importance to the young, of a great amount of exercise—free, spontaneous, and unrestrained. It is a principle of their natures, absolutely essential to their well-being, and we must not permit the artificial customs or restraints of society to prevent it.

Our remarks apply with more force to cities than

to the country, for in the former everything is forced and unnatural: children are born into hot-houses, and reared in dwellings heated with Lehigh coal, to the temperature of 75 or 80 degrees Fahrenheit. Here do these unfortunates pass the best part of their existence, encompassed by everything which is unnatural and artificial, and inhaling an atmosphere deprived of a portion of its oxygen, and impregnated with carbonic and other noxious gases, until, while yet young in years, they arrive at the conditions of old age, satiated with the displays and luxuries of life, and reduced to a miserable state of physical inefficiency.

It has been well remarked by physiologists, that if the large cities were not constantly supplied with healthy recruits from the country, they would soon become desert wastes. This remark is, beyond question, true, and it is only necessary to look into any of our large towns and behold the numerous worn-out and impotent wrecks of the wealthy families who have been inhabitants for two or three generations, to be convinced of the fact.

The second means which we should advise to secure health would be, a correct system of dietetics. The use of all kinds of animal and vegetable substances which are perfectly pure, digestible, and healthy, should be rigidly prohibited. In order to accomplish this object, we do not believe that better rules could be adopted, than those instituted and commanded by Moses for the Jews. Amongst the articles forbidden in the dietetic regulations of the great Hebrew lawgiver, we find pork excluded, from the supposition that the swine is unclean and unhealthy. When we consider how frequently the animal is affected with that dreadful malady, scrofula, and also how filthy and disgusting are its habits, it is not surprising that any person who is at all particular as to the quality of the food he consumes, and who possesses ordinary powers of observation, should denounce this nasty, offensive, and diseased animal, as unfit for food. But this abominable stuff in all its different forms, is consumed by christians everywhere. Lard constitutes the culinary expletive which serves to connect the ingredients of almost every dish in one greasy union.

Whether the uses of pork and its preparations, have any agency in causing scrofula, we leave for others to determine. An argument, however, which tends to establish the affirmative, is in the fact, that amongst the strict Jews, and all of those nations where the animal is not used as food, this malady is scarcely known, while in every country where it constitutes an article of diet, scrofula abounds.

In a word, care in regard to the selection of proper articles of food, suitable methods of cookery, avoidance of fat and condiments, stimulant, narcotic, and hot drinks, and regularity in partaking of meals, will enable mankind to preserve the integrity and health of those organs which are concerned in digestion and assimilation, and thus avoid the numerous evils which accrue from errors in diet.

Finally, we would recommend the establishment of such a state of society as should recognise no pursuit or custom as legal or respectable, except such as should conduce directly to the health, morals, and general welfare of the community.

MIASMATA, &C.

Numerous experiments have been made for the purpose of arriving at the chemical and physical properties of miasmata, and contagious and epidemic effluvia, but as yet, all investigations upon this subject have proved futile. We only know that when animal or vegetable substances undergo decomposition, a principle is set free which diffuses itself in the atmosphere, and which possesses the power when absorbed into the system, of producing certain specific effects upon the extreme nerves, which generate fever. The portion which is thus liberated by the aid of heat and moisture, constitutes, without doubt, the *active principle* of the original crude substance, in its purest form and most perfect state of development. This *active principle* is as imponderable and attenuated as the preparations of homœopathy, and a few inhalations under favourable circumstances are capable of causing fever: it is also as specific and uniform in its operation and effects upon the economy, as remedial agents themselves.

CHAPTER XIV.

INTERMITTENT FEVER.

We have observed that each type of fever is marked by certain symptoms which distinguish it from all other varieties. The type under consideration presents its characteristics in a very striking manner. Indeed, so great is the difference between intermittent and other fevers, that some writers have withdrawn it from the list of febrile diseases, and ranked it with those connected with derangement of the cerebro-spinal system. The regularity and distinctness of the paroxysms, and the complete state of apyrexia between the periods of attack, certainly offer some reason for this course; but, on the other hand, as the combination of symptoms termed fever, is universally present during the paroxysms, and since upon the whole it bears a closer resemblance to *febrile* than *neuralgic*, or *ganglionic* affections, we shall continue to adopt the old classification.

In the different forms of intermittent fever, the interval which elapses between the commencement of one paroxysm and another, varies; some cases having an interval of 24, some 48, and others 72 hours from one attack to another. From this circumstance the different types have been designated—*quotidian*, or 24 hour type; *tertian*, or 48 hour type; *quartan*, or 72 hour type. These have also been subdivided into *double quartan*, *double tertian*, &c.

Diagnosis. A paroxysm of intermittent fever is composed of three stages, viz.: first, the *cold*; second the *hot*; third, the *sweating stages*.

Preceding the cold stage, there usually occur general feelings of lassitude, debility, uneasiness, and pains in the head, back, or loins, and sometimes slight sensations of external or internal cold. There is also a loss of appetite, disinclination to bodily or mental exertion, and a constant disposition to stretch or yawn.

As the *cold stage* actually commences, the extremities feel cold and contracted; the surface becomes pale, shrunken, rough, with diminished sensibility; a sensation of cold along the spine, extending into the thorax and abdomen; the coldness soon diffuses itself throughout the whole body; universal tremors, external and internal; chattering of the teeth; respiration laborious, rapid, and imperfect; oppression at the præcordia; countenance pale, leaden, earthy, or livid, shrunken, and expressive of anguish; eyes dull and sunken; lips livid; general sense of physical and mental prostration.

The *pulse* is variable: it may be slow, rapid, weak, oppressed, or intermitting.

The *temperature* of the body is usually natural, with the exception of the extremities.

The *duration* of this stage is exceedingly various; sometimes terminating in ten minutes, at other times, lasting four or five hours.

Paroxysms occasionally occur without any well marked cold stage, a slight trembling only being experienced previous to the hot stage; at other times neuralgic or rheumatic pains, or coma, precede the second stage.

Hot Stage. As soon as the chills begin to abate, flushes of heat commence passing over the body, until, in a short time, the hot stage is fully developed.

This stage is characterized by hot and dry skin; countenance flushed and full; mouth dry, tongue parched; urgent thirst; headache; respiration rapid and anxious; general restlessness; pains in different parts of the body; more or less disturbance of the mind; pulse usually rapid, sharp, and bounding.

This stage also varies very much in duration, it rarely terminating in less than four, and often continuing twelve, and sixteen hours. In some instances the hot stage even continues several days, when it becomes a *continued* fever; or it may assume the *remittent* form.

Sweating Stage. After the hot stage has run its course, a perspiration makes its appearance upon the forehead and extremities, which is soon diffused over the whole body. As the sweating becomes more and more profuse, the febrile symptoms, with the pains and uneasy sensations, gradually subside, until the paroxysm terminates in a perfect state of *apyrexia* or *convalescence*.

The above is a general description of the ordinary course of an intermittent paroxysm; but in some instances these stages are reversed, or one or more of them may be absent, or if present, only a few of the symptoms enumerated will be recognised.

Writers have divided intermittents into four varieties, viz., first, the *inflammatory;* second, the *congestive;* third, the *gastric;* fourth, the *malignant* intermittents.

This division is made from the fact that the different types, under certain circumstances, partake of the general character which these terms indicate. Thus, the *inflammatory* variety generally occurs during the winter and spring. *Quotidians* are more prone to partake of this modification than *tertians* or *quartans*. Patients labouring under this variety, rarely enjoy perfect intermissions between the paroxysms, and they are often left with permanent disorders of the liver, lungs, &c.

The *congestive* variety is very uncommon. It seldom attacks any except those of feeble, relaxed, and exhausted constitutions, in whom there is not sufficient vigour to accomplish a perfect reaction. The brain is the organ which usually suffers most, and coma often supervenes during the cold stage, which ends in death.

The *gastric* variety presents prominent symptoms of gastric derangement from the first, a superabundance of the biliary secretion, furred and bitter tongue, with nausea and vomiting. It is peculiar to temperate latitudes, and usually occurs in the autumn. In this variety the liver is much affected, and therefore we find chronic enlargements of this organ often remaining after the paroxysms have been subdued.

The *malignant* intermittents are peculiar to hot latitudes. They are attended with extreme debility from the onset; respiration is feebly and imperfectly performed, the blood is only partially oxygenated, diarrhœa now and then ensues, and a rapid prostration of the powers of the system usually occurs, which, in many instances, speedily proves fatal.

It has been noticed that chronic enlargements and indurations of the liver and spleen, affections of the lungs, dyspepsia, scirrhous indurations, &c., often succeed fever and ague. These affections have been looked upon as secondary consequences of the fever, while, in point of fact, they are *medicinal* diseases, superinduced by the abuse of mercury and bark.

These drugs are empyrically employed by the allopath, for the cure of this malady in all its various forms: Whether inflammatory symptoms predominate, whether there is congestion of the brain, lungs, or liver, or whether the system is exhausted by previous debilitating causes, *quinine* and *calomel* in large doses are the grand, and we might almost say, the only remedies of allopathy. But do these violent drugs actually *cure* the malady? When the paroxysms are arrested by the use of these herculean doses, are the seeds of the disease eradicated, and is there no danger of a relapse? Let the candid practitioner of the old school answer.

It is the opinion even of some eminent allopaths, that large doses of quinine often suspend chills and fever, by superinducing in the liver or some other important viscus, a serious medicinal inflammation or congestion which usurps, temporarily, the place of the intermittent. The effect of this truly allopathic measure is, however, only of short duration, for the paroxysms return again as soon as the artificial disease has somewhat abated, or from some slight exciting cause. Thus will the paroxysms repeatedly return, and be as often temporarily suspended, until finally some permanent chronic malady will become fastened upon the system and thus supersede the original affection.

Is there a man in existence sufficiently robust to swallow *with impunity* the quantities of antimony, calomel, bark and quinine, which are usually prescribed by the old school in fever and ague? Must not some part of the organism necessarily succumb before such formidable quantities of powerful medicines? Let the stoutest allopath presume to try the experiment upon his own person, and if he escapes without inflammation of the stomach and intestines, serious disease of the liver, lungs, spleen, or some other organ, we will confess our error, and say that large doses of quinine are innocent and harmless, and that the preparations of mercury are manageable, mild, and safe, when admitted into the human stomach.

Causes.—The most common cause of intermittent fever is a peculiar miasm which arises during the progress of vegetable decomposition, and which some authors have termed *koino miasmata.* The term *marsh miasm* is often used, but we deem it improper, as the miasms generated in *elevated* locations, are as capable of causing the disease, as those formed in low and *marshy* ground. The decomposition of vegetable matters, by the aid of solar heat and moisture, is the only condition requisite to develop the morbific principle.

Other causes occasionally give rise to fever and ague, as intestinal irritation from indigestible food, and worms, sudden suppression of old discharges, and atmospheric vicissitudes.

Therapeutics.—The remedies most commonly made use of in this malady, are *china* and *arsenicum.* The following will also be found appropriate in many instances:—*ipecacuanha, bryonia, eupatorium, perfoliatum, nux vomica, veratrum alb., belladonna, carbo veg., pulsatilla, antimonium crud., ignatia, cocculus, lachesis, sabadilla, sulphur, cina, natrum mur., capsicum.*

China.—*External indications.*—Yellowish colour of the skin and face; during the chill and heat, redness of the face, and distention of the veins of the face and head. "During the chill, bilious vomiting; palpitation of the heart; short cough."—(*Hartlaub*). "During the intermission, yellowish, clay-coloured countenance; weak eyes; fulness of the abdomen; cough; anasarca. In tertian fever, with thick, brown, yellow-coated tongue: countenance palish yellow during the paroxysm and intermission; swelling in the region of the spleen; eyes red and sensitive."—(*Knorre.*) Quotidian fevers, with pale countenance: cold and pale hands and feet, and retching up of mucus during the chill; while during the fever there are, red face, full quick pulse, dry spasmodic cough.

Physical Sensations.—Paroxysm preceded by palpitation of the heart, sneezing, anguish, nausea, thirst, bulimia, headache and colic. Thirst *before* and *after* the shiverings, or *during the sweating stage;* coldness of the body, with congestion to the head; soreness in the region of the liver; easy perspiration during sleep, or when moving; short cough; for the most part no thirst during the *cold* or *hot* stages. Hartlaub has cured chills, external or internal, without thirst, followed by heat with thirst; and followed, or not, by sweat; or chills in some parts of the body, with shuddering and heat in the head, terminating in fever, intermingled with chills, attended with thirst and followed by sweat; or no chills, but fever with urgent thirst, and afterwards with perspiration. Hartmann advises china, when we have during the paroxysm throbbing pain in the head, extending to the orbits; vertigo; nausea; pain in the region of the liver; sharp pain in the chest; short cough; aching pain in the abdomen during the chill; pains in the loins and legs. During the intermission, confusion of the head; transient vertigo; variable appetite; thirst; drowsiness after meals; uneasy sensation in the pit of the stomach; nausea; constipation; general debility. Knorre has cured the *quotidian* type, with vertigo; pale and cold hands and feet, and retching of mucus, during the chill; and pains in the head, both sides, and pit of the stomach; dry and jarring cough, and drowsiness during the fever, which is protracted and violent. Also, *tertian* fevers, with violent chills, heat, and thirst, followed by perspiration. During the paroxysm and intermission, there were bitter taste, eructations, and vomiting; aching pains in the pit of the stomach, and in the region of the spleen; yellow and sickly aspect. Also in *tertian* fever, when the chill is short and slight, but followed by violent aching pain in the forehead, in the right temple, and around the right eye; general heat; intense thirst; eyes hot, painful, and sensitive to the light; paroxysm commences in the forenoon, lasts until evening, and is succeeded by perspiration during the night.

Mental and moral symptoms.—Confusion of ideas and drowsiness during the paroxysm and intermission; anxiety; discouragement; great activity of the mind; sometimes delirium.

Administration.—One drop of the third dilution in a teaspoonful of water, may be given previous to the chill, and during the forming stage. Should this prove insufficient to remove the symptoms, the dose may be repeated every four hours during the intermissions.

Arsenicum.—*External indications.*—Face puffed and earthy; or countenance anxious, sunken, and of a yellow tint; pendiculations and drawing in the limbs during the cold stage; pungent and burning feel of the skin during the fever; dropsical swellings; trembling of the limbs during the sweating stage; pulse irregular, or quick, weak, small, and frequent, or suppressed and trembling; tongue bluish, white, or bright red; diminished urine; night-sweats; face red during the fever, but pale and sunken during the intermission.

Physical sensations.—Aggravation of existing symptoms just previous to, or during the attack; paroxysms imperfectly developed; chills and heat alternating; periods of attack regular, and generally in the morning or evening; burning thirst, or adypsia; fever of either type; burning in the stomach, sharp pains in the limbs, chest, back and head, during the heat, with difficulty of breathing; during the sweating stage, heaviness of the head, buzzing and ringing in the ears; between the cold and hot stage, drowsiness, languor, thirst, nausea, vomiting and hiccup; sweats during sleep, or on waking in the morning. Dr. Watzke has cured chills and thirst, followed by high fever, urgent thirst, dizziness, confusion in the head, and, finally, profuse perspiration without thirst. During the apyrexia, pains in the chest and head; weakness and faintness; small appetite; abdomen swollen, and affected with occasional colic pains. Dr. Hartlaub has cured chills without thirst, followed by fever with or without thirst, and then by perspiration:

before the chill, vertigo; fainting; pains in the side, chest, abdomen and back; stretching and yawning: *during the chill*, anxiety; pains in the head, back, limbs, and pit of the stomach; stretching and yawning; prostration; nausea; vomiting; coldness of the abdomen, oppression of the chest: *during the fever*, delirium; pain in the head; vertigo on rising; nausea; bitter taste; aching pain in the region of the liver; aching and burning, extending from the pit of the stomach to the left hypochondrium; oppression of the chest: *during the intermission*, pale countenance; white tongue; swelling of the hypochondrium and abdomen; cold, clammy sweat; throbbing pain in the forehead; thirst; no appetite; nausea; extreme debility; pains in the head, chest, back, and limbs.

Mental and moral symptoms.—Depression of spirits, and irritability previous to the attack; anxiety, uneasiness, confusion of ideas, which gradually increase until the sweating commences; occasionally delirium during the hot stage.

Administration.—Two drops of the sixth dilution in an ounce of water,—a dessert spoonful once in six hours during the apyrexia, until the symptoms have disappeared. One dose of this remedy will often prove successful where allopathic doses of crude cinchona, and other articles, have produced no effect. I have, in two instances, succeeded in curing cases which have resisted the old school method for months, with a *single drop* of the *thirtieth* attenuation.

Remarks.—Arsenicum is appropriate in any type of fever and ague, provided the symptoms correspond, although several authors especially commend it in the *tertian* and *quartan* forms. Fleischmann employs from the third to the sixth attenuation; Watzke generally gives the second, third and fourth dilutions. Unless the patient is unusually susceptible, we prefer the third to the sixth.

Ipecacuanha.—External indications.—Before the shiverings, uneasiness, stretching and lassitude, with cold sweat on the forehead; tongue clean or loaded; during the apyrexia, countenance pale or yellowish.

Physical sensations.—Slight chills, followed by much heat; or, severe chills with little heat; aggravation of the rigours from external heat; thirst only during the chill; nausea, vomiting, and other signs of *gastric disturbance*, manifest during the heat; also, constriction of the chest. Watzke advises *ipecac.*, when the *chills* are attended with thirst, confusion of ideas, and dull pains in the head; the *hot stage*, with thirst, and sharp pains in the head; the *sweating stage*, with but little or no thirst; the *apyrexia*, with want of appetite, bitter taste, oppression at stomach, and pale face. Hartlaub has cured slight and short chills, without thirst, followed with violent fever with thirst, and succeeded by profuse perspiration, or without perspiration. *Before* the chill, pain in the back: *during the paroxysm*, headache, dulness of intellect, gastric derangement, nausea and vomiting, oppression, contraction, pain in the chest, and cough: *during the intermission*, bitter taste of food, much saliva, loss of appetite, vomiting after eating, lassitude, sleeplessness.

Mental and moral symptoms.—Before the chill, dulness of intellect and sleeplessness: during the chill, confusion of ideas, irritability, impatience, and indisposition to mental effort.

Administration.—Same as *china.*

Remarks.—This remedy has been most frequently used in fevers of the *quotidian* and *tertian* types. Lobethal, Hartmann, Boenninghausen, Schmid, Fleischmann, Watzke, Madden, Trinks, Elwert and Rummel, have expressed themselves strongly in favour of the low dilutions of *ipecac.* in this disease.

Bryonia.—*External indications.*—During the shiverings, trembling and redness of the face: during the heat, nausea, and tendency to keep the recumbent posture: during the sweating period, frequent sighing and cough.

Physical sensations.—Preceding the cold stage, vertigo, headache, and lassitude; first stage, ushered in with severe chills and trembling, with heat in the head; chilly stage, more violent than the hot, or, slight but protracted chills, and some thirst; second stage, ushered in with flushes of heat and slight chills, in alternation in the first instance, afterwards burning heat and thirst; universal dry heat, external and internal; spasmodic cough; vertigo and headache during the fever; shooting pains in the side and abdomen; after the heat, profuse sweat; oppression in the chest, with dry cough; tendency to sweat night and morning; during the apyrexia, constipation, thirst, unhealthy yellowish complexion, and night sweats.

Mental and moral symptoms.—Irascibility, and disposition to look on the dark side of affairs.

Administration.—Two drops of the third dilution in an ounce of water,—a dessert spoonful two or three times during the apyrexy.

Eupatorium perfoliatum.—This is a remedy which we have found highly serviceable in many cases which have been complicated by the abuse of calomel and quinine. It is particularly indicated when the liver is much implicated. An intelligent friend of mine, who resides at the West, in a fever and ague district, informs me that he has for many years past made use of a very small quantity of an exceedingly *weak infusion* of this agent, as a prophylactic against the disease, in his own family, and with complete success. He also assures me, that he has often cured with astonishing facility, cases which had baffled for months the ordinary treatment, with a dose or two of an infusion very slightly bitter.

The *external indications* are, yellow tinge of the skin and eyes; eyes dull, heavy and sunken; lips pale or bluish, dry and cracked.

Physical sensations.—Irregular development of the paroxysms; frequent slight chills previous to the commencement of the first stage; partial chills in the back and extremities; dizziness, heaviness and ringing in the head, during the cold stage; hot stage ushered in with slight chills, alternating with flushes of heat, until in a short time the heat becomes general, attended with headache, nausea, vomiting, pains in the chest and stomach; pains in the bones; tenderness of the abdomen on pressure; loss of appetite; sensation of fatigue, languor and debility; constant inclination to sleep; nocturnal sweats.

Dr. Williamson advises *eupatorium* in the *quotidian* and *tertian* types, when the following symptoms are present: paroxysm commencing in the morning; thirst several hours before the chill, continuing during the chill and heat; stiffness of the fingers during the chill; soreness in the bones; aching pain with moaning, throughout the cold stage; a greater amount of shivering during the chill than is warranted by the degree of coldness; retching and vomiting of bile from drinking; vomiting after every draught; vomiting at the conclusion of the chill; distressing pain in the scorbiculus cordis throughout the chill and heat; chill beginning at nine o'clock in the morning; throbbing headache during the chill and heat; violent pain in the head and back before the chill; inconsiderable perspiration, or none at all; fever in the forenoon, preceded by thirst early in the morning, but no chill; attended by fatiguing cough and not followed by sweat; loose cough in the intermission; cough in the night previous to the paroxysm; yellowness of the skin.

Mental and moral symptoms.—During the paroxysm, confusion of ideas and ringing in the ears; discouragement; indifference to life; dull of conception, and discontented during the apyrexy.

Administration.—One drop of the first dilution in a spoonful of water, during the apyrexy. As a prophylactic against intermittents, one drop of the tincture two or three times a week.

Nux vomica.—External indications.— During the chills, skin, hands, feet, face and nails are cold and bluish; redness of one or both cheeks; spasmodic contractions in the limbs; yawnings and stretchings. Sweat profuse, sometimes with a disagreeable acid smell; partial or one-sided sweat; pulse hard, full and frequent, or small, quick, or feeble, or intermittent; dryness of the lips; tongue coated white or yellow.

Physical sensations.—First stage preceded by external and internal cold and yawning; chills usually *at night*, or in *the morning;* aggravated by motion, drinking, or excitement; pain and heat in the head; thirst for beer; pains in the back and loins; during the hot stage, headache, vertigo, thirst, nausea, pains in the chest; shivering on motion; debility; during the sweating stage the symptoms are mitigated; sweat and chills alternately.

Watzke gives us the following indications: chills

with thirst; headache, loss of consciousness, or delirium, painful and inflexible limbs, contracted feel of the muscles. Chills last four or five hours, and not followed by heat or perspiration. After the chill, exhaustion; pains in the hypochondria from distention; thirst and want of appetite; tongue white; feet swollen; sensation of heaviness when walking. Or, chills followed by heat and sweats; with thirst; anxiety; headache; slight cough, with burning sensation in the chest, worse during the chills and heat; constipated bowels; loss of appetite; craving for beer; weakness and faintness. Hartlaub has cured chills with or without external coldness, and without thirst; followed by fever with thirst, and succeeded or not by perspiration. The chill may be slight and short, or violent and protracted, with shaking and chattering of the teeth, and blue nails; fever attended with perspiration about the head and neck. Or, shaking chills with thirst, followed by fever with thirst, and by perspiration; chill preceded by thirst, coldness increased by drinking. Or, alternating chill and fever; motion during the fever or sweat causes chills; *during the chill*, pain in the back (sacrum); *during the fever*, headache, vertigo, red face, pain in the chest, vomiting of water, bile, slime and food; red urine; *during the intermission*, headache; vertigo; trembling of the head on motion; pain in the forehead; acid eructations; bad taste in the mouth, loss of appetite, disgust for food; much thirst; pain in the pit of the stomach after eating; distention and pain of the belly; constipation; pressing at the neck of the bladder after urinating; drawing in the limbs; weakness. Hartmann employs it when, at the commencement of the paroxysm, there are paralytic weakness of the limbs; disordered stomach; vertigo, and sudden prostration of strength.

Mental and moral symptoms.—During the chills, stupid or delirious; during the fever, anxious, melancholy, sad, timid, apprehensive of death. Occasionally monomania during the progress of the disease.

Administration.—Two drops of the twelfth dilution in an ounce of water—a dessert spoonful each night. If a cure is not effected at the end of a week, give a drop of the first dilution once in six hours, until the symptoms disappear.

Remarks.—*Nux* is particularly applicable to the quotidian and tertian types. If the individual has been a hard drinker, or luxurious and sedentary in his habits, the indications are still stronger.

Arnica.—*External indications.*—Inclination to remain quiet.

Physical sensations.—Chills occur in the evening; thirst; contraction of the features. In the hot stage, pain in the back and limbs; shiverings from the slightest exposure; the hot and sweating stages slight and of short duration. In the apyrexia, pain in the stomach; loss of appetite and general appearance of wretchedness and debility.

Mental and moral symptoms.—Obstinate; reckless; quarrelsome.

Administration.—My friend Dr. Shue, has been accustomed to exhibit this remedy in alternation with *ipecacuanha*, with marked benefit. It may be given at the first attenuation—a few drops every four hours during the apyrexy.

Veratrum album.—*External indications.*—Cold and clammy perspirations on the forehead; shuddering. In the hot stage, coma and red or purplish cheeks; pulse slow, and almost extinct, or small, quick, and intermittent; tongue red and dry.

Physical sensations.—General coldness of the whole body; cold stage of short duration, and attended with shivering; vertigo; nausea; pains in the back and loins; thirst for cold water; the second stage more protracted, and accompanied with headache; short dry cough; fever with external coldness; urine dark coloured; diarrhœa or constipation; coma; in the third stage, profuse perspiration, with thirst and drowsiness.

Hermann prescribes *veratrum*, when the chills are followed by sweat, and afterwards coldness. Or, chills alternating with fever, with thirst; vertigo; nausea, and pain in the back, succeeded by fever with delirium; flushed face, and tendency to sleep. After the paroxysm, morbid appetite. Or, cold stage, without the hot or sweating stage.

Mental and moral symptoms.—In the cold stage, confusion of ideas; in the hot stage, coma; during the apyrexy, restlessness, and sometimes mental alienation.

Administration.—One drop of the first dilution in an ounce of water—a table spoonful two or three times between the paroxysms.

Belladonna.—*External indications.*—Face pale and bloated during the cold fit: eyes red and injected; face red; pulsations of the carotids; veins of the forehead swollen; and some perspiration during the heat.

Physical sensations.—Shiverings and heat alternating; rigours followed by heat; during the fever, burning thirst; headache; shootings in the temples; great sensibility to impressions; delirium; sweat of the parts covered only; stitches in the chest; dimness of sight.

Mental and moral symptoms. Quarrelsome and passionate during the paroxysm; or, great agitation; mistrustful; constant dread of evil; visions of frightful or ludicrous objects; delirium.

Administration.—A drop of the third dilution in water, every four hours between the paroxysms.

Carbo veg.—*External indications:* Before the chill, pale face; cold feet and hands; during the fever, red face; during the intermission, nocturnal sweat; cold sweat on the face and limbs.

Physical sensations.—Tertian type, kept up by roused psora; rigours, preceded by throbbing of the temples; rending in the teeth and bones; and attended with thirst and sense of prostration; hot stage, attended with thirst, or absence of thirst; headache; vertigo; impaired vision; nausea; pains in the stomach and chest; acid sweats in the morning: in the intermission, paleness; emaciation; distention of the stomach; headache; loss of appetite; lassitude and disturbed sleep.

Mental and moral symptoms.—Anxiety and fear in the evening; intellect dull.

Administration.—One grain of the third trituration in two ounces of water, a tablespoonful once in four hours during the apyrexia.

Remarks.—This remedy was supposed by Hahnemann to be of especial service, in those old and obstinate cases of intermittent fever, which appeared to be connected with a psoric miasm lurking in the system. Hartlaub has found it curative in similar cases. It is adapted to the tertian type.

Pulsatilla.—*External indications.*—Face pale during the cold stage; face red and bloated in the hot stage, sometimes with sweat on the face; swelling of the veins; anxious and rapid respiration; eyes dull, and cloudy; inclination to remain in the recumbent posture; pulse quick and small, or full and slow, or feeble and suppressed; tongue coated, whitish, grayish, or yellowish.

Physical sensations.—Chills in the evening or afternoon; vertigo, pain and heaviness in the head; sensation of cold from slight exposure; irregular diffusion of heat, chiefly in the face, or on one side; absence of thirst: after the paroxysm, headache, oppression of the chest, moist cough, bitter taste.

Or, according to Lobethal, Hartmann and Watzke, chills without thirst; fever, with thirst, and dull headache; sweating very slight. Or, chills commencing with vomiting, with slight thirst during the cold, hot and sweating stages; diarrhœa; loss of appetite.

Mental and moral symptoms.—During the paroxysm, anxiety; sadness; taciturn; apprehension; dread of sudden death: great depression of spirits during the apyrexia.

Administration.—Two drops of the first dilution in an ounce of water,—a dessert spoonful three or four times during the apyrexia.

Remarks.—When the attacks have been incited by abuse of fat and indigestible food, or are connected with any derangement of the menstrual function, pulsatilla is appropriate. It has been most frequently employed in the *quartan* type.

Antimonium crudum.—*External indications.*—Face and eyes of a yellowish hue; yellow or whitish fur upon the tongue; pulse quick or slow.

Physical sensations.—Tertian type; short chills, followed by fever, with pain in the chest and pit of the stomach; predominance of gastric or bilious symptoms; frequent nausea and vomiting; bitter taste in the mouth; thirst; diarrhœa; distention of the stomach.

Mental and moral symptoms.—During the apyrexy, indifference to life; during the paroxysm, peevish; dread of misfortune; out of humour.

Administration.—Two drops of the third dilution in an ounce of water,—a tablespoonful once in six hours during the intermission.

Ignatia.—*External indications.*—During the chill, pale or sunken face; bilious vomiting: during the second stage, pale face, or one cheek red and the other pale: during the intermission, lips dry and cracked; countenance pale; hard, dry stools; nettle-rash; pulse variable; tongue white.

Physical sensations.—Rigours, with thirst for cold water; nausea and vomiting; pain in the back and limbs; oppression at the chest; loose, short cough; coldness, relieved by external heat; heat general during the second stage; vertigo; headache; pain in the back and limbs; drowsy; absence of thirst during the hot and sweating period; during the intermission, pressing and shooting pains in the head, back, and limbs; loss of appetite.

Mental and moral symptoms.—Occasionally delirious during the fever; suppressed grief, with sighing; timid, sad, irresolute, and inclined to weep during the apyrexy.

Administration.—Same as *belladonna.*

Cocculus.—*External indications.*—Trembling during the first stage; redness of the cheeks during the heat; pulse full, hard and frequent; tongue clean or loaded.

Physical sensations.—Transient chills; skin hot to the touch, in the first stage; burning heat in the cheeks; cramps in the loins and stomach, and but slight fever in the second stage; apyrexy, accompanied with vertigo; dull pain in the head, and general debility.

Mental and moral symptoms.—Apprehension of approaching evil; fear of death, during the paroxysm; sadness and discouragement during the apyrexy.

Administration.—Two drops of the third dilution, in

an ounce of water—a tablespoonful every four hours between the paroxysms.

Lachesis.—External indications.—Face pale, or leaden, discoloured or yellowish, during the cold stage and the intermission; red spots on the cheeks while the fever is on; blue circle round the eyes; red swelling of the face; agitation and tossing in the cold and hot stages; pulse intermittent, or feeble and frequent; tongue dry in the second stage.

Physical sensations.—Most of the time, icy coldness of the limbs; rigours only partial; pains in the limbs; fever at night or in the evening, with headache and great debility; oppression at the chest; severe pains in the limbs; thirst, and sometimes bilious vomiting.

Mental and moral symptoms.—In the apyrexy, melancholy, violent jealousy; weakness of memory: during the paroxysm, delirium; loquacity; irritability.

Administration.—One grain of the third trituration in two ounces of water—a dessert spoonful every twelve hours until the desired effect is obtained.

Sabadilla.—External indications.—In the cold stage, trembling of the limbs, spasmodic cough: in the hot stage, yawning and stretching; pulse variable; tongue natural.

Physical sensations.—The different stages imperfectly developed; external coldness with shivering; dry cough, pains in the chest, limbs and bones in the first stage: during the apyrexia, dull pains, with sense of fatigue.

Mental and moral symptoms.—During the paroxysm, inability to collect or arrange the thoughts; delusions of the imagination with respect to oneself; delirium.

Remarks.—This remedy is useful when the malady has been preceded for some time by gastric derangement, or in cases complicated by abuse of quinine.

Administration.—Same as *veratrum.*

Sulphur.—External indications.—Countenance pale or hot during the first stage; circumscribed redness of the cheeks during the second stage; sweat upon the head, face, and hands; eruptions or scabs upon the face, hands, or limbs; pulse hard, full and quick; tongue natural.

Physical sensations.—Previous to the first stage,

thirst and lassitude; chilliness in the *evening* or at *night*, and sometimes in the *afternoon;* shiverings in the back, chest and arms, with coldness of the hands, feet and nose; heat attended with thirst; burning sensation in the hands and feet; bruised and tired feelings in the limbs; palpitation of the heart; perspiration easily excited in the head, neck, hands, &c.

Mental and moral symptoms.—In the apyrexy, sadness, with frequent inclination to weep; during the paroxysm, irritable and peevish; thoughts incline to religious subjects.

Administration.—One grain of the first trituration in four parts—a powder every twelve or twenty-four hours until decided amendment or aggravation of symptoms ensue.

Remarks.—Sulphur has most often been employed in the quotidian type. In many cases of fever and ague occurring in psoric subjects, it will also prove eminently serviceable.

Cina.—Hermann and Gross have found *cina* curative when during the paroxysm there are, pale countenance; canine appetite; headache; nausea; foul breath: during the intermission, cold surface; morbid appetite; lassitude; occasional sweats.

Hartlaub advises *capsicum* in chills with thirst; headache; mucous vomiting; flow of saliva; great and painful swelling of the spleen; rending pains in the back, loins, and knees; yawning and stretching; fever, with or without thirst; headache; bad taste; cutting pains in the belly; pains in the chest, back, and legs; after the fever, slight or profuse sweat; in the intermission, ash-coloured countenance; swelling of the spleen and the feet; constant chilliness and coldness; drawing pains in different parts when in the air; useful in relapses after abuse of quinine.

The same writer commends *natrum mur*, in chills with little or no thirst; sharp pains in the forehead, back, and bones; short breath; yawning and sleepiness, followed by fever, with great thirst; severe rending or throbbing pains in the head and forehead; in the intermission, yellowish face; white tongue; hard and scanty stools; swollen stomach; headache; weak eyes; bitter taste; no appetite; great thirst;

pit of the stomach painful to the touch; sleepy in the day time, but sleepless at night; lassitude and debility. It also cures *tertian* and *quotidian* types, with chills only.

Administration.—A drop of the first dilution once in four hours between the paroxysms.

CHAPTER XVI.

YELLOW FEVER.

This fever is exceedingly uncertain in its course, violence, and duration. It may strike its victim suddenly prostrate, overwhelming in its severity the whole system, and thus preventing a single rally of the circulatory vessels; or it may advance mildly, differing but little from an ordinary attack of remitting fever. In some instances it bears a strong resemblance to the higher grades of bilious fever. Much depends upon the peculiar circumstances of the individual attacked. If he is recently from a temperate climate, and unaccustomed to hot regions, he will be more susceptible to the action of the poison than if he had been previously acclimated.

Medical men have supposed that after a certain period of exposure, the system becomes so completely accustomed to the miasm, that it loses all susceptibility to its influence, and in this manner the process of acclimation is accomplished. There is doubtless some truth in this idea, but there are other causes which exercise quite as important an influence in this process. Those persons who abandon a temperate for a residence in a tropical climate, do so in that physical condition which the requirements, habits, and regimen of the former naturally generate. In a previous chapter we have seen, that in cold regions, where the atmosphere is highly condensed, a large amount of animal food is requisite to supply the system with sufficient carbon and hydrogen to resist and neutralize the action of the inspired oxygen. With these habits, appropriate only where a condensed atmosphere is respired, individuals seek the tropics, with bodies abounding in carbon, and continuing, in most instances, their accustomed regimen of animal food and stimulants, thus burdening their systems with an amount of the elements of nutrition far greater than the oxygen contained in the rarefied air which they inhale can decompose.

It is probable, therefore, that one of the chief predisposing causes of yellow fever, is the presence of a greater amount of carbon in the system than the inspired air can properly act upon. The exact equilibrium between the supply of the elements of the food and the absorbed oxygen, is disturbed; the carbon predominates, and all of those derangements which proceed from a superabundance of this agent, necessarily ensue.

The inhabitants of tropical latitudes have comparatively but little desire for animal food, but prefer farinaceous diet, vegetables and fruits: in this manner naturally securing to themselves a due proportion between the elements assimilated and the oxygen absorbed; while the inhabitants of the north find it necessary to consume large quantities of meat and other articles abounding in the elements of nutrition, in order to preserve a healthy equilibrium. We therefore most strongly urge it upon those who remove from cold to hot climates, to adapt their systems by appropriate regimen, and strict temperance in all things, for the change, and we confidently predict that they will enjoy as great an immunity from this dreadful scourge, as the natives themselves.

Diagnosis. The premonitory symptoms of yellow fever are giddiness, wandering pains in the back and limbs, slight chills, nausea, and frequent sensations of faintness.

After these symptoms have continued a few hours, a decided reaction occurs: the circulation becomes excited, the face flushed, the eyes red, there are violent pains in the head, back, loins, and extremities, distress of stomach, and vomiting of acid bilious matters, the surface becomes dry and burning hot, mouth and throat dry, with intense thirst, and sometimes delirium.

The duration of this paroxysm is usually about twenty-four hours, although occasionally it continues two or three days, after which there is a remission of all the symptoms, except a distressed sensation in the stomach, with nausea and vomiting. The patient remains in this state with a considerable degree of comfort for a few hours, when there is a recurrence of many of the former symptoms in an aggravated form. The stomach now becomes extremely painful and sensitive, vomiting is violent and incessant, the fluids ejected are of a darker colour, the skin and eyes acquire a yellow tinge, and the mind becomes confused and wandering.

The duration of this second stage varies from twelve to forty-eight hours, with sometimes slight remissions towards the termination of the paroxysm, when the third or last stage sets in. This stage is characterized by the complete development of the dreaded "*black vomit.*" At this period, the powers of the system all sink rapidly; the pulse flags, and perhaps intermits; the tongue becomes dry, black and shrivelled; the breathing irregular and laborious; cramps seize the calves of the legs and the bowels; the whole countenance loses its natural, lifelike expression; the extremities become cold; colliquative sweats, diarrhœa, hæmorrhages, and loss of intellect occur, and, finally, dissolution ends the scene.

This is only a brief outline of the more ordinary symptoms and course of the malady, and will, we trust, serve to aid the inexperienced practitioner in his diagnosis. Each case, however, must necessarily present modifications according to the predisposition, habits, and peculiar circumstances of the individual attacked.

Causes.—When animal and vegetable matters are submitted, for a considerable length of time, to the daily influence of intense solar heat, and a certain amount of moisture in the crowded and filthy streets of cities, or other confined places, a miasm is generated, which, under favourable circumstances, will cause yellow fever. Concerning the nature of this miasm we know nothing; but it is evident, that the continued high degree of temperature to which these substances are exposed, and the confinement of their noxious emanations within the walls of crowded cities developes a more virulent morbific agent than is the case when the same matters are exposed in the open country, or to a more irregular and less intense heat, such as usually occurs in more temperate localities.

There are several other causes which act as powerful predisposing influences, one of the most important of which, as before mentioned, is the too free use of animal food and stimulants. We may also include in this category, irregular habits, mental anxiety, depression of spirits, fear, grief, exposure to night air or to a burning sun, and, indeed, whatever else tends to debilitate the organism.

Therapeutics.—The remedies most commonly applicable to the treatment of this affection are, *ipecacuanha, belladonna, bryonia, rhus, arsenicum,* and *aconite.* The other medicines likely to prove serviceable are, *nux vomica, mercurius, veratrum, china, sulphur, cantharides, carbo veg.,* and *crotalus.* The late and much lamented Dr. Taft, of New Orleans, was eminently successful in his treatment of the yellow fever as it occurred in that city. Sometime since, we had the pleasure of perusing a letter from a highly intelligent gentleman of New Orleans, in which he states, that the success of Dr. T. was so great in this malady, as to attract the marked attention of a large number of citizens; and the writer expresses a deliberate opinion, that a new and favourable era would soon have occurred in the management of this formidable affection, if the able and accomplished Taft had survived. The remedies which this physician found most successful, and upon which he chiefly relied, were *aconite, ipecacuanha, belladonna,* and *bryonia,* in the *first,* and sometimes *second* stages; in the second and third stages, in addition to the above, *rhus tox., arsenicum, veratrum, cantharides, carbo veg., nux vom.* These medicines were usually employed at the first attenuation, and frequently repeated, either singly or in alternation, as the circumstances of each case appeared to require.

When the first symptoms declare themselves, as dizziness, slight chills, pains in the back and limbs, uneasy sensations at the epigastrium, with nausea, vomiting, and sensation of faintness, *ipecacuanha*, at the third attenuation, should be immediately exhibited. This remedy may also be found serviceable during the second and third stages, in alternation with some other article. Should the malady continue to progress, the following medicines should be considered, and, in proper cases, promptly administered.

Belladonna.—External indications.—Glowing redness and bloated appearance of the face; eyes red and sparkling, or fixed, glistening, and prominent; tongue loaded with whitish mucus, or yellowish, or brownish; pulse variable.

Physical sensations.—Dry burning heat; sharp, darting and shooting pains in the head; violent throbbings in the head; burning thirst; painful heaviness and cramp-like pains in the back, loins, and legs; pressure, cramp-like, and contractive pains in the stomach; inclination to vomit, or violent vomitings.

Mental and moral symptoms.—During the remission, melancholy; dejection: when reaction comes on, great agitation, with continual tossing and anguish.

Administration.—*Belladonna* is for the most part applicable to the first stage of yellow fever. One drop of the third potency may be given once in one, two, three, or four hours, according to the violence of the symptoms.

Bryonia.—External indications.—Skin yellow; eyes red, or dull and glassy, or sparkling and filled with tears; tongue dry, and loaded with a white or yellow coating; pulse rapid, and full, or weak and rapid.

Physical sensations.—Severe pain and burning sensation in the stomach; vomiting, particularly after drinking; burning thirst; pains in the back and limbs; headache aggravated by movement; eyes painful on motion; sense of fulness and oppression in the stomach and intestines.

Mental and moral symptoms.—Anxiety, with dread and apprehension respecting the future; loss of memory; delirium.

Administration.—Two drops of the first dilution in

an ounce of water,—a dessert spoonful every two hours until an impression is produced.

Rhus.—External indications.—Surface of a dirty yellow colour; eyes glazed and sunken; tongue dry and black; lips dry and brownish; pulse quick and small; loquacious delirium, or coma with stertorous breathing; constant moaning.

Physical sensations.—Distressing pain and burning in the stomach; nausea and vomiting; paralysis of the lower extremities; spasms in the abdomen; want of power over the abdominal muscles; colic; diarrhœa; difficulty in deglutition, and pain on swallowing.

Mental and moral symptoms.—Intellect dull and clouded; constant uneasiness; delirium.

Administration.—Two drops of the third dilution in an ounce of water,—a dessert spoonful at a dose, and repeated as the symptoms require. In cases where this dilution is not sufficiently prompt or active, the first dilution may be substituted in drop doses.

Arsenicum.—External indications.—Face of a yellowish or bluish colour; eyes dull and sunken, with a dark mark under them; sclerotica yellow; nose pointed; coldness of the body, with cold and clammy sweat; lips and tongue brown or black; colliquative sweats; pulse irregular, or quick, weak, small and frequent, or suppressed and trembling.

Physical sensations.—Sense of extreme debility; dull, throbbing, stunning, or shooting pains in the head; burning or sharp and darting in the epigastrium, or in the region of the liver; limbs feel stiff and useless; frequent evacuations, with tenesmus, or painless and involuntary; oppression at the chest, with rapid and anxious respiration; cramps in the calves of the legs; great oppression at the stomach, with violent vomiting, especially after drinking; drawing and cramp-like pains in the abdomen; sensation as if a weight was pressing upon the abdomen.

Mental and moral symptoms.—Indifference; weakness of memory; stupidity; delirium, with great flow of ideas; loss of consciousness and of sense; raving.

Administration.—In urgent cases, a drop of the third dilution may be exhibited every half hour, until some change is produced in the symptoms. In less dangerous instances, the intervals of administration may be lengthened as circumstances require.

Aconite.—External indications.—Suitable in the first and second stages, when there are burning and dry skin; red cheeks; full and rapid pulse; red and sensitive eyes; tongue natural or covered with a whitish slimy coat; lips and mouth dry; vomiting of mucus and bile; urine dark red.

Physical sensations.—Violent febrile reaction; sensation of intense heat; great thirst; acute pains in the temples, forehead, or on one side of the head; vertigo on rising, eyes weak and sensitive to light; pains and soreness in the back and limbs; nausea; general sense of debility; great heat and irritability of the stomach; short and anxious respiration.

Mental and moral symptoms.—When the fever is on, great anguish, anxiety, and restlessness; for the most part nightly delirium.

Administration.—A drop of the first dilution may be given in water every two hours, until the active febrile symptoms abate. *Aconite* and *belladonna* may sometimes be alternated with benefit in the first period of the disease.

Remarks.—In a majority of cases, a few doses of this remedy will be found indispensable, during the first reaction. This corresponds with the experience of several physicians with whom we have communicated upon the subject, and whose opportunities of observation have been ample. Dr. Hempel thinks it probable that *aconite* is the only specific for this disease.

Nux vomica.—External indications.—Skin yellow; face pale or yellowish, especially round the nose and mouth; lower part of the sclerotica yellow; eyes inflamed with redness of the conjunctiva; eyes surrounded with a dark circle and full of tears; tongue with a thick white or yellow fur, or dry, cracked, and brown, with red edges; pulse variable.

Physical sensations.—Burning pains in the stomach; pressure or cramp-like pains in the epigastrium; vomiting of acid, bilious, or mucous matters; frequent and violent hiccough; eyes sensitive to light; vertigo, or pains in the head; tremours of the limbs; cramps in different parts; thirst for beer, brandy, or some stimulant; contraction of the abdominal muscles; loose discharges of slimy or bilious matters or blood; burning pains at the neck of the bladder, with difficulty in urinating; coldness, paralysis, and cramps in the legs; feet benumbed and cramped.

Mental and moral symptoms.—Excessive anxiety, uneasiness, fear of death; despair, or loss of consciousness and delirium, with moaning or muttering.

Administration.—Two drops of the third dilution in an ounce of water,—a dessert spoonful once in from two to six hours.

Mercurius.—*External indications.*—Yellow colour of the skin; eyes red, blood vessels of sclerotica injected; eyes sensitive to light; paralysis of one or more limbs; tongue with moist thick white fur, or dry and brown mucus; fæces variable; pulse irregular, or quick, strong, and intermittent, or weak and trembling.

Physical sensations.—Excessive inclination to sleep, or restlessness from nervous irritation; sense of fatigue and debility; rapid loss of strength; dizziness, or violent pain in the head; violent convulsive vomiting of mucous and bilious matters; burning pain and tenderness of the stomach; constipation, or diarrhœa with discharges of mucus, bile, or blood; coldness of the arms and legs, with cramps; excitability and sensibility of all the organs.

Mental and moral symptoms.—Anguish and agitation; weakness of memory; apprehensions; discouragement; moroseness; raving.

Administration.—A grain of the third trituration in an ounce of water—a dessert spoonful every two, four or six hours.

Veratrum alb. External indications.—Face of a yellowish or bluish colour, cold and covered with cold perspiration; eyes dull, clouded, yellowish and watery; lips and tongue dry, brown, and cracked; hiccough; coldness of the hands and feet; trembling and cramps of the feet, hands, and legs; evacuations loose, blackish or yellowish; pulse slow and almost extinct, or small, quick, and intermittent.

Physical sensations.—General prostration of strength;

confusion of head, or vertigo; deafness; difficult deglutition; intense thirst; violent vomiting of green bile and mucus, or black bile and blood; burning in the stomach; great exhaustion; cramps in the stomach, abdomen, and limbs; diarrhœa.

Mental and moral symptoms.—Timid; despondent; restless; loss of sense; coma or violent delirium.

Administration.—A drop of the third dilution in an ounce of water; a dessert spoonful frequently repeated, until an effect is apparent.

Sulphur.—*External indications.*—Face pale, or yellowish; eyes red, or yellowish; aphthæ in the mouth; tongue dry, rough, and reddish, or with white or brownish coat; pulse hard, quick, and full; fæces whitish, greenish, or brownish, bloody or purulent.

Physical sensations.—Dizziness, or sharp pains in the head; itching and burning pain in the eyes; roaring in the ears; nausea, with trembling and weakness; vomiting of bilious, acid, bloody, or blackish matters; pressure and pain in the stomach; pains in the back and loins.

Mental and moral symptoms.—Melancholy; sad; timid; undecided; wandering.

Administration.—A grain of the third trituration in an ounce of water; a dessert spoonful every four or six hours, extending or diminishing the intervals according to the exigencies of the case.

Cantharides is sometimes indicated in the third stage with complete insensibility, cramps in the abdominal muscles and legs, suppression of urine, hæmorrhages from the stomach and bowels, and cold sweat on the hands and feet. It may be employed at the first dilution, a drop every half hour, until a decided impression is produced.

Carbo veg. and *crotalus*, have both proved curative in the third stage of yellow fever, and should always receive due attention in grave cases.

CHAPTER XVII.

INFANTILE REMITTENT.

This is a disease peculiar to childhood, and is usually caused by the use of unhealthy and indigestible food, the irritation of teething, worms, repelled eruptions, sudden drying up of ulcers, discharges, &c. The affection is characterized by prominent disorder of the stomach and intestines, in most instances, but occasionally the brain or lungs seem to be chiefly affected. In all cases, however, whichever part the disease may seize upon, there occur regular *remissions* and *exacerbations.*

Diagnosis.—The malady under consideration makes its appearance with the premonitory symptoms of ordinary fever, as slight chills, restlessness, thirst, and wandering pains in the back, bowels, and limbs. When the hot stage is fully developed, the patient refers most of his sufferings to the stomach and intestines: they become painful, tender upon pressure, and there is either obstinate constipation or diarrhœa. The evacuations are usually darkish, offensive, and indicative of a deficiency of bile. When the disease is concentrated in the stomach, there is burning thirst, with vomiting of liquids as soon as swallowed; the tongue is usually covered with a moist, whitish fur, and red at the edges. If the inflammation be not promptly arrested, but is permitted to progress without the aid of appropriate remedies, lesions will occur in the digestive tube, or disorder of the brain or lungs will be very likely to supervene.

Causes.—Undue exposure to cold, sudden changes of temperature, improper food, worms, teething, repelled eruptions, abrupt suppression of accustomed discharges, and the injudicious use of irritating medicines.

Therapeutics.—The remedies suitable for the treatment of this affection, are, in the first instance, the higher dilutions of *aconite*, followed by those medicines which accord with the peculiar symptoms of each case. As soon as the fever has been sufficiently subdued by the former medicine, some of the following articles may be resorted to with advantage: *ipecacuanha, cina, chamomila, mercurius, belladonna, arsenicum, pulsatilla, nux vomica, spigelia, sulphur.*

Since in most instances the gastro-intestinal mucous membrane is the seat of the malady, it will be necessary to make a free use of *ipecac., merc., puls., nux, cham., dulc.* Should the brain or lungs become involved, *belladonna, bryon., nux, opium,* and *stramon.,* will prove efficient remedies.

Dr. Drysdale has found this fever, as it occurs in England, exceedingly intractable, notwithstanding the most assiduous care and attention on the part of both physician and friends. In children of scrofulous constitutions, Dr. D. has known the disease to persist for months, in spite of every remedial measure. In cases of this description, he advises *sulphur, calcarea, arsenicum,* and *silicea.*

In highly impressible and irritable children, we have often witnessed an almost constant tendency to febrile attacks, during dentition. The alimentary canal, the brain, and the nervous system, appear to remain in such a condition of erethism, that the slightest exciting causes, as errors in diet, worms, suddenly checked perspiration, &c., serve to develop the affection. In instances of this kind, *aconite, belladonna,* and *chamomela* are peculiarly appropriate, and will generally enable us to subdue permanently this morbid excitability. These remedies should be given in drop doses of the twelfth to the sixteenth dilution, once in twelve hours, until every sign of undue irritability has disappeared. Hartmann commends a few doses of *coffea cruda,* or of *cal. carb.* when this erethism is obstinate, and has continued for a long time.

If the febrile attack has already made considerable progress, with excessive irritability of the stomach, and immediate ejection of every thing which enters it, however simple; distention, pain, and tenderness of the stomach and bowels upon pressure; hot and dry skin; burning thirst; tongue covered with a whitish fur, and red at the edges; great restlessness and irritability ; loathing of food ; dark, yellow, slimy, or green diarrhœa, we may give a grain of the third trituration of *ipecacuanha*, or a drop of the sixth dilution of *chamomela*, once in two hours, as long as is deemed necessary.

If the disease is still farther advanced, and the countenance has assumed a pale, or dingy, sunken and cadaverous aspect ; dark and puffy appearance under the eyes ; coldness and dryness of the skin, or cold clammy sweat ; burning pains in the stomach and intestines ; thirst ; constant nausea ; the smallest quantity of food or drink, increasing the burning and distress, until they are rejected ; watery diarrhœa, with smarting and tenesmus ; great prostration ; frightful dreams, anguish and uneasiness, especially at night ; dark, dry and trembling tongue ; black and dry lips ; grinding of the teeth, we should employ *arsenicum* at the twelfth dilution—a drop in a teaspoonful of water every two hours, until the requisite effect is produced.

When in addition to the symptoms enumerated above, the child is exceedingly restless, and sensitive to light on the slightest noise ; with flushed cheeks ; red, glistening and protruded eyes ; hot head ; constant raising of the hands to the head ; rolling of the head from side to side ; sudden starts from sleep, with screams ; spasmodic twitches in different parts ; dilated or contracted pupils ; short and oppressed respiration, we should administer *belladonna* at the twelfth dilution—a drop in water, every two hours, until a decided impression is evident.

When the fever is accompanied by obstinate constipation ; frequent desire to urinate ; burning heat of the whole body ; morning exacerbations ; rigidity of the limbs ; or drawing, contractive sensations through the body ; occasional spasms ; frequent trembling both sleeping and after an exertion ; shudderings and chills from the least contact of cold air ; great sensitiveness of the whole body ; unpleasant symptoms often excited by motion or contact ; and indications of gastric or bilious disorder, we may employ *nux vom.* at the twelfth dilution—a drop in water, every two, three, or four hours, as circumstances require.

When the malady has been caused by the irritation

of worms, it will be necessary to use *cina* or *spigelia*. These medicines may be employed at the third attenuation, and a dose given three or four times daily until the morbid disposition of the alimentary canal is corrected.

Bryonia is applicable in cases attended with disorder of the pulmonary tissues. In addition to biliary and gastric derangement, there should be dry racking cough; stitches in the chest and sides; painful, anxious, and hurried respiration; bruised pains, and soreness in the limbs; pains aggravated by motion or contact; hot skin; thirst; alternating heat and chills; nightly delirium; irritable and quarrelsome. This remedy may be used at the sixth dilution—a drop once in two to four hours.

Dulcamara is the specific when the fever can be traced to exposure to wet and cold, which has caused a sudden check to the perspiration. In these cases, the force of the disease is expended upon the mucous membranes of the digestive and respiratory organs, as is indicated by watery diarrhœa, pains in the stomach and bowels, oppression at the chest, dry coryza, cough, and difficult respiration. Its administration is the same as *bryonia*.

If the attack is attributable to abuse of fat, crude and indigestible food, and is accompanied with prominent gastric derangement, *pulsatilla* should be employed at the sixth dilution—a drop every four hours until the disturbance is corrected.

CHAPTER XVII.

CONTINUED FEVER.

In this class of fevers may be included those arising from *functional derangement*, from *inflammation*, from *congestion*, and *typhus*.

FEVER FROM FUNCTIONAL DERANGEMENT.

Diagnosis.—This is generally the mildest and least dangerous of all the continued fevers. It commences with slight chills, alternating with flushes of heat, lassitude, restless nights, wandering pains in the head, back and limbs, which are soon succeeded by increased action of the heart and arteries, dry and hot skin, thirst, furred tongue, scanty and high-coloured urine, and moderate derangement of almost every function. If the malady is met at the onset with suitable remedies, its progress is cut short, and immediate convalescence ensues; but if it be allowed to continue unopposed, although it occasionally subsides spontaneously, it generally terminates in one of the other forms of continued fever.

Causes.—Overloading the stomach with fat, crude, and indigestible food, insufficient clothing, irregular habits, dwelling in damp and ill-ventilated houses, and the habitual and intemperate use of coffee, tea, and tobacco.

Therapeutics.—*Aconite*, from the first to the third dilution, if administered early, is sufficient to cure most cases of this form of fever; but if the disorder is neglected until inflammation or congestion occurs in some structure, then those medicines which operate specifically upon the parts affected, are to be employed, selecting those, of course, the pathogenetic symptoms of which cover the most perfectly those of the malady.

FEVER FROM INFLAMMATION. (*Synocha.*)

Diagnosis.—In this form of fever the general symptoms, as hot and dry skin, rapid and full pulse, dyspnœa, thirst, nausea, oppression at the epigastrium, restlessness, furred and dry tongue, are present; but the symptoms which more particularly characterize the disease, are determined by the organ which is prominently affected.

When the inflammation is located in the membranes of the brain, the face becomes flushed, the eyes red and sparkling or protruded, staring, and distorted, the carotids throb violently, pupils contracted or dilated, expression unnatural, furious delirium, pulse full, rapid, and bounding, and finally if the disorder progresses, sopor, muttering delirium, subsultus tendinum, and convulsions.

If the disease attacks the lungs, we shall have rapid, anxious, and oppressed respiration, shooting pains in the thorax, troublesome cough, with difficult expectoration, pain and soreness during inspiration, and perhaps other symptoms pertaining to inflammation of the pulmonic structures.

If the gastro-intestinal membrane be affected, we shall have the signs peculiar to inflammation of this tissue, as nausea and vomiting, pains in the bowels, increased on pressure, tongue red, countenance expressive of anguish, thirst, bowels hot and swollen.

Causes.—Atmospheric vicissitudes, extremes of cold or heat, errors in diet, and over-exertion. Inflammatory fever often succeeds neglected or mismanaged fevers from functional derangement, especially in cases where some organ has been previously debilitated, and in this manner rendered susceptible to inflammatory action. Indeed, it is probable that inflammations seldom occur in parts which are perfectly healthy and vigorous, but that when the exciting causes of fever operate in these cases, they merely give rise to slight and easily remedied functional derangements. Whenever, therefore, any structure of the organism is in a state of unnatural irritation or debility, this constitutes a powerful predisposing cause of inflammatory fever, which only requires some farther morbific influence to ensure its full development.

Therapeutics.—As in this form of fever there is an exaltation of most of the functions, and particularly of the circulatory vessels, *aconite* is an indispensable remedy, always in the onset and frequently during the course of the malady. This remedy, as all are aware, exerts a peculiar power over the action of the heart and arteries, and is, therefore, particularly appropriate in those cases distinguished from the first, by full and rapid pulse, hot and dry skin, thirst, &c.

In those instances where cerebral disorder predominates, *belladonna, opium*, and *stramon.*° will be found essential in the treatment, either alone, or in alternation with *aconite.*

If the pulmonary tissues are inflamed, suitable remedies may be found in *bryon., tart. ant., ipecac.*, and *phosphorus.*

For gastro-enteritic inflammation, recourse must be had to one or more of the following medicines, viz.: *merc., nux, ipecac., puls., dulc., cham., ars.*, and *verat.*

Administration.—In the selection of remedies, much depends upon the age, sex, temperament, as well as the peculiarities of each particular case. For children and adults who are very impressible, we advise the higher potencies; while in cases of vigorous and unsusceptible persons, the very lowest attenuations will prove most efficient.

In regard to the repetition of doses, no definite rules can be prescribed beforehand; everything must of necessity depend upon the nature and violence of the disease, and the effect which each particular dose produces.

FEVER FROM CONGESTION.

Diagnosis.—The precursory stage of congestive fever is characterized by restlessness, irritability, indisposition to mental or bodily exertion, fatigue from the slightest exercise, vertigo, giddiness, apprehension, pulse often below the natural standard. This stage continues from a few hours to six or seven days, when the second period fully developes itself.

The symptoms will now be modified in accordance with the organ which sustains the violence of the attack. If the brain be the suffering structure, the patient will complain of headache, oppression or tightness in the head, pupils contracted or dilated, the ideas confused, the pulse slow and labouring, and, finally, coma, paralysis, and convulsions may supervene.

When the bowels are the seat of the congestion, we shall observe an anxious and distressed expression of countenance, eyes sunken and glazed, more or less nausea and vomiting, bowels burning hot, and tender on pressure, while the extremities are cold; tongue slightly coated with a whitish or reddish fur; uneasiness, with constant desire to change position; frequent sighing; bowels constipated or relaxed; and, finally, spasms and stupor, with stertorous breathing.

If the disease concentrates in the lungs, there will be rapid, laborious, and obstructed respiration; pulse irregular or intermitting; cough; face and skin purple from imperfect decarbonization of the blood; surface cold, and pains in the chest.

In all of these varieties of congestion, the physical and mental energies of the system are below the natural standard, the pulse is generally unusually slow and feeble, the function of the lungs is imperfectly executed, there is an unequal distribution of heat, and diminution of sensibility throughout the body.

Causes.—Excessive cold, atmospheric changes, drinking large quantities of cold water when the body is heated, insufficient clothing, improper food, severe mental or physical exertion, sudden news, grief, fear, depression, disappointment, mortification, &c.

Therapeutics.—The remedies which have been used with most success in congestive fever, are, for the cerebral form, *bell.*, *acon.*, *op.*, *stram.*, *hyos.*, *conium mac.*, *coff.*, *mosch.*, and *camph.*

For the abdominal form, *ipecac.*, *verat.*, *ars.*, *nux*, *cuprum*, *merc.*, *phos.*, *carb. v.*, *secale cor.*

For the pulmonary form, *bryon.*, *acon.*, *phos.*, *lach.*, *seneg.*, *rhus tox.*, *tart. em.*, *hyos.*, *ammon. carb.*

Administration.—Congestive fevers often attack the organism suddenly and violently, and if not promptly arrested, run on to a speedy and fatal termination. In severe cases, therefore, as soon as the remedy has been selected which is homœopathic to the malady, it should be repeated at short intervals until a decided impression is made upon the symptoms. After a reasonable time, if no effects are apparent, give a still stronger dose, or change the medicine.

Let it be remembered, in all violent maladies, that our object is, to produce a specific effect upon the diseased structure as soon as possible, in order that we may supersede the morbid by a healthy medicinal action. We need have no fear in this fever of creating too great a medicinal aggravation, for there is a low grade of erethism and impressibility of the whole organism, and we can readily apply an antidote to any over-action which may be excited, and thus control its influence, while, if we permit the natural affection to make progress from a too timid and sparing an exhibition of remedies, disorganization will be likely to ensue.

In this form of fever, we generally employ the first, second, and third attenuations,—the dilutions in drop, and the triturations in grain doses.

CHAPTER XVIII.

TYPHUS.

Few diseases have attracted more attention and been the cause of more bitter controversies in the medical world, than typhus fever. While some have maintained that it is a malady peculiar to the cold seasons of temperate latitudes, and caused by exhalations of animal or vegetable matters in a state of putrefaction,* others assert with equal confidence that it occurs in all climates, at all seasons, at every period from infancy to old age; and that it does not arise

* Dewees, Bancroft, &c.

from any specific cause (sui generis), but may proceed from marsh miasms, animal exhalations, intense cold, errors in diet, over-exercise, and a variety of other causes.* Some suppose it contagious, and others non-contagious.

Respecting its nature and seat, it has had the honour of being located by different medical writers in every part of the body, from the crown of the head to the soles of the feet. At one time the whole world placed it in the blood : then another generation of theorists arose who seated it in the solids : at another period all the world, of France, made the discovery that its place was the gastro-intestinal mucous membrane, and that Hippocrates, Galen, Celsus, Stahl, Boerhaave, Cullen, Hoffman, Brown, *et omne id genus*, had been labouring under a succession of errors upon the subject for more than two thousand years. Still later, some theorists have found out that its position is in the brain and nervous system, while a few very sensible persons have arrived at the conclusion that the exact nature and seat of typhus is yet involved in obscurity.

At the present moment there are a great variety of opinions respecting it. One class of medical men suppose it to be a disease affecting principally the brain and ganglionic system of nerves. Another class suppose its action to be in "the mucous membranes and lymphatic glands, especially those of the ileum, whence it has been termed *typhus abdominalis*."† Others still suppose it to be a disease of a dynamic character, or an affection of the "vital properties" of the system. In regard to this last supposition, it cannot be refuted, because it means nothing at all. It is as senseless and absurd as it would be to attribute it to a derangement of the electric, magnetic, galvanic, or any other "properties" which we may *assume* that the organism possesses.

The malady assumes different characteristics according to the predisposition of the individual when exposed to the influence of the contagion. If his sys-

* Natham Smith, Macintosh, &c. † Hartmann.

tem has been debilitated by over-exertion of body or mind, by grief, care, misfortune, disappointment or shame, the brain and nervous system will be prominently affected, and we shall be presented with that variety termed *cerebral typhus.*

Should the stomach and intestines happen to be in a state of irritation and debility, when the contagion is absorbed, they will receive the impression, and we shall have what is denominated *abdominal typhus.*

If the organ predisposed be the lungs, the morbific agent will spend its effects at this point, and *pneumo typhus* be the result.

So long, however, as the whole organism remains in a perfectly sound and vigorous condition, with the mind cheerful and moderately active, it will be able to resist the influence of the miasm, and in all probability escape the malady. The law is fundamental, and cannot be too often inculcated, that just in proportion as the organism, or any part of it, diverges from the normal standard, in the same ratio will the susceptibility of such affected structures to morbific or remedial influences, be increased.

Diagnosis.—The symptoms which appear at the commencement of typhus, are, lassitude, debility, sense of fatigue, impaired memory, slight chills, alternating with flushes of heat, dull pains in the head, back and limbs, loss of appetite, and melancholy. These symptoms often continue one or two weeks, the patient not feeling sick enough to take his bed, or sufficiently well to attend to his occupation, when he becomes more restless during the night, delirium sets in, he is obliged to keep his bed from debility, his tongue, which was at first coated with a thin, white fur, becomes dark, dry, and cracked, and as the disease advances, the old fur passes off, leaving the surface red, glazed, and dry. As the disease progresses, the eyes become suffused, the countenance loses its natural expression, the muscles are weak and tremulous, a viscid saliva is secreted, which collects and dries upon the lips and teeth, the surface acquires a dingy colour, there are subsultus tendinum, defective vision, partial loss of hearing, a tendency to slide down to the foot of the bed, involuntary discharges from the bowels and bladder, picking at the bedclothes, low muttering delirium, and, finally, coma, convulsions and death.

The symptoms and course of the complaint will, of course, be modified in accordance with the severity of the attack, the part affected, and the plan of treatment pursued.

If we may be allowed to judge from the opinions which have from time to time been expressed by some of the eldest, most experienced, and distinguished members of the old school, upon this subject, we will say, that the course of treatment ordinarily recommended and pursued by allopathists, is productive of far more injury than benefit, in typhus. In proof of this, we quote from a monograph upon typhus fever, by the late Professor Nathan Smith, of Yale College, published in 1831.

After commenting upon the various contradictory methods of treatment advised by different authors, as the antiphlogistic, stimulant, tonic, derivative, &c., he asserts: "I am clearly of opinion, that we had better leave the disease (typhus) to cure itself, as remedies, especially powerful ones, are more likely to do harm than good."

In another place he declares: that "the use of powerful means, with a view of curing this disease, is liable to do great mischief."

These are not the hasty opinions of a mere theoretical man of books, but they are the matured sentiments of one who enjoyed an immense practice in several of the different New England states, for a period of more than forty years. Many other more recent authors have not hesitated to avow similar views, and, although they do not yet admit the truths of the new law of cure, they entertain an entire lack of confidence in the therapeutical doctrines of the old system, so far as typhus, and many other maladies, are concerned.

It may, then, with much propriety be affirmed, that serious injury is often inflicted in typhus by allopathic treatment, and that many of the symptoms above enumerated are aggravated, if not actually superinduced, by blood-letting, counter-irritants, and powerful drugs.

Causes.—The presumption is very strong, that the cause of typhus is a specific agent, *sui generis*, and that it is set free from the animal body during the course of a fever, or when a number of individuals are crowded together in close, filthy, and ill-ventilated apartments. This specific poison rarely, if ever, makes a serious impression, unless the organism is previously predisposed to its influence. When all of the organs are in a normal condition, and operate in a healthy manner, an equilibrium is maintained throughout the system which enables it to resist the action of noxious agents. The ideas which we have here advanced in regard to the specific nature of typhus contagion, were maintained by a number of medical men many years ago, amongst whom may be named the distinguished gentleman to whom we have before alluded, Dr. Nathan Smith.

The reasons adduced by this careful observer of nature in support of his opinion, are as follows: "On the Connecticut river, for two hundred miles from north to south, and on all its tributary streams on both sides, for an hundred miles in width, there has been no instance of any person's having contracted the intermitting fever, from the first settlement of the country to the present time; and yet the typhus fever has prevailed, more or less, in every township within that tract of country."

If, as many writers assert, the miasms of intermittent, yellow, and typhus fevers are analogous, should we not constantly witness these maladies running into each other, or assuming indiscriminately these different forms in the same location?

But a still stronger reason is brought forward by Dr. Smith to sustain his position: he asserts that "there is a remarkable odour arising from a person affected with this disease, so peculiar, that I feel assured, that upon entering a room blindfolded, where a person has been confined for some length of time, I should be able to distinguish it from all other febrile affections. This is an additional circumstance in favour of the existence of the specific cause assigned above, as several other diseases which arise from contagion are attended by an odour peculiar to each, which, when once fixed in the mind, enables a person to recognise their presence ever after. This is strongly evinced in smallpox, measles, malignant sore throat, &c."

It is also a fact worthy of note, and one which bears strongly upon this point, that typhus fever was entirely unknown to the savage tribes of America, previous to the settlement of the whites; and, even at the present time, those bands which have not been contaminated by the *civilizing* aggressions of the usurpers of the soil, but continue their wild, roving, active and simple modes of life, are not at all subject to this fever. The moment, however, they forsake their simple and primitive customs, and adopt our dissipated and enervating habits, enclosing themselves in close, ill-ventilated, and heated apartments, and stuffing themselves with spirits, greasy and indigestible food, coffee, tea, condiments, and tobacco, they become affected with contagious and miasmatic disorders, and often die in great numbers. This fact goes to prove that typhus is a disease pertaining exclusively to civilized life, and that it requires the unnatural and artificial customs and habits of the white race to ensure its generation.

But as the constituents of animal and vegetable substances are so nearly identical, it is highly probable that the typhus poison may also arise from vegetable decomposition in close and heated apartments. Of one thing we may be assured, respecting both animal and vegetable matters: that when decomposition occurs in dark, damp, and confined places, a far more active and virulent miasm is generated, than when the same substances undergo transformations in the open air.

Therapeutics.—In the management of inflammatory typhus, the liberal use of *cold water*, both internally and externally, will be found highly beneficial. This important agent has been hitherto quite too much overlooked in the treatment of fevers, for there is no doubt of its immense power as a curative agent, when judiciously employed. This is by no means a modern remedy, as many suppose, but its frequent use was strenuously recommended and actually adopted for many years, by one of the most eminent and successful * physicians of New England, as long ago as 1796. The following quotations will show the views then entertained respecting this agent.

"The most effectual method of reducing the temperature of the body, is by the use of cold water, which may be taken internally, or applied externally."

"The only effectual method of cooling the body in these cases (hot stage of typhus), is by the use of cold water applied externally; by this means we can lessen the heat to any degree we please."

"The method which I have adopted, is to turn down the bed clothes, and to dash from a pint to a gallon of cold water on the patient's head, face and body, so as to wet both the bed and body linen thoroughly. As soon as the linen and bed clothes are dry, if the heat returns again, the water should be again and again applied until the heat is subdued."

We are aware that physicians have been deterred from the free external use of cold water in fevers, through fear of aggravating existing inflammations, causing metastases, congestions, &c., by repelling the blood from the surface to the internal organs, but the danger from this cause is purely imaginary: for cold water, externally applied, not only operates by abstracting the superfluous heat, and reducing the animal temperature, but it also acts as a *tonic*, imparting tone and vigour to the debilitated and relaxed capillaries in which the morbid action is supposed to reside.

In slight cases, frequent sponging of the surface will be sufficient to accomplish our object; but in more severe instances, the method adopted by Prof. Smith may be resorted to.

By adopting this course of treatment, while at the same time we administer appropriate remedies, the disease will run a milder course, and most of those grave symptoms which are too often witnessed, will be absent. It has been a question whether typhus

* Treatise on Typhus, by N. Smith.

can ever be cut short by remedies; some maintaining that it may be broken up in the first stage, while others are of opinion, that it must have its course. Upon this point, Dr. Drysdale observes as follows: "We do not believe it possible to *cure* typhus; all we can do is, to conduct it to a favourable termination by carefully watching, and curing all the intercurrent affections so apt to appear in it, by judicious management. At the same time we have always given the remedies usually recommended, especially *rhus, bryonia* and *arsenicum;* and we believe that the convalescence will be much hastened by judicious treatment." Dr. D. advises the use of brandy and wine in addition to our remedies during the stage of collapse; "especially when there is great want of animal heat, and the pulse is very quick and small, attended with much trembling of the hands and constant muttering delirium."

The appropriate medicines will be determined by the form which the malady assumes, *and the exact nature of each particular case.*

TYPHUS CEREBRALIS.

Belladonna, bryonia, aconite, opium, and *rhus*, will cover most of the symptoms which are ordinarily present in this form. The following are the indications for these medicines.

Belladonna. — *External indications.* — Countenance flushed and bloated; eyes red and sparkling, or dull and turbid; or pale, brownish and glassy; wild expression, stupid, fixed, or wandering look; visible pulsation of the carotids; respiration irregular, short and quick, or slow and deep; pupils contracted or dilated, generally immovable; pulse variable, but generally quick and resisting; tongue red, moist or dry, or yellowish white; breath offensive; urine brownish or red; spasms; distortion of the face and eyes; head very hot, while the extremities are cool.

Physical sensations. — Fulness and heavy pain in the head; vertigo; dizziness; violent throbbings in the head; strong pulsation of the carotids, and arteries of the head; double vision, sparks before the eyes, or weak sight; humming in the ears; inflammation of the throat, chest, and abdomen; pains, heaviness, or numbness of the limbs; palpitation of the heart; pressure and cramp-like pains in the stomach; dryness of the mouth; adypsia, or thirst; continued watchfulness or lethargy; constipation, or diarrhœa with tenesmus; constant moaning.

Mental and moral symptoms.—State of mind apathetic; or irritability of temper; illusions of the senses, and frightful visions; or gloomy, suspicious; constant moaning, or drowsiness; profound coma.

Administration.— A drop of the third dilution in water once in two hours, until the desired impression is produced.

Remarks.— Belladonna is indicated in typhus, presenting a sub-synochal character. It is contra-indicated in great depression of the cerebral and nervous energy; but applies in vascular and nervous erethism.

Bryonia.— *External indications.*— Face red, burning, and swollen; eyes red and swollen, or dull, glassy, turbid, or sparkling and suffused; dryness of the nose; groans; respiration difficult, short, rapid, anxious, or sighing; thick and tenacious expectoration; petechiæ; mouth dry; tongue dry, and coated with a dirty or yellowish fur; lips brown and dry; trembling of the limbs, and appearance of great weariness and debility; pulse variable; urine pale, or brownish and without sediment.

Physical sensations.—Fulness, heaviness, and pressure in the head, from within outwards, worse on movement; confusion and dull pains in the head; vertigo; buzzing in the ears; dulness or acuteness of hearing; sensation of dryness in the throat; profuse sweat during the heat; bitter, sour, or putrid taste; thirst; nausea; hiccough, or pressure at the stomach; constipation; abdomen inflated; weariness and pains in the back, loins, and limbs, aggravated by motion; abdominal pains; drowsy during the *day;* restless in the *night,* with delirium.

Mental and moral symptoms.—Irascibility; passion; fear of the future; anxiety; fear; stupidity; delirium, with raving respecting business; visions on closing the eyes.

Administration.—Same as *belladonna.*

Remarks.—Bryonia is applicable in the cerebral and abdominal varieties, and in typhoid pneumonia, especially in the first period before the muscular and nervous strength have become materially depressed. After the system is reduced to a certain extent, it may be alternated with one of the other remedies with benefit. *Bryonia* may often follow belladonna with propriety.

Aconite.—In the first stages of this, as well as in most other maladies in which there is excessive action of the circulatory vessels, aconite is an indispensable remedy. Its properties and uses are so well known, that we shall add nothing respecting it in this place, excepting a simple caution to the inexperienced practitioner, that while endeavouring to reduce the force of the general circulation, he should not neglect important local inflammations. It may be administered in the same manner as belladonna.

Opium.—*External indications.*—Face dark red, or brownish, hot and bloated; pupils dilated and immovable; lower jaw hanging from relaxation; lethargy, with snoring; mouth and eyes open; irregular and slow respiration; pulse slow or suppressed; bluish colour of the skin; convulsive movements of the limbs; offensive black fæces; involuntary evacuations; urine scanty, high coloured, depositing a brick-dust sediment.

Physical sensations.—Sensation of great heaviness in the head, vertigo, dizziness, buzzing in the ears; general diminution, or entire loss of sensibility; cloudiness of sight; paralysis of the tongue; sensation of weight and pulsations in the stomach and abdomen; difficulty in evacuating the bladder; great oppression at the chest; hoarse, dry cough, with bloody expectoration; troublesome itching of the skin; convulsions.

Mental and moral symptoms.—Stupor; loss of consciousness; delirium; frightful visions.

Administration.—A drop of the third dilution in an ounce of water—a table spoonful once in two hours, until a medicinal aggravation or an amendment occurs,—afterwards repeat according to the exigencies of the case.

Rhus tox.—This remedy is particularly adapted to the nervous forms of typhus, and may often be used with advantage in cerebral typhus after *bryonia* or *aconite*, or in ganglionic typhus, when the following symptoms present themselves :

External indications.—Petechiæ ; face red and swollen ; blue circle around the eyes ; nose pointed ; lips dry, brownish or black ; eyes red, with viscid secretion at the angles ; eyes fixed and dull ; nose dry, swollen, and tender when touched ; tongue dry, red, or dark ; mouth filled with viscid mucus, which collects upon the teeth, forming sordes ; constipation or diarrhœa ; teeth white, dry, and shining ; colour and consistence of fæces variable ; retention or incontinence of urine ; clear, red, or turbid urine ; paralysis of the lower extremities ; pulse quick and small ; coma, with snoring or moaning.

Physical sensations—Stupefaction ; vertigo ; dizziness ; bruised sensation within the head ; soreness of the scalp ; painful oppression in the stomach ; pulsations in the epigastric region ; spasms and pinchings in the abdomen ; pains in different parts as if from a bruise, worse during repose, or at night, and relieved by movement ; great weakness ; tendency to faintness ; pain and difficulty in swallowing ; tenesmus, with loose, slimy, frothy, sanguineous, white, yellow, or red evacuations ; constant and pressing desire to urinate ; oppression at the chest, with difficult respiration ; soreness in the limbs, back, and neck, when touched or at rest ; raw feeling in the throat and chest ; excessive weakness, tremblings, sweats.

Mental and moral symptoms.—Muttering delirium, or coma somnolentum, with snoring ; anguish and dejection in the evening and at night ; inclination to weep ; fear of death ; frequent sighing.

Administration.—A drop of the first dilution in an ounce of water ; a dessert spoonful every two or four hours. If no decided effect ensues after a reasonable time, give a drop of the mother tincture in a tablespoonful of water, repeating as may be necessary.

Mercurius vivus has been successfully employed in cases where there is great weakness, rapid sinking of strength, profuse perspiration, fainting fits, trembling and numbness of the limbs, cramps, and convulsive movements, great agitation and uneasiness of body and mind.

PNEUMO TYPHUS.

The medicines which have proved most efficient in this form of typhus, are, *aconite, bryonia, phosphorus, ammonia, carb., acid phosph.*, and *mercurius viv.*

When the affection is characterized by accelerated circulation, great heat of skin, thirst, difficult, anxious, short and rapid breathing, with painful stitches in the chest and side when inspiring; cough on motion; full, hard, and rapid pulse, *aconite* should be exhibited. A dose of the third dilution every hour or two, until an impression is made upon the symptoms.

After aconite has been administered, and symptoms remain unsubdued, it will be necessary to resort to some of the following remedies, the indications for which we proceed to describe.

Bryonia.—External indications.—Same as under *cerebral typhus.*

Physical sensations.—Confusion, fulness, heaviness, and swimming in the head; headache, aggravated by movement or opening the eyes; respiration difficult, short, anxious, rapid, or sighing; oppression of the chest; stinging in the chest when coughing, or breathing deeply. Shooting pains in the chest, side, and abdomen; pains in the limbs on movement; nose swollen, dry, and painful to the touch; throat dry, with sharp pains when touched or in motion; nausea and oppression at the stomach; constipation and diarrhœa alternating, the one in the night, and the other during the day; urine scanty and high coloured; cough, with stingings or stitches in the chest and side, with yellowish or bloody expectoration, or pains in the head; shooting pains under the left shoulder-blade when coughing; tongue dry, contracted, dark, or yellow; pulse rapid and full, or quick, weak, and irregular.

Mental and moral symptoms.—Same as under *cerebral typhus.*

Administration.—Same as under *cerebral typhus.*

Phosphorus.—*External indications.*—Yellow, brown, coppery, or bluish spots upon the skin ; viscid secretion about the eyes, particularly at night ; quivering of the eyelids ; dryness and obstruction of the nose ; face pale, dingy, or red and bloated ; eyes sunken and surrounded by a dark circle ; lips dry and bluish ; ulcers at the corners of the mouth ; tongue with a dry and dark, or whitish fur ; respiration irregular, laborious, noisy, or panting ; pulse quick and hard.

Physical sensations.—Stunning headache, vertigo, and dizziness, worse in the morning ; smarting or burning sensation in the eyes ; throbbing in the ears ; deafness ; offensive discharge from the nose ; dryness and raw sensation in the throat ; nausea and pains in the stomach ; uneasiness and painful contraction of the abdomen ; stitches and roughness in the chest ; expectoration of mucus, slimy, sanguineous, or purulent matter ; sharp pains in the shoulder-blades ; stiffness of the neck ; trembling, coldness, and numbness of the limbs ; great oppression at the chest, with distressed and anxious respiration.

Mental and moral symptoms.—Despondency, anguish, and fear, especially at night ; disposition to weep or laugh.

Administration.—A drop of the third dilution in an ounce of water ; a dessert spoonful once in two to six hours, until an effect is perceptible.

Ammonium carb. — *External indications.* — Miliary eruptions, or redness of the skin ; eyes dry ; nose obstructed with dry coryza ; face pale and bloated ; lips dry and dark-coloured ; fæces in small, hard lumps ; respiration short and anxious ; breath offensive ; tongue covered with slime or vesicles ; pulse weak and rapid.

Physical sensations.—Great restlessness at night ; drowsy during the day ; disturbed sleep at night, with frightful dreams ; pains in the head ; nausea ; ringing in the ears, worse at night ; sensation of excoriation in the mouth and throat ; constant thirst ; constipation and itching at the anus ; frequent desire to urinate during the night; hoarse, or short dry cough, with tickling and roughness in the throat; mucous and sanguineous expectoration; sharp pains in the chest and sides, on coughing, breathing, or moving; drawing pains in the nape of the neck and small of the back; extremities stiff and numb; cramps, coldness, and swelling of the feet; excessive weakness of the limbs; right side worse than the left.

Mental and moral symptoms. — Discouragement; anxiety; apprehension; anguish; sad, weak, timid; mental distress, worse at night.

Administration.—A grain of the first trituration every two, four, or six hours, as the nature of the case requires.

Acid Phosphoric.—External indications.—Eruption of small pimples on the skin; redness of the skin; coma; eyes dull, glassy, fixed, with pupils dilated; coryza, with redness of the nostrils; face pale, or covered with pimples; teeth yellow; gums swollen and bleeding; tongue covered with thick and adhesive mucus; fæces hard, knotted, and slimy; urine clear or white, depositing a white sediment; pulse quick and weak.

Physical sensations.—Great physical and mental prostration; pains in the chest, abdomen, and head, worse *during repose*, relieved by motion; head confused, bewildered with pains when moving it; eyes weak and sensitive to candle-light; music painful to the ears; cheeks hot and burning; nausea and oppression at the stomach; diarrhœa, frequent inclination to urinate; tightness and oppression in the chest; cough, with purulent expectoration; sharp pains in the chest; burning sensation in the hands and feet.

Mental and moral symptoms.—Indifferent; taciturn; peevish; stupid.

Administration.—Suitable in some cases of advanced pneumo typhus. A dose of the third dilution may be given once in four to six hours.

The following medicines should be named as appropriate under certain circumstances, in pneumo typhus, viz., *lachesis, tart., emet., senega, merc., lobel. inflat.*

TYPHUS ABDOMINALIS.

From the close analogy of appearances produced upon the intestinal canal, by fatal doses of *arsenicum* and by fatal abdominal typhus, it would be a natural conclusion that arsenicum is for this disease a valuable homœopathic remedy. There has been, however, a wide difference of opinion upon this question, between some of our most eminent practitioners. Many, like Hausmann, Fleishmann, Gumpendorf, Staph, Jahr, Henderson, Laurie, Currie, and Hartmann, have eulogized *arsenicum* for this form of typhus, in the most enthusiastic manner; at the same time a very few, as Wurmb, Lorentz, &c., have denied that it possesses any special curative properties in any stage of the malady.

But the weight of testimony is so much in favour of the advocates of *arsenicum* in abdominal typhus, that we shall not enter into any discussion of the question, but simply express the opinion, that in all cases of the genuine forms of this disease, *arsenicum*, when exhibited judiciously, will prove a remedy of immense importance. Indeed, we believe in those cases of ulceration of the mucous membrane of the ileum, Peyer's glands, &c., and in those instances where the blood becomes congested in different parts of the intestinal canal, giving rise eventually to sphacelation if unopposed, that *arsenicum* is a specific of positive and decided power. In support of this opinion, we refer with full confidence to the numerous hospital and private reports, which have been presented to the public in the last few years.

In relation to the *cause* or *causes* of the ulcers so often discovered by the Hippocratics in autopsical examinations of those who have died of typhus abdominalis, an allopathic* physician of forty years' standing in Massachusetts, makes the following very pertinent inquiries in a late number of the Boston Medical and Surgical Journal: After expressing himself as "fully persuaded that one of the great secrets of curing patients is not to kill them," he proceeds:—"I should like to be informed whether there is not danger in giving

* Silas Brown, M. D.

inwardly, in any quantity, strychnia, creosote, prussic acid, nitrate of silver, and a host of other virulent caustic poisons; and whether some of them would not have a tendency to cauterize or constringe the delicate absorbents and other vessels of the digestive organs; and whether such medicines have congeniality or affinity enough with the membranous and vascular portions with which they come in contact, to become sanative medical agents; or whether they would not have a tendency to *produce obstructions and those ulcers which we meet with in* the *post-mortem examinations* of *those subjects who die of typhus fever*." He requests an answer, and we venture the suggestion that if he adopts an *affirmative* one, he will be in little danger of error. But to proceed with our description:

Arsenicum.—*External indications.*—Skin dry or yellowish, or cold and bluish; reddish or dark spots on the skin; petechiæ; eyes dull, glazed, and sunken; pupils contracted; face shrunken, hollow, pale, and cadaverous, or yellowish, bluish, or leaden coloured; expression of countenance distorted and unnatural; cold sweat on the forehead; lips dark, dry, and cracked; teeth dry, white, and shining; sordes upon the teeth; tongue dry, shrivelled, bluish or black, with trembling and inability to protrude it; fæces variable, generally loose, darkish, or greenish, and fetid; involuntary discharges of fæces and urine; urine reddish, brownish, yellow, or turbid; tympanitis; guggling noise of liquids swallowed; respiration short and anxious; cramps in the legs; pulse irregular, or quick, weak, small, and frequent, or feeble and trembling; voice sepulchral and tremulous; coma or low muttering delirium; trembling of the limbs; subsultus tendinum; sometimes deafness; hippocratic countenance; colliquative sweats.

Physical sensations.—Extreme debility or complete prostration; burning and heat at the pit of the stomach and epigastrium; nausea, and vomiting, especially after eating or drinking; violent pains and burnings in the abdomen, generally on the left side; sometimes only pain on *pressure;* pains in the right hypochondrium; stitches in the side with anxious and difficult breathing; universal loss of strength, and excessive restlessness; stools dark, greenish, putrid, fetid and involuntary; head painful, weak, confused, as if stunned; distention of the abdomen; stiffness of the limbs.

Mental and moral symptoms. The patient is dissatisfied, restless, anxious, discouraged; or muttering; delirious; sleep disturbed, with unpleasant visions.

Administration. In extreme cases, a grain of the second or third trituration may be given every half hour, gradually lengthening the intervals as circumstances require.

Remarks. Arsenicum is especially serviceable in the third stage of abdominal typhus, when ulcers have formed. It will also frequently apply in the second stage, when the bowels become relaxed.

Carbo vegetabilis, is also a remedy of importance in the last stages of abdominal, and in all stages of putrid typhus. In the former, it may sometimes be exhibited in alternation with *arsenicum*, with good effect. The following are the *external indications*:—hippocratic countenance; face pale, yellowish, or dingy; eyes sunken and glazed, with nocturnal agglutination; lips dry and cracked; tongue dry, dark, and tremulous; position upon the back; cold, clammy sweat; pulse rapid, trembling, and almost imperceptible; tremblings and jerkings of the limbs; urine red and high-coloured; fæces putrid and offensive.

Physical sensations.—An entire prostration of the animal powers; heavy, pressing, or drawing pains in the head; ulceration and bleeding of the gums; rattling in the throat; cramp-like, pressing, or burning pains in the stomach and intestines; burning pains and oppression at the chest; rigidity, or complete paralysis and relaxation of the nape of the neck and limbs; bowels swollen and tender on pressure; feet, legs, and hands cold; numbness of the limbs.

Mental and moral symptoms.—Coma, or sleeplessness, with muttering delirium; mind dull, confused, wandering, or stupid.

Administration.—A dose of the third trituration may be given in water, every half hour, in extreme cases, until the necessary impression is made.

Hartmann speaks in high terms of *staphysagria* in

the first stage of the disease, when the following symptoms appear: "Sordes on the teeth, pale and bleeding gums, with painful swelling of the gums, and rapid decay of the teeth; vanishing of thoughts and ideas, weakness of memory, dulness of mind, great indifference and ill humour; vertigo, with stupifying headache; dimness of the eyes, itching, stinging, and heat in the canthi; fulness in the pit of the stomach, with frequent hiccough and vomiting; tension across the hypochondria, oppressing the breathing; pressure, weight, and tension in the abdomen; cutting pain in the bowels, with nausea; copious diarrhœic stools."

Muriatic acid is a highly important remedy in many cases of advanced typhus, when the patient is stupid, unconscious of surrounding occurrences, and extremely prostrate. Other symptoms are, constant tendency to settle down towards the foot of the bed, low muttering delirium, groaning in sleep, moaning, picking at the bed-clothes; inability to protrude the tongue, dry heat, with transient and partial sweats, general uneasiness, "depression of the lower jaw, digging with the head into the pillow, turning up of the whites of the eyes, slavering, &c." (*Hempel.*) We may employ the first to the third dilution—a drop in a drachm of water, every two hours as long as necessary.

Dr. Kidd found *phosphorus* a valuable remedy in the treatment of the typhus which devastated Ireland during 1847 and 48. *Rhus tox.*, *bryonia* and *arsenicum* are likewise highly commended by the doctor, when, "from the very commencement, the heat of skin and acceleration of pulse are very inconsiderable, and in the middle and latter stages, are almost invariably below the natural standard. For two or three days the patient would labour under lassitude and languor, with loss of appetite and of sleep, the tongue being generally the first index of the probable mischief in store. About the fourth or fifth day, the disease being generally well marked, with a very slight heat of skin, which felt soft and clammy, being covered with moisture, (not like the ordinary feel of a perspiring skin, but as if the skin were damped, and by some contrivance all evaporation prevented,) the pulse very little, if at all altered, except in strength, which even at this period would be somewhat deficient; the tongue presented a most characteristic appearance: in general dry, hard, and glazed, like brown leather, or deeply covered with brown or blackish fur. In some cases it appeared soft, moist, and tremulous, covered with a perfect and uniform layer of pure white paste or mucus, (this in general omened a very severe and dangerous form of the disease,) the gums and teeth became covered with brownish incrustations, thirst being incessant and insatiable, with nausea and vomiting; in many cases abdominal symptoms, as tension and tympanitic resonance of the abdominal walls, with tenderness and shooting pain over either iliac region, (in general the right;) bowels seldom costive, in general relaxed, with or without pain; urine in a few cases suppressed, in most unchanged; head in general implicated: in most from the beginning, with aching and heaviness at the forehead, throbbing at the temples, vertigo, sense of emptiness and bewilderment; delirium, mostly at night, with low muttering, or with stupid, heavy insensibility, and incoherence of speech. The eyes appeared dull, inanimate, and listless, with the head instinctively turned from the light. In a few cases, towards their termination, a peculiar sort of stolid deafness supervened, which gradually disappeared as convalescence advanced.

"Almost invariably the lower extremities were complained of as being dead and numbed, rendering the least motion impossible, (but without any actual pain,) the feet and legs feeling cold and damp.

"General debility and prostration set in early in the disease, and proved the most obstinate of the symptoms."*

Dr. K. relied upon the four medicines above named, in this form of the malady, and the results show a mortality of less than two per cent. His success in the numerous cases of continued fever which came under his care, was no less gratifying. The low dilutions were employed for the most part; but in a few cases drop doses of the tinctures were deemed necessary.

* Truths and their Reception, &c., by J. Kidd, M. D., London, 1849.

The other medicines necessary in the treatment of certain stages of this, as well as the other forms of typhus, are: *rhus tox., acid. nit., nux vom., secale cor., merc., op., camph., china, nux mos., valer., stram., hyos., and lach.* These remedies will all occasionally be called into requisition, so that their effects upon the human system should be well understood and appreciated.

It will be observed that we have divided typhus into but three varieties. Other authors add a *typhus putridus, typhus contagiosus, typhus lentus, typhus petechialis,* &c. In practice, however, we seldom find any one of these forms distinct and unmixed; but the brain, nervous system, lungs, and abdominal viscera partake more or less in the general disturbance, causing each particular case to present peculiar and diverse symptoms. So in regard to the treatment of this fever, it will often be found, from its commencement to its termination, to require one or more of the medicines which we have placed under each form of the malady. The sympathetic connections are so strongly pronounced, between the important organs in which the different varieties of typhus are located, that one cannot be affected without imparting disorder to the others.

Physiologists note it as a curious fact, that no two human faces are exactly alike, and it may be asserted with equal safety, that no two instances of typhus fever ever presented, from first to last, *precisely the same symptoms.* Therefore it is, that in all cases of this, as well as of other maladies, we must trust to *symptoms alone,* and be guided by them in the application of our remedies, rather than by the *name* of the disease. Our nomenclatures and classifications unquestionably facilitate the investigations and diagnosis of complicated cases, but they can be of very little importance in the practical exhibition of medicines.

CHAPTER XIX.

HECTIC FEVER.

Diagnosis.—The ordinary symptoms of this fever, are: daily febrile paroxysms, general debility, emaciation, skin pale, face often tinged with the "hectic flush," irritable stomach, loss of appetite, moderate thirst, night sweats, tendency to perspire through the day, diarrhœa, pulse quick, small, and sharp.

Causes.—The combination of symptoms denominated hectic fever, in most cases, proceed from long continued and profuse suppuration; but they may arise from protracted local irritation without suppuration. Some writers suppose that hectic can only proceed from the absorption of pus, but this is erroneous, as the symptoms of hectic often make their appearance before suppuration occurs. In nearly all instances, it is a secondary affection consequent upon either protracted disease in some vital part, some of the joints, or of some extensive surface. It proceeds more readily from diseases of the "bones, ligaments, and tendons, than from those of the muscles, skin, cellular membrane, &c." *

It may, then, be considered as a constitutional disturbance, originated and kept up by some previous local disease, and which cannot be permanently cured until the original cause upon which it is dependent, is eradicated or removed.

In those cases where it is kept up by incurable diseases of the joints, bones of the extremities, or other parts which can be safely removed by the surgeon, amputation or excision should be at once resorted to, and the hectic symptoms will speedily disappear. Mr. Hunter remarks, that "a hectic pulse at one hundred and twenty has been known to sink to ninety in a few hours after the removal of the hectic cause." Several instances have occurred in my own practice, in which an almost immediate and entire cessation

* Sir A. Cooper.

of the hectic symptoms, such as sleepless nights, febrile paroxysms, night sweats, diarrhœa, rapid pulse, &c., has resulted from amputation or excision of the offending parts.

When the original cause is a suppuration of some important organ like the lungs, liver, stomach, &c., our prognosis must generally be unfavourable. In these instances it is of the utmost importance to the homœopathic practitioner that he makes a thorough investigation of all remote causes, in order to arrive at an accurate knowledge of the latent and original sources of the malady. He will thus be able to direct his remedial applications with judgment, and afford to his patients the only possible chance of cure.

Therapeutics.—In the selection of remedies, every thing must of necessity depend upon the original cause,—its seat, nature, and violence; and upon the secondary consequences to which it gives rise. It should always be a prime object, to direct our most potent remedies with perseverance against the local affection; and if any latent or apparent influences exist, against these also.

If we are called to a case of hectic fever, proceeding from an inflammation of a scrofulous character, advantage will be derived from the use of some of the following medicines: *sulphur, aurum mur., calcarea, china, iodine, ol. jecor., asel., acid. nit., acid. mur., acid. phos., phos., arsenicum, silicea,* and *mercurius.*

In cases proceeding from syphilitic or mercurial diseases of the bones, ligaments, &c., the medicines adapted to the cure of these disorders should be selected.

If a chronic miasm, whether psoric or otherwise, has originated the disturbance, then strike deeply at the original cause with *antipsorics,* as well as at present symptoms, and good results may accrue in apparently desperate cases.

CHAPTER XX.

OF THE FEBRILE CUTANEOUS DISEASES.

EXANTHEMATA.

These fevers, like some of those heretofore described, can only arise from certain specific morbific contagions which give rise to uniform and readily recognised symptoms. They all commence with general febrile disturbance, followed sooner or later by eruptions, and other characteristic symptoms, which serve to distinguish each particular variety.

A peculiarity attending this class of diseases, is, that a single attack usually renders the subject safe against any future action of the morbific poison. I have, however, witnessed two or three well marked examples of second attacks of scarlatina in the same individuals.

The maladies which we shall notice under this head, are, *Scarlatina, Rubeola, Variola, Varicella, Miliary fever, Roseola, Urticaria, Erysipelas, Plague.*

SECTION I.

SCARLATINA. — SCARLET FEVER.

This fever has been divided into three varieties, namely: first, *Scarlatina simplex;* second, *Scarlatina anginosa;* third, *Scarlatina maligna.*

In its simple form, scarlet fever is not attended with danger, but runs its course mildly like a simple continued fever, and terminates in five or six days in convalescence.

In the other varieties, however, inflammations and congestions often supervene soon after the attack, and if not promptly met by suitable remedies, gangrene, sloughing, and fatal disorganizations occur in the throat, larynx, and other important parts of the organism.

Scarlet fever is of much more frequent occurrence

in the fall and winter, than during the summer months. Its attacks are usually confined to children passed the nursing period, and persons under twenty years of age; but it may occur at all ages from infancy to old age.

1. SCARLATINA SIMPLEX.

Diagnosis.—Shiverings, succeeded by heat, moderate thirst, frequent pulse, slight soreness of the throat, nausea, loss of appetite, headache: — After these symptoms have continued about forty-eight hours, a scarlet eruption makes its appearance upon the face, extending gradually downwards to the neck, trunk, and extremities. This eruption consists of an immense number of fine pimples (aptly compared by Dr. Armstrong to a boiled lobster shell), either running together and diffusing themselves uniformly over the skin, or appearing in patches in different parts of the body. Upon the appearance of this eruption, many of the unpleasant symptoms, like nausea, oppression at the stomach, dyspnœa, &c., abate, and the case thus progresses until the fourth or fifth day of the fever, when desquamation of the cuticle takes place, and a happy convalescence usually ensues.

2. SCARLATINA ANGINOSA.

Diagnosis. — The anginose variety of scarlet fever is ushered in with chilliness and shiverings, succeeded by intense heat and pungency of the skin, frequent and hard pulse, nausea, vomiting, headache, sore throat, painful deglutition, intense thirst, pain and tenderness of the epigastrium, abdomen tender, pain and stiffness in the neck, tongue covered with a whitish or yellowish fur, through which the papillæ are seen red, inflamed, and prominent; fauces, throat, and tonsils swollen, deep red, inflamed, or ulcerated; eyes red and injected, voice thick and hoarse, sometimes dyspnœa and cough, and universal tenderness of the whole surface.

These symptoms continue an indefinite period, varying from two to five days, when the eruption shows itself, either uniformly diffused over the body, or in irregular blotches. If the disease progresses favourably, the skin desquamates in from six to eight days from the commencement of the fever, the febrile symptoms all subside, the ulcers in the throat granulate kindly, and a speedy convalescence obtains. On the contrary, if the eruption prematurely disappears from the surface, the ulcers assume a foul and unhealthy appearance, secreting an acrid and highly irritating fluid; while the fever continues to rage with unabated severity. We may have a supervention of abdominal, bronchial, or cerebral inflammation, which will complicate the malady in a serious and perhaps fatal manner.

"In this fever, the temperature, as indicated by the thermometer, rises several degrees higher than in any other."* The pulse is also more rapid and strong than in almost any other fever, indicating conclusively that it is an affection of an inflammatory character.

3.—SCARLATINA MALIGNA.

Diagnosis.—Scarlatina maligna was formerly known under the name of "putrid sore throat," and is at present designated by some writers as *scarlatina typhoides.* It is unquestionably one of the most dangerous maladies with which the physician has to contend. It generally commences with the common precursory symptoms of the anginose form, which, however, very soon give way for a train of symptoms bearing a close resemblance to typhus. The eruption is either entirely wanting, or makes its appearance only partially, in irregular blotches of a pale colour; the heat of the skin often subsides below the natural standard; the pulse becomes very frequent and weak; the countenance assumes a besotted expression; the eyes become dull and suffused; the throat is filled with ash-coloured ulcers; fauces, larynx, and bronchia inflamed and swollen; an acrid discharge issues from the nostrils; the tongue, at first red, soon becomes dry and black; the surface, in the advanced stages, acquires a dark red or mahogany colour, and petechiæ, diarrhœa, and hæmorrhages finally ensue. The ulcers in the throat

* Southwood Smith, on Fever.

often slough and extend in all directions, involving in their ravages the cartilages of the larynx and the soft parts within the nostrils.

If the disease seizes particularly upon the brain, lungs, or abdominal viscera, there will be a predominance of those symptoms which characterize the disorders of these particular parts. From the tendency of this malady to these different organs, some authors have subdivided scarlatina maligna into the *inflammatory*, *congestive*, and *mixed* varieties. Examples have occasionally occurred in my own practice, in which, in the very onset of the malady, those symptoms have appeared, indicating congestion of the brain,—as coma ; slow, oppressed, and noisy respiration; sighing; face pale or livid, skin cold, pulse slow and irregular, pupils contracted or dilated. In these cases, the eruption seldom comes out well, but is of a pale colour, and shows itself irregularly in different parts of the body.

In other instances the inflammation seizes upon the laryngeal, bronchial, or intestinal mucous membranes, thus often deciding the case against the patient, when the local affection of the throat seemed to be progressing favourably.

Causes.—Scarlatina can only proceed from a specific morbific contagion, respecting the *nature* of which we are entirely ignorant. Whether this contagion is generated and diffused solely by those suffering under the disease, or whether, as some pathologists assert, it may be generated in the atmosphere independently of the animal body, is a question which admits of discussion, although we entertain the former opinion. Of this we are confident, that when the agent is *infinitesimally* diffused in the air, it is capable of being absorbed into the circulation, and of producing its specific morbific effects upon the organism.

Some have doubted the contagiousness of this affection, because certain individuals of families occasionally escape, while others are affected ; but let it be remembered, that this happens now and then in smallpox, plague, typhus, and all other maladies which are universally deemed contagious.

We have before observed, that the contagion of typhus cannot make a serious impression upon the organism, so long as every part is in a perfect state of health and vigour. The same remark will apply with equal truth to the disease under consideration. In these cases, the tissues on which the poison operates, are stronger than the noxious influence, and are thus enabled to resist its action until some cause predisposes the system to receive the impression.

Therapeutics.—The provings of *belladonna* upon the healthy subject, as well as the numerous successful experiments made at the bedside of the sick, have stamped it as a remedy of distinguished importance in the treatment of scarlet fever. It has even been extolled by eminent practitioners of the old school, and in some instances adopted, both as a remedy in this disease, and as a valuable prophylactic against it.

In the *scarlatina simplex*, an occasional dose of this medicine at the third attenuation, will suffice to conduct the patient safely through the malady. Should the febrile symptoms run high, the *belladonna* may be advantageously preceded by *aconite.*

In the *anginose* form, where there is intense inflammatory excitement, swelling and soreness of the throat, painful deglutition, quick pulse, burning hot skin, nausea, tenderness at the epigastrium, *belladonna* is still the grand remedy. If the fever assumes a violent character, evincing a tendency to excite inflammatory action in any particular structure, *aconite* may here also be administered with advantage, either by itself, or in alternation with *belladonna.* So long as the local inflammation in the throat is retained within due bounds, and the eruption shows itself in a proper manner, remaining out a sufficient length of time, we shall receive ample aid from these potent remedies. We take the liberty of introducing the following special symptoms of *belladonna*, from Drs. Curre, Hermann, Laurie, &c. :

External indications.—Spots of a scarlet or deep red colour on the face, or other parts of the body; swelling of the submaxillary glands, and those of the neck; eyes red, sparkling, and convulsed, or fixed, shining, and prominent; pupils dilated or contracted; tongue red, hot, and dry, or white in the centre, with red edges; throat, tonsils, uvula, and velum-palati dry, inflamed and swollen; suppuration of the tonsils; strong pulsations of the temporal arteries; inflammation of the stomach and abdomen; constipation, or involuntary evacuations; urine turbid, of a brownish red or yellow colour, with a red or whitish sediment; pulse small and quick, or strong and quick, or full and slow, or small and slow, or hard and tense; pulsations of the carotids; face hot, red, and bloated; sweat with the heat, or after it.

Physical sensations.—Vertigo, confusion, fulness, heaviness, pressure; shooting or expansive pain in the head, aggravated by motion of the head or eyes, by contact, and by cold air, mitigated by holding the head back, and by supporting it; mouth dry and hot; dryness and burning in the throat, with painful and difficult deglutition; loss of appetite; nausea and vomiting; great thirst; sense of fulness and distention in the stomach and abdomen after eating; drawing pains in the back and shoulders; difficult respiration; violent cough; shiverings, alternating with heat, or followed by heat, worse in the evening or night; adypsia, or excessive thirst; dry, burning heat.

Mental and moral symptoms.—Great agitation and tossing about; anguish and inquietude in the afternoon and night; delirium, with muttering, groans, and cries; vivid and frightful dreams; starting from sleep with fright, groans, and cries; ill humour and irritability.

The same writers give us the following special indications for the employment of *aconite:*

External indications.—Face red, hot, and bloated, or alternately red and pale; skin dry and hot; forehead cold, and tips of the ears hot; deep redness of the throat; bilious or mucous vomitings; urine scanty, deep red, with brick-coloured sediment; pulse hard, frequent, and accelerated; respiration rapid and difficult.

Physical sensations.—Oppressive or throbbing pains in the head, aggravated by motion; talking, rising up, &c.; better in the open air; great sensibility of the affected parts to the touch, or on movement; pains in the joints and limbs; fainting and weakness; extreme thirst; coldness of the surface, with internal heat, or burning over the whole body; pain in the throat, and difficult deglutition; burning and prickling in the throat in swallowing; bitter or putrid taste; loss of appetite; sense of swelling, weight, or pressure in the præcordial region; hot and burning urine; bruised pains in the loins, back, and nape of the neck.

Mental and moral symptoms.—Discouragement and agitation; noise appears insupportable; humour changeable: at one time sad, depressed, irritable, contradictory, despairing, at other times excited, gay, and full of hope; inquietude under disease, and even despair respecting a cure.

If there is slight fever through the day, but an increase in the evening, with sleeplessness, sadness, despondency, and tears, *ipecacuanha* is our remedy. The following are the particular symptoms which point to this medicine:

External indications.—Face pale, sallow, yellowish, and bloated, with livid circles round the eyes; tongue loaded with a white or yellowish fur; profuse secretion of saliva; vomiting of green, bilious, acid, slimy, or gelatinous matter; sweat; fetid breath; turbid urine, with sediment like brickdust.

Physical sensations.—Nausea and vomiting of drinks or food; no appetite; insipid and clammy taste; adypsia; violent itching of the skin; empty risings; great uneasiness in the stomach and epigastrium; feeling of emptiness and flaccidity in the stomach; sensation of debility in the bowels, worse on motion; colic, with agitation; tossing, with cries; diarrhœa, with nausea; griping and vomiting.

Mental and moral symptoms.—Anxiety and fear of death; moroseness; cries, and howling; vague desire for different things.

When the disease commences with prominent derangement of the stomach and bowels, headache, vertigo, shiverings, weakness, nausea, and nose-bleed, soon succeeded by hasty, anxious, and oppressed respiration, mucous vomiting, taste of food, longing for acids, spirits, or beer; flatulence; adypsia, or great thirst; constant anxiety, moaning, or sighing, and disturbed sleep, *pulsatilla* is appropriate.

Scarlatina occurring in individuals of decidedly *scrofulous* dyscrasias, will sometimes require the employment of *sulphur*, or *calcarea carb.*

Dr. Elb, of Dresden, advises *zinc* in those cases where paralysis of the brain is threatened, or when it already exists. He has likewise used it with success in the malignant form, with violent delirium, alternating with sopor; icy coldness of the skin from sunken vitality; small and frequent pulse, and fixed and stupid expression of the eyes. Dr. E. usually employs the first trituration in grain doses every two to six hours.

Occasionally, troublesome ulcers form in the mouth, throat, and upon the tonsils, covered with ash-coloured sloughs; deglutition becomes exceedingly difficult, and is attended with a stinging pain; the fluids which the patient attempts to swallow, often escaping through his mouth and nose, with perhaps an acrid discharge from the nostrils, and profuse secretion of saliva. Under these circumstances, *mercurius* is a proper remedy.

In *malignant* scarlet fever, where, in addition to the above symptoms, we have inflamed, swollen, and tender salivary glands, dark-coloured ulcers, with a decided tendency to slough and extend, together with great debility, lassitude, tremours, obtuseness of intellect, cold extremities, and other signs of a typhoid condition, *muriatic*, or *nitric acid*, from the first to the third dilution, should be exhibited.

If, at the same time, there should be present a considerable amount of *pulmonary* or *cerebral* excitement, indicated by delirium, restlessness, contracted or dilated pupils, heaviness and dull pain in the head on motion, difficult, anxious, and sighing respiration, sensation of weight and pressure upon the chest, troublesome, hacking cough, with soreness and sensitiveness of the whole surface, *bryonia*, third dilution, may be called into requisition.

Arsenicum is a remedy of great power in the advanced stages of malignant scarlatina, where there are extreme prostration, pain in the stomach and abdomen, diarrhœa, eruption of a livid or mahogany colour, ulcers dark and foul, tongue and lips dry and black, pulse extremely frequent and weak, cold, clammy sweats, hippocratic countenance. This remedy has often rescued patients from the grave who have been given over in despair by physicians of the old school.

Should profound coma supervene during the course of the malady, with snoring and open mouth, open and convulsed eyes, red and puffed face, hanging jaw, difficult, slow, or intermittent respiration, convulsive movements of different muscles, retention of urine, &c., *opium* will be found the best specific. We are satisfied that this is an agent which will rarely disappoint our expectations in instances of this description.

When the rash suddenly disappears during the eruptive stage, Drs. Schmidt, Hartmann, and others, recommend very highly *acetat, cuprum* as a specific against this symptom. *Sulphur, iodine, bryonia, phosphorus*, and *belladonna* also deserve consideration, and will, in some cases, promptly restore eruptions which have been prematurely repelled.

The other remedies which may be consulted in cases where those above described do not accord with the symptoms, are, *ipecac., nux v., carb. veg., rhus tox., stram., phos., kreosote, hyos.*

For the troublesome *sequela* which sometimes follow scarlet fever, as *dropsical affections, purulent otorrhœa, deafness, furunculi, enlargements* and *suppuration* of the glands of the neck, axilla, and groin, appropriate remedies may be found in *apis., mel., ars., dig., hellebore, sulph., hep., senega, cham., aur. mur.,* and *merc.*

Administration.—We most commonly employ the first, second, and third attenuations; but in young and impressible children, we often resort to the higher dilutions with the most satisfactory results. Some cases are characterized from the commencement by a high state of vascular and nervous excitement, while others evince a loss of vascular and nervous power, and a very low grade of impressibility. The propriety, therefore, of the employment of both the high and low attenuations, in different instances, is evident. If dilutions are used, a drop may be given at a dose, in a drachm of water; but if the triturations are selected, one grain is a suitable dose, given dry or in water. We advise a frequent repetition of the dose until decided changes arise from the remedy, or until we are satisfied that it is not producing the required effect upon the disordered structures.

SECTION II.

RUBEOLA.—MEASLES.

Formerly, measles and scarlet fever were described and treated as one and the same disease, the differences which were observed in different cases being ascribed to modifications originating from peculiarities of constitution, the state of the atmosphere, and other accidental causes. About fifty years ago, however, Withering, and several other writers, recognised a distinction between them; and measles, for the first time, was accurately described and ranked as a distinct malady.

As it generally occurs, it is unattended with danger, unless interfered with by purgatives, emetics, and infusions. Fortunately, it is confined for the most part to children, for when adults are the subjects of attack, it is far more severe and dangerous. Like scarlatina, one attack renders the subject secure against any future operation of the contagion.

Diagnosis.—The precursory symptoms of measles are similar to those of ordinary catarrhal fever: as lassitude, chilliness, sneezing, coryza, red and watery eyes, headache, nausea, slight soreness of the throat, short, hoarse cough, pain and soreness in the chest; dyspnœa, heat, and thirst. These symptoms continue with more or less severity for four or five days, when the eruption makes its appearance, commencing at the forehead, and proceeding gradually downwards to the neck, breast, arms, body, and lower extremities. About the period of the eruptive stage, there is usually an increase of the febrile symptoms, which continue for four or five days, when a bran-like scurf is cast off from the surface, and the fever subsides. During the fever, the cough is often very trublesome, and sometimes terminates in inflammation of the bronchia or lungs. Schroen thus describes the malady: "Small, scattered, red spots, in the centre of which we generally find a small pimple. These spots soon become confluent, and spread over the whole body, after being preceded by *catarrhal fever*, for three or four days, attended with redness of the mucous membrane of the mouth, with cough, catarrh, dread of light, and flow of tears. They disappear upon pressure, and develope themselves again from the centre towards the periphery, after the pressure is removed. The pimple becomes a small yellow prominence in the course of sixteen hours, when a scurfy desquamation commences."

The attentive observer will have no difficulty in distinguishing this malady from scarlatina, by the following marks of difference: the *primary* symptoms of measles are red and watery eyes, sneezing, fluent coryza, short cough and some hoarseness. These signs, which are almost uniformly present in this disease, are usually wanting in scarlet fever. In the general character and appearance of the eruption also there is a marked difference. The scarlatina rash is composed of innumerable fine pimples, resembling in appearance the shell of a boiled lobster, uniformly diffused over the surface, and of a *bright scarlet colour*. The eruption of measles appears in spots (sometimes papular) resembling flea-bites, which run together and form semi-lunar patches. There is a roughness or elevation where the eruption exists, perceptible to the touch: and which is not usually observed in scarlatina. But one of the best marks of distinction is the difference in the colour of the rash, that of measles being a *purplish*, or *darkish scarlet*, while that of scarlet fever is a *light scarlet*.

Measles is a disease which, under different circumstances, assumes a great variety of forms, both as to its general character and violence. During some seasons it prevails as a mild and simple affection, requiring little or no treatment; while at other periods it assumes a highly inflammatory, congestive, or typhous character. Sometimes almost all cases seem to have a tendency to run on to pneumonia; at other times cerebral or typhoid symptoms predominate; in still other instances, gastric disorder prevails ; but in the great mass of cases, the malady is mild and tractable.

In contemplating the numerous varieties of this, as well as of most other diseases, the impartial physician must acknowledge the utter uncertainty and empyricism of prescriptions guided only by the *name* of a disease.

Causes.—In common with the other contagious disorders, measles arises from a specific morbific contagion. This has been amply proved by Home, Dewees, Speranza, and Majendie, who, in numerous instances, succeeded in communicating this affection by inoculation. The season of the year, the condition of the atmosphere, and the peculiar circumstances of the individuals exposed, exercise a powerful and perhaps controlling influence, in determining the character of the epidemic. When measles prevail during seasons of *influenza, typhus,* or *dysentery,* the disease will partake of the peculiar character of the existing epidemic, and its course be modified accordingly.

Therapeutics.—The most common medicines in the treatment of measles, are, *acon.,* and *puls.:* next in importance stand *bry., bell., ipecac., merc., sulph., cup. ac., rhus, ac., phos., ars., cham., &c.*

Schroen recognises five different varieties of measles, founded upon the characteristic symptoms present in each given case: viz., first, the *simple* or *erethistic,* in which *aconite* is the appropriate remedy; second, the *inflammatory,* requiring the use of *aconite, bryonia,* and *belladonna;* third, the *gastric,* demanding the employment of *pulsatilla, chamomela, ipecacuanha,* and *veratrum;* fourth, the *typhus,* or *irregular,* calling for *rhus tox., china, nux vom.,* and *belladonna;* fifth, the *septic,* or *malignant,* corresponding with *acid. phos., acid. sulph., acid. mur., opii,* and *arsenicum.*

At the commencement of an attack, when heat, thirst, quick pulse, red, inflamed, and watery eyes, sneezing, fluent coryza, cough, dyspnœa, oppression at the chest, and sore throat are present, *aconite* at the third potency is the most suitable remedy. So long as the disease progresses mildly, running through its regular stages in due form, no other medicine will be requisite to complete the cure. Even in those complications which call for the use of other medicines, as pneumonia, croup, cerebral or gastric disturbance, whether occurring before, during, or subsequent to the eruption, should the inflammatory excitement run high, *aconite* will still be required. Its repetition must, of course, be subject to the circumstances of each particular case.

When there exists a predominance of catarrhal symptoms, and a tardiness in the appearance of the eruption, we have an appropriate remedy in *pulsatilla.* This medicine may often succeed *aconite* with peculiar advantage in the catarrhal forms of more than ordinary severity. In these cases, some writers claim for this agent important prophylactic properties. It is also a valuable in retrocession of measles, attended with one or more of the following symptoms: hoarseness, swelling of the parotids, puffiness of the face, pain in the ears, discharges from the ears, hardness of hearing, dry short cough, great restlessness, pains in the head, back, and loins, and mucous diarrhœa.

Dr. Croserio believes *pulsatilla* to be especially adapted to measles, not only as a remedy, but as a prophylactic. He asserts that "it is to this disease, almost what *belladonna* is to scarlet fever. The precursory symptoms of measles accord perfectly with the febrile symptoms of *pulsatilla,* viz., chills, heat, lassitude, throbbing pains in the head, anxiety, nausea, vomiting of bile or glairy mucus, violent coryza, red eyes, lachrymation, photophobia, &c. Then follow pricking of the skin, red spots like flea-bites, excoriation and creeping in the throat, difficult deglutition, dry, fatiguing cough, epistaxis, &c. If given in the precursory stage, I have often seen the disease terminate in abundant perspiration in twenty-four hours."

Belladonna is indicated when the throat is much inflamed and swollen, with very painful and difficult deglutition, short, hacking, throat cough, inflamed eyes, nervous, uneasy and sometimes delirious, hurried respiration, headache, intense thirst, dry hot skin, and signs of cerebral disturbance. It has likewise been recommended in cases of sudden disappearance of the eruption after having been out one or two days.

"When the eruption suddenly disappears and is succeeded by fever, violent headache and breathlessness, great benefit will be derived from the administration of *aconite* and *arsenicum* alternately; and afterwards, when the head appears to be the chief point of attack, indicated by excruciating headache, screaming or moaning during the night, *belladonna* and *cuprum aceticum*, repeated every hour or two, will afford marked relief."—(*British Jour. of Hom.*, No. xxiv., p. 232.)

Bryonia will apply in cases attended with marked pectoral symptoms, like stitches or darting pains in the side and chest, anxious, sighing, difficult and painful respiration, and very great general uneasiness.

Hartmann says, that *bryonia* "is also a powerful remedy in *retrocessent measles*, in reproducing the eruption on the surface, or in rendering its disappearance harmless. In these cases I give *bryonia* in the fifteenth dilution, and notice that it is chiefly indicated, if after the retrocession of the eruption, a morbid affection of the eyes supervenes, which resembles that which I lately noticed when speaking of ophthalmia."

Ipecacuanha should be administered when there is gastric disorder, indicated by nausea, vomiting, pain and oppression in the stomach, and inability to retain food or drinks.

For the ulcers which sometimes form in the mouth and throat, also the glandular swellings which occur in the neck, *mercurius* is a valuable specific.

As a remedy for the restoration of retrocessent measles, as well as for the inflammatory affections of the eyes, which now and then remain as sequela of this malady, *sulphur* is sometimes a remedy of the highest importance. Many cases, after having apparently ran their courses in a mild and regular manner, leave the patient with some annoying *dreg*, like discharges from the ears, weak eyes, eruptions of various kinds, or chronic cough, with profuse expectoration, which are attributable to some miasm which has been roused during the course of the disease. For the cure of cases of this description, *sulphur* is an indispensable agent.

We occasionally meet with nervous or typhoid symptoms which render the use of *ars.*, *rhus tox.*, *stram.*, *op.*, and *phos.* necessary. Whatever symptoms present themselves, the judicious physician will be able to select from the great number of medicines of which the pure effects are known, those that are precisely homœopathic to the malady.

Administration.—In cases of children, we employ from the third to the sixth attenuations; and in those of adults, from the first to the third. Our repetitions must be governed by the nature of the case, and the effects produced by the medicine.

SECTION III.

VARIOLA.—SMALLPOX.

Two varieties of this disease have generally been recognised by pathologists; one termed *distinct* and the other *confluent.* The former is more mild and less dangerous than the latter, being attended with less severe constitutional disturbance, and having detached, distinct, and fewer pustules, which are surrounded by a pale red areola. The *confluent* variety, by the pustules running together and meeting each other, presents the appearance of a uniform and homogeneous swelling, from which it has derived its name.

Diagnosis.—Smallpox may, with propriety, be divided into the following stages or periods, viz.: 1, *the primary fever;* 2, *the eruptive stage;* 3, *the maturing period;* 4, *the period of exsiccation.*

The *primary fever* in the *distinct* variety is ushered in with lassitude, rigours, pains in the head, back, and loins, slight sore throat, soon followed by *nausea* and *vomiting, pain at the epigastrium,* often severe, *with tenderness on pressure.* hot and dry skin, thirst, scanty and high-coloured urine; these symptoms continue for about three days, when there is a supervention of the

Eruptive stage.—The eruption first comes out in small red spots or points, which, in the course of forty-eight hours, become rounded into pimples with vesicles upon their tops and slight depressions in the centre. They show themselves first upon the face, and then in regular succession upon the scalp, neck, arms, breast, body, and lower extremities, requiring about twenty-four hours for the full development of the eruption. After this period, there is a marked remission of all the febrile symptoms, which continues for three or four days, when the

Maturing or *suppurative period* commences. There is now a renewal of the febrile disturbance still more violent than at first, which commonly continues during the remaining course of the disease. This period continues from three to five days, when the serous fluid within the pustules acquires a purulent character, becoming thick and yellow. On the tenth or eleventh day, the pustules burst, giving vent to the matter which collects upon the surface of the pock, forming hard dark scabs or crusts, which in a few days fall off, leaving the skin scurfy and sometimes pitted.

Now commences the *period of exsiccation*, which occupies from three to five days; after which, if the malady has pursued a moderate course, the morbid symptoms all subside, and convalescence ensues. Thus it will be perceived, that the regular course of the disease occupies about fifteen days; this course, however, is subject to modifications from a great variety of causes, such as the supervention of pneumonia, bronchitis, ophthalmia, abdominal inflammations, disease of the glands, retrocession of the eruption, &c.

In the *confluent variety*, the primary fever is of a more violent character, the eruptive period more irregular, usually commencing at the end of two days from the onset of the malady; there are often spasmodic twitchings of the muscles, at or previous to the appearance of the pustules, the secondary or suppurative fever frequently assumes a typhoid form, salivation occurs about the period of the eruption, after which the tongue, mouth and throat become dry and dark, pocks form in the mouth, throat, larynx, pharynx, rectum, and urethra, and occasionally symptoms manifest themselves which indicate a high degree of malignancy. The face is often much swollen and disfigured from the pustules running into each other, so that the eyes become entirely closed, and the nostrils obstructed. The matter of the pustules is of a dusky colour, and is sometimes so acrid as to irritate the surrounding skin.

What has been denominated *varioloid*, is nothing

more or less than an exceedingly mild form of small pox, modified by previous vaccination, or some other accidental influence. The primary fever is very mild, the eruption distributed over the body in patches, the suppurating process slight and imperfect, attended with little or no secondary fever.

Causes.—All agree that variola proceeds from a specific morbific poison, *sui generis.* There are, however, causes constantly in operation, which exert a powerful influence in modifying or aggravating the character of the malady, respecting the nature of which, authors are not so well acquainted. At some periods, smallpox is characterized by a high degree of putridity, the symptoms assuming a low typhoid form, and a majority of the cases proving speedily fatal in spite of all remedial measures. At other seasons we may have a predominance of pulmonary or cerebral symptoms, attended with a high grade of synochal fever, and requiring a very different course of treatment from the form above mentioned. Again it may run its course in a regular and moderate manner, without serious complication from disturbance of any capital organ, and demanding but little aid from remedial agents.

Some writers have supposed that these different modifications were owing to certain occult conditions in the atmosphere, and also that the existence at the same time of other epidemics, has a material influence over the character and progress of smallpox. This is doubtless true; but there are other causes more under our control, which are of no less importance, as predisposing agents to the more violent forms of the malady. The most prominent of these, are, small and ill-ventilated dwellings, a lack of healthy and nutritious food, want of cleanliness, insufficient clothing, immoderate use of ales, and impure liquors, and the pernicious custom of crowding together in the same apartments, a number of individuals, who thus inhale, a good part of the time, a vitiated and unhealthy air.

The fatality of the disorder, when it seizes upon this degraded class, indicates the importance of the influences just enumerated, in aggravating the character of the malady. Does it not, then, behoove the guardians of the public health, during the prevalence of contagious affections, to look well to these deleterious agencies, and purge their towns of the filth, the dissipation, and the other corruptions of these hot-beds of contagion?

Therapeutics.—The following are the ordinary medicines used in the treatment of smallpox, namely, *aconite, belladonna, rhus tox., vaccinin, variolin, sulphur, opium, mercurius, bryonia, pulsatilla, nux vom., carbo veg., arsenicum.*

Aconite, second or third dilution, is the proper medicine during the primary fever, provided the attack is regular, and there exists no tendency to inflammation or congestion of any important organ.

In case the eruption is slow in making its appearance, or the process should be attended with great internal oppression, either *rhus* or *sulphur,* at the third attenuation, may be exhibited—a dose every three or four hours.

Belladonna is the specific, when, during any part of the malady, inflammation or congestion attacks the brain. In cases of this description, this remedy exercises a two-fold effect; first, by its special action upon the cerebral organs, and second, by its power of forcing and of retaining the eruption upon the surface. The third dilution may be used in these instances—one drop every two hours until amelioration of the symptoms is evident.

Dr. Liedbeck of Stockholm considers *tart. antim.* our most valuable remedy in smallpox. When taken in large doses, it produces dryness, heat and redness in the throat, internal eruptions, large pustules (with depressions in their centres) in the mouth, throat, larynx, and trachea: therefore, Dr. L. infers, that "it is as much the specific remedy for the smallpox, according to homœopathic principles, as *mercury* is that for syphilis." The second trituration may be used—one grain every two to six hours, as circumstances require.

Sulphur at the commencement of the attack, and about the period of desiccation, will often prove exceedingly serviceable in determining the eruption to the surface, and in disposing it to progress kindly. In individuals who suffer from a psoric taint, it cannot well be dispensed with. It may be administered at the third trituration, in grain doses, and repeated sufficiently often to ensure the kindly progress of the eruption.

Vaccinin and *variolin* have been highly extolled within the past three or four years, as a remedy in all stages of this affection. It is said, that, by the use of these agents, variola is rendered a very mild and harmless disease. It is claimed by those who have made considerable use of them, that all of the stages of the malady are shortened in duration, and that a majority of the cases thus treated, resemble varioloid more than real smallpox. These medicines may be used in the form of trituration, of the third attenuation.

Bryonia will be called for if pneumonic symptoms obtain. This remedy will also prove serviceable in typhoid forms, attended with gastric or biliary derangements.

Bryonia may be administered in mild cases, at the third dilution, and in severe congestive forms at the first—a drop every two or three hours in water.

Mercurius viv., third trituration, should be administered, if salivation, ulcerated throat, or diarrhœa with bloody stools, and tenesmus, occur. It is also a remedy of value during the suppurative stage, and in the ophthalmias which often accompany and succeed the variolous attack.

Opium, at the third dilution, will always be appropriate whenever coma, and nervous sensibility, stertorous respiration, convulsive movements, and impaired muscular action supervene during the progress of the malady.

In cases of great malignancy, with a gangrenous tendency, and other symptoms evincing a low typhus grade, *carbo veg.*, *acid. nit.*, *acid. mur.*, or *arsenicum*, may prove serviceable when all hopes from other remedies have been abandoned. From the first to the third attenuations should be employed in these instances. The age, sex, temperament, and the peculiar circumstances connected with each particular case, must determine the proper strength of the medicine and the frequency of its repetition.

SECTION IV.

VARICELLA.—CHICKENPOX.

Diagnosis.—There are a few points of similarity between the milder cases of smallpox and the more severe forms of varicella, which require an acute observer to discriminate between them during the early part of an attack. Both diseases commence with a similar primary fever, which continues until the eruption makes its appearance; the pustules in both instances resemble each other; both are likewise contagious, and communicable by inoculation.

At the eruptive period, however, an attentive observer will perceive that the resemblance usually ceases, for the pustules of variola make their appearance in a uniform manner, first on the face, then successively upon the neck, arms, breast, body, and lower extremities, occupying usually but twenty-four hours for the completion of the eruption, while the pustules of varicella come out in repeated series, first upon the breast, then upon the face, head, arms, body, and lower extremities, and require three or four days before the eruption is complete. Therefore, we often observe during the progress of the latter, some vesicles drying up, some in a state of partial development, while others are but making their first appearance. The vesicles of chickenpox contain a whitish or yellowish lymph, which seldom advances far towards the suppurating stage; and even in those cases where pus is formed, there is never any secondary or suppurative fever, as in variola.

Causes.—Varicella, like the other contagious disorders, is a distinct affection, and proceeds from a peculiar specific cause. This is apparent, from the fact that inoculation with varicellous matter never gives rise to any other malady than varicella itself.

It is not only a much milder disease than smallpox, or varioloid, but is of much shorter duration, running its course generally in six or seven days, when the pocks all disappear, leaving smooth surfaces.

Therapeutics.—Varicella, as it commonly occurs, requires no medicinal treatment: a due regard to diet, and avoidance of exposure to cold, dampness, &c., being only necessary to ensure its safe progress.

In cases where the malady assumes unusual severity, manifested by a high grade of febrile excitement, determinations of blood to the brain, lungs, or abdominal organs, then the medicines which are homœopathic to the existing symptoms may be administered. The remedies which have been most frequently used in these cases, are, *acon.*, *coff.*, *bell.*, *merc.*, *rhus tox.*, and *sulph.* The strength of the medicines, as well as the repetitions of doses, the same as under modified smallpox.

SECTION V.

MILIARIA.—MILIARY FEVER.

Diagnosis.—This disease is ushered in with lassitude, slight creeping chills, pain in the loins and lower extremities, oppression at the precordia, cough, general uneasiness, more or less heat and thirst, rapid pulse, and high-coloured urine. These precursory symptoms continue about five days, when a very fine eruption, resembling millet seeds, makes its appearance on different parts of the body. The little vesicles which compose this eruption are round, hard, and transparent, becoming after a time opaque. As they are about coming out, there is an itching, stinging, and burning sensation in the skin, the oppression at the chest and stomach is increased in severity, and, in general, a profuse perspiration of a disagreeable, sour odour, breaks out over the whole surface. After two or three days the vesicles become opaque, then soon dry up and fall off in the form of scurf.

Some writers consider miliary fever as a purely *symptomatic* affection, while others, with equal tenacity, maintain that it often occurs *idiopathically*. According to my own opinion, it is not at all improbable that it may be dependent upon some latent miasm, which only requires an exciting cause, like puerperal fever, heating and stimulating ptisans, undue exposure in heated and close rooms, &c., to call it into action. I am confirmed in this opinion from the fact, that in nearly every case with which I have been made acquainted, where the eruption has retroceded, whether by improper use of external lotions, or otherwise, there has been a supervention of some serious internal disorder.

If this view of the cause of the malady be correct, the therapeutical indications are evident, and the prudent physician will use every effort which our specific medicines afford, to aid nature in casting off the poison from the system through the medium of the skin.

Therapeutics.—In conjunction with our internal remedies, it is essential that the patient be kept in a dry apartment, of uniform temperature, and be confined to a strict dietetic regimen. By these means, we shall prevent the retrocession of the rash from the sudden application of external cold, and avoid those unpleasant complications which errors in diet are so apt to induce.

A strict adherence to the above rules, with an occasional dose of *aconite*, third dilution, will generally suffice for the cure of this complaint.

After the eruption has manifested itself, if the patient is troubled with a train of nervous symptoms, like sleeplessness, general uneasiness, partial loss of power over the voluntary muscles, spasmodic twitchings, and constant desire to change position, a dose of the sixth dilution of *hyoscyamus* may be given, and repeated as circumstances require.

Should the brain become affected in any stage of the disease, *belladonna* may be exhibited in the same manner as advised under measles.

Chamomela, at the tenth potency, should always be administered when infants and children are the subjects of attack. If the malady commences with strong febrile excitement, this medicine may be preceded by *aconite.*

Bryonia is also highly recommended in cases of miliaria in infants and parturient women. It may be administered in the same manner as *bell.*

Ipecacuanha will apply when the eruption is accompanied with laborious and noisy respiration, nausea, or vomiting, groaning, aversion to food, chilliness, alternating with flushes of heat, and sweet, insipid taste. The third trituration should be employed —one grain every four or six hours until the symptoms yield.

SECTION VI.

ROSEOLA.

Diagnosis.—This is one of the mildest and least dangerous of all the eruptive fevers. It is characterized by an eruption or efflorescence of a rose colour, preceded and accompanied by some slight symptoms of febrile disturbance. The rash shows itself on the third or fourth day of the fever, and comes out in distinct and irregular spots upon different parts of the surface, or the spots run together, giving to the skin an almost uniform redness. The cuticle is neither elevated, nor is there any appearance of papulæ; but a simple blush of a rose colour, characterizes the eruption, and serves as a mark of distinction between it and that of other diseases of this kind. The appearance of the rash is often attended with itching and tingling, which are present more or less until the eruption vanishes, which is usually in five or six days, without desquamation of the cuticle or any unpleasant after symptoms.

Causes.—Roseola is for the most part confined to infants and females. It arises from undue exposure to cold, after having been confined in a warm room, indigestible food, dentition, gastro-intestinal irritation, and the abuse of stimulating infusions, cathartics, &c.

Therapeutics.—Rigid dietetic regulations, a moderate, dry, and equal temperature, mental and physical rest and quietness, and an entire exclusion of all "herb teas," and such other "domestic remedies," so called, as are commonly suggested by the officious ignorance of old women. A regard to these rules will suffice to secure the patient from any ill consequence of this naturally mild and simple affection.

SECTION VII.

URTICARIA.—NETTLE RASH.

Diagnosis.—The primary symptoms of urticaria are, languor, oppression, and sickness at stomach, foul tongue, bitter taste, giddiness, creeping chills, succeeded by preternatural heat of skin and thirst. During the early period of the disease, elevated, circular, and florid spots or weals, each with a whitish spot or point in its centre, appear, sometimes in only one part of the body, at other times generally diffused over the whole surface. These weals are attended with an exceedingly annoying itching, stinging, and burning sensation, somewhat resembling the stings of nettles. The itching, as well as the febrile excitement, is always worse in the evening or during the night; but when the eruption is upon the surface, the nausea and distress at the stomach abate, and do not return until another eruptive period, unless there is a sudden retrocession of the weals.

In some instances the eruption appears suddenly without any febrile or other premonitory symptoms, and without any apparent exciting cause. At other times, certain articles of food, like shell-fish, porgies, esculent vegetables, acid fruits, or stimulants like wine, spirits, hot ptisans, condiments, or frictions upon the skin, seem to become its exciting causes. It usually terminates in a few days, but now and then it persists many months, sometimes apparent upon the skin, at others suppressed.

"Its sudden disappearance without leaving a trace behind, and its equally sudden reappearance, are quite characteristic. Inclination is also present in all the varieties of this disease, and vomiting frequently occurs as a crisis."—(*Schroen.*)

Some nosologists have divided this malady into two, and some into four varieties; and others, like Bateman, and a few of the older writers, have gone so far as to recognise and describe seven: but these fine and arbitrary distinctions are not founded in nature, and therefore offer no aid in diagnosis; while, on the other hand, there is danger that they may confuse and embarrass the inexperienced practitioner. We know that the eruption is very irregular in regard to the periods of its appearance, and also in the size, form, general aspect, and diffusion of the weals, yet, we see no necessity for complicating our classification with so many varieties, for we might with as much propriety go on with divisions, *ad infinitum,* as to stop after having described six or seven genera, since the most acute nosologist will scarcely be able to discover any two cases presenting precisely the same symptoms in all respects.

If, however, we were to adopt any classification, it would be that of Schroen, who distinguishes two forms of the malady, the *acute* and the *chronic.* Under the first form, he includes: first, *urticaria maculosa,* or spots of different degrees of redness, attended with sensation of formication and intense itching; second, *urticaria vesicularis,* or vesicular prominences, with empty and almost transparent apices; third, *urticaria tuberosa,* or hard, tense, and painful tuberosities, generally appearing in the night. Amongst the *chronic* varieties, he ranks *urticaria evanida,* resembling the *urticaria tuberosa,* appearing on exposure to cold, and disappearing on the application of warmth. This variety sometimes continues for weeks, and even months.

Causes.—We entertain the opinion that the remote cause of nettle rash consists of a specific miasm, either generated within the organism, or introduced from without, and which is liable to be roused into action by numerous exciting causes. The proofs of this are numerous, and we think satisfactory; for if it were merely an effect or symptom of one of the various exciting causes, like indigestible food, certain kinds of fish, acid fruits, vegetables, wines, liquors, &c., it would disappear as soon as the exciting cause was withdrawn, and all irritation from this source obviated; but in very many instances no such result takes place, and after the noxious article has been entirely removed, and the part previously deranged restored to its usual normal condition, there is a persistence of the urticaria for months, and even years; it appearing and disappearing at frequent intervals, without the slightest apparent reason.

Another fact which sustains the position we have advanced, is, that if the eruption be suddenly repelled by the use of lotions, or cathartics, serious internal disorders frequently supervene as a consequence of the retrocession, which terminate, if the weals are not reproduced either spontaneously or artificially, in dissolution. A painful case, illustrative of this position, came under my observation a few years since. The patient was a lovely and highly interesting young lady, who from some slight exciting cause was afflicted with urticaria, although previously she had remained for many years in excellent health. The malady annoyed her by turns for more than three months, when, from the application of a lead-water lotion, the external symptoms suddenly vanished, leaving in their place wandering pains in the chest and side, some cough, fits of oppression at the chest, and difficulty of breathing. These symptoms of pulmonary disturbance continued to increase until she was pronounced by two eminent physicians of a neighbouring city to be past cure, with tubercular consumption. About this period the case came under my charge, in what seemed to be the last stages of consumption. Notwithstanding, however, the unpromising condition of affairs, my patient slowly but gradually recruited, so that in six or seven months the abscess which had existed in one lobe of her lungs was healed, and the lungs, with her whole system, were restored to a comparatively sound and healthy state. In this condition she continued for nearly two years, when a second attack of urticaria supervened, affording still farther relief for a few days, from all remaining difficulties, when the rash permanently disappeared. From this time her symptoms were all aggravated, her old complaints returned, the lungs became again ulcerated, so that in a few months the malady advanced to a fatal termination. Is this an isolated instance? Without doubt, the experience of almost every physician could furnish one or more cases of the same description.

This example offers conclusive proof to my own mind, that an intimate connection existed between the two diseases, and that whenever the rash was upon the surface, nothing disturbed the lungs; while the moment retrocession ensued, pulmonary symptoms manifested themselves. If urticaria is a purely local disease, depending upon a distention or spasm of the extreme cutaneous vessels, how can the suppression of such local inflammation affect so seriously internal organs?

It must be confessed, that our knowledge respecting the causes and intimate nature of cutaneous affections, is at present quite limited; but when we take into consideration the fact that so many internal constitutional maladies take their exit through the surface in the form of eruption, we are constrained to believe that this is almost uniformly only a symptom of some internal constitutional disorder.

Therapeutics.—As it is of the first importance in all cutaneous diseases, that the eruption should be urged and retained upon the surface, in order that the miasm may not fall upon any vital organ, we should select our remedies chiefly from those which exercise a specific action upon the skin.

Another point of no less importance in the management of eruptive fevers, consists in securing for the patient a dry, moderate, and equable temperature. This precaution, combined with cleanliness, and a placid and composed frame of mind, will always aid us materially in our therapeutical measures.

The medicines which are the most appropriate for the treatment of this complaint are, *acon.*, *sulph.*, *dulc.*, *rhus.*, *calc.*, *carb.*, *lycop.*, *nat. mur.*, *acid. nit.*, *puls.*, *ignat.*, *ipecac.*

Aconite will only be required in those cases which are attended with undue febrile action. It may be administered as advised, under measles.

Sulphur.—This medicine should always be prescribed in cases occurring in individuals of a marked scrofulous dyscrasia, when the following symptoms obtain.

External Indications.—General appearance of debility; pale, sallow, and sickly expression of face; redness of the margins of the eyelids; swellings of the glands of the neck.

Physical Sensations.—Eruption and violent itchings occurring in the night, from the heat of the bed, and occasionally from exposure to cold air; great sensitiveness to cold; dizziness and pains in the head; spasmodic twitchings of the eyelids; bad taste in the mouth; nausea; pyrosis; weakness and oppression at the chest.

Mental and moral symptoms.—Melancholy; sadness; irritability.

Administration.—One grain of the third trituration in two ounces of distilled water,—a dessert spoonful once in twelve hours.

Dulcamara is useful in urticaria, which proceeds from taking cold, and is attended with nausea, vomiting, oppression at the stomach, heat of skin, thirst, bitter taste, diarrhœa, and great general uneasiness. The symptoms are aggravated at night, during repose, and by the heat of a room; but they disappear in the open air.

Administration.—A drop of the third dilution, in a small quantity of water, may be given once in six to twelve hours.

Rhus tox.—Eruption, attended with itching and burning during inaction, or on entering a room from the open air; disappearance of the weals, on exercise, followed by shifting rheumatic pains, pains and pressure in the stomach, difficult respiration, short breath in the evening, agitation and anguish. This medicine is particularly applicable in *urticaria vesicularis.*

Administration.—Same as *dulcamara.*

Calcarea carbonica is indicated in cases where the rash vanishes on going into the fresh air, and excited by the application of cold water: face yellow, upper lip swollen, skin rough and covered with goose pimples, stunning lateral pains in the head, with nausea and vertigo at night, or in the morning, on waking, with faintness; anxiety, anguish, apprehension.

Remarks.—*Calcarea carbonica* is suitable in obstinate *chronic* urticaria, especially when occurring in scrofulous or cachectic constitutions. It is sometimes necessary to persist in the use of this remedy for several weeks.

Administration.—A drop of the third dilution in an ounce of water,—a dessert spoonful once or twice in the twenty-four hours.

Lycopodium.—Rash and itching during repose, headache in the afternoon or at night, smarting of the eyes by candle-light, nausea when in a hot room, relieved in the air, silent and peevish.

Administration.—Same as *calcarea carbonica.*

Natrum mur., at the sixth potency, may be prescribed, when there are languor, uneasiness, nausea, headache, weakness when lying down at night, relieved on rising in the morning, eruption coming out after violent exercise.

Nitric acid, third dilution, will be proper for patients of a consumptive or scrofulous habit, afflicted with debilitating night sweats, weak, enfeebled, subject to hæmorrhages from the bowels, lungs, nose, &c., and rash caused by exposure to cold air. A drop should be prescribed two or three times daily.

Pulsatilla, sixth dilution, when the elevations are redder than the skin, when the itching is of a burning or pricking character, worse at night in bed, in a hot room, or by scratching; better in the open air; worse every other evening; heaviness and disposition to numbness in the limbs; great sensibility to the open air.

Ignatia, sixth dilution, is particularly adapted to attacks occurring in nervous and hysterical females: the eruption is brought out by exercise, and is often preceded by nervous symptoms; there is also fulness and pressure of the head, with sparks before the eyes; also sighing, and irregular respirations.

Ipecacuanha, third trituration, is useful in cases attended with excessive vomiting, oppression at the chest, and dyspnœa; it is also a valuable remedy in asthma from suppressed urticarias.

Other remedies worthy of consideration are, *arsenicum, balsam copaïbæ, iodine* and *bryonia* in the *chronic* forms; and in the *acute* varieties, *clematis, staphysagria,* and *belladonna,* for *urticaria vesicularis; urtica* and *hepar sulphur,* for *urticaria tuberosa; mercurius, iodine, aurum mur.* and *sepia,* for *urticaria maculosa.*

Administration.—The above remedies may be given dissolved in pure water. They may be repeated in six, eight, or twelve hours, according to the urgency of the symptoms. In all cases of this description, where a latent miasm is suspected to exist, a persevering and judicious course of anti-psoric treatment, should be adopted, after the eruption has disappeared and the acute symptoms have subsided.

SECTION VIII.

ERYSIPELAS.—ST. ANTHONY'S FIRE.

Erysipelas presents itself under so many different aspects, and so often makes its appearance in connection with other morbid conditions of the system, that any description which shall cover all its various phases, is scarcely possible. The structures upon which it seizes are the skin, the cellular-tissue, and the internal organs, especially the brain and the lungs. It may exist in a *chronic* form, unattended by febrile, or other constitutional disturbance, and persist for a long period—displaying itself at intervals, upon the surface, in the form of slight superficial inflammations; or sometimes passing to an internal organ, and producing temporary derangement of function; while at other times it will remain latent and inactive. But it very frequently appears in an *acute* form, either as an *idiopathic* or a *symptomatic* affection. It is in this active condition that erysipelas has proved so formidable to the old-school physician and surgeon. It was in this form of the malady, that the late celebrated Liston, conscious of the inefficiency of allopathic remedies, was induced to adopt homœopathic treatment in the numerous symptomatic cases, from surgical operations, wounds, &c., which came under his care; the results of which were so highly satisfactory to Mr. Liston and the friends of homœopathy.*

Erysipelas prevails most commonly in the spring and autumn, and not unfrequently it assumes an epidemic character. Females are likewise more subject to its attacks than males.

The circumstances which operate to modify the character and course of the malady are very numerous. In some instances a peculiar state of the atmosphere exists, which serves to develop the affection in a highly malignant form, in those who are predisposed to its influence. At other times, the effluvia arising from

* See Reports of North London Hospital, 1836, 7 and 8.

those who are suffering from the disease, appears to possess contagious qualities, and to be capable of communicating the morbid influence to those who come within its reach. Cases of this kind, are usually severe and malignant—attacking the cellular-tissue with a low grade of inflammation, which is exceedingly prone to terminate in gangrene, and not unfrequently to extend its ravages to the brain and lungs. The habits and constitution of the individual likewise exercise an important influence in determining the character of the disease. Excessive indulgence in malt liquors, and impure spirits, and the exclusive use of fresh meat, reduce the system to a condition peculiarly favourable to the generation of malignant erysipelas, whenever slight exciting causes operate. So also, general debility, a dropsical tendency, a scrofulous or scorbutic habit, or any other dyscrasy, will be likely to determine a dangerous form of the complaint.

Diagnosis.—Erysipelas is sometimes preceded by general lassitude, depression of spirits, and protracted rigours, followed by accelerated circulation, hot skin, thirst, headache, wandering pains in the back and limbs, and general restlessness ; or it may make its appearance without any premonitory symptoms, except, perhaps, slight chills, succeeded in a few days by fever ; or it may occur during an attack of pneumonia, typhus, bilious, or gastric fever ; or after wounds, or other injuries, in different parts of the body, especially of the scalp ; or it may arise suddenly from violent mental emotions, as terror, joy, anger, &c. When the inflammation is confined to the skin, the malady runs its course in a mild and simple manner, and the accompanying symptoms will be merely stiff, heavy, burning, or pungent sensation in the part affected, impaired appetite, slight febrile disturbance, and nocturnal restlessness. The inflammation generally comes out in blotches, which sometimes run together, and after a few days, are covered with vesicles filled with a limpid or yellowish fluid. These blotches vary from a light red, to a dark red, or purplish colour, becoming white under pressure, but again resuming their original appearance as soon as the pressure is removed. As the disease is about subsiding, the colour of these spots changes to a pale or dirty yellow, after which desquamation of the cuticle takes place.

When the malady is complicated by gastric or biliary derangement, we may have a high grade of febrile excitement, and the other phenomena which usually attend affections of this kind. In these instances, the erysipelatous inflammation is apt to be more violent, and to extend deeper, than when no complications exist. The tumefaction is more extensive, and deep-seated, the inflammation is more intense, the hardness greater, and the pain more profound, in this variety, than in that first described. Some authors have designated this variety the *erysipelas phlegmonodes.* The most common seat of this phlegmon is in the face and head, although it occasionally attacks other parts of the body.

Another and highly malignant variety of erysipelas prevails at certain seasons, and attacking more particularly females after confinement, and individuals who have already been enfeebled by other diseases. The tumefaction in these instances is more soft and spongy than in the preceding varieties—often pitting on pressure; the skin assumes a pale, waxen, or sallow colour; the temperature of the parts is sometimes above and at other times below the natural standard; the skin of the affected parts presents a smooth and glossy appearance; vesicles, containing a limpid or yellowish serum, are diffused over the swelling; sensations of stiffness, weight, and deep-seated burning pains are experienced; followed, if the disease advances, by nausea, vomiting, obtusion of the senses, rapid and feeble, or slow and full pulse; constant inclination to sleep, and finally profound coma; stertorous respiration; contracted or dilated pupils, either partially or wholly insensible to light; protrusion of the lips at each expiration; frothing at the mouth; diminished temperature of the skin; livid and inactive appearance of the diseased part, and general and rapid abasement of the energies of the system. This form of erysipelas has been recognised under the term *erysipelas œdematodes,* from the resemblance of the affected parts to dropsical swellings.

There is another form of the disease which evinces a strong disposition, from the commencement, to gangrenous degeneration. The inflammation is confined principally to the sub-cutaneous cellular tissue; the swelling is hard and inelastic; the colour of the skin is dark-red or purple; large vesicles filled with an acrid fluid, form on the surface, presenting a sluggish and gangrenous tendency; the accompanying fever is of a low typhoid character; the muscular and nervous energies are below the natural standard; delirium or coma are for the most part present, and suppuration, gangrene, and sloughing soon supervene. This form of the malady has been termed *erysipelas gangrenosum.*

Another form attacks newly born children. The inflammation is generally confined to the lower part of the body in the first instance, but sometimes extends over the whole surface. The character of the attack depends much upon the constitution and predisposition of the child; although, commonly, the inflammation is of a high grade, the swollen parts very painful and tender, and disposed to suppurate and slough. The course of the complaint varies from two to four weeks. This variety is called *erysipelas neanatorum.*

Another, and very common kind, may be observed in old people and in cachectic and intemperate persons. It is unattended with febrile disturbance, or much pain: but as it is apt to make its appearance from very slight exciting causes, it becomes a constant annoyance. When the inflammation is upon the surface, the subject feels well; but on its disappearance, there often occur internal pains, congestions, and numerous unpleasant symptoms, which lead to the inference that the disorder is dependent on some internal miasm. Frank terms this form, *habitual erysipelas.*

A number of other varieties have been described, founded upon the disease as it has prevailed in different localities and climates, and as modified by various forms of disease which may have accompanied it; but as we only aim to give a general outline of the complaint, with its characteristic phenomena, we shall refrain from entering here into a more minute enumeration of symptoms.

Causes.—There is much difference of opinion respecting the causes of erysipelas. Some attribute it to a local cutaneous vice; some to a degeneration of the blood in consequence of improper food, abuse of stimulants, &c.; some to a derangement of the biliary organs; some to atmospheric influences; while others entertain the opinion that it is dependent upon a peculiar dyscrasia which is constantly present as a predisposing cause. This opinion appears to us reasonable; but whether this dyscrasia is in all instances hereditary, or whether it may be acquired by intemperance, unwholesome food, or from contaminated air, we are as yet unable to determine.

The more common exciting causes of erysipelas are, debility and loss of resisting power, from disease, abuse of stimulants, violent emotions of the mind, undue exposure to cold, certain states of the atmosphere, accouchement, disordered stomach and bowels, confinement in close and crowded apartments, and wounds.

Eberle asserts that "the inflammation which is produced by the recent leaves of the *rhus toxicodendron*, is strictly of an erysipelatous character." This, however, is an error, for although a close similarity exists between the two inflammations, the careful observer will be able to distinguish decided marks of difference.

Therapeutics.—The important medicines in the treatment of erysipelas, are, *rhus toxicodendron, belladonna, aconite, sulphur, opium, graph., arsenicum, carbo vegetabilis, merc., phosphorus, pulsatilla, acid phosphorus, acid nitric, sil., china, hep. sulph., lach., bryonia, chamomela, clem.*, and *euphorb.*

Rhus toxicodendron. — *External indications.*—Inflammation confined to the skin; numerous vesicular blotches, attended with itching and burning sensation; swelling and redness of the face, worse in the eyelids, around the eyes, and in the lobules of the ears, attended with burning and itching; swelling in the scalp; erysipelatous inflammation of the scrotum in new-born children; distinct or confluent vesicles, containing an acrid, limpid, or yellowish fluid, with redness of the skin over the whole surface of the body; partial or entire closure of the eyelids; swelling and hardness of the *alæ nasi;* gangrenous ulcers; hot and dry skin; rapid and full pulse; urine small in quantity, dark and turbid.

Physical sensations.—Burning, itching, and stinging of the affected parts, aggravated by scratching; irritation and sometimes excoriation of the skin from contact of the vesicular discharge; the itching and burning sensations worse in the evening; stiffness and sense of immobility in the swollen parts; bruised feeling in the limbs and back; general sensation of heat, both externally and internally, occasionally interrupted by slight rigours; mouth filled with saliva, or dry, with or without thirst; dryness and obstruction of the nose, relieved by drafts of cold air, or by being fanned; painful pulsations in the internal ears, when resting on the affected side; scalp swollen and painful to the touch; eyes painful on motion; dull heavy pain in the head, aggravated by motion or stooping.

Mental and moral symptoms.—Obtuseness of intellect, stupefaction, and weakness of memory; sadness, anxiety, and despondency towards evening, and during the night; nightly delirium.

Administration.—A drop of the second or third dilution in water, once in two to four hours.

Remarks.—Ruoff and Schroen consider *rhus* particularly applicable in vesicular erysipelas which is confined to the skin; but if symptoms indicative of serious cerebral disorder are present, they prefer *belladonna.* It has been used with success in infantile erysipelas.

Belladonna.—External indications.—Skin swollen, red, hot, and painful; cheeks, eyelids, nose, lips, and forehead, swollen, tense, shining, and painful to the touch; eyes red, prominent, and glistening, or dull and cloudy; pupils dilated or contracted; whole head swollen and painful; obstruction of the nostrils; inflammation and enlargement of the parotid glands; hardness of hearing; redness and swelling of the tonsils and throat; urine scanty, dark, yellow, or reddish, clear or turbid; vesicular inflammation, with intense febrile excitement; tongue and lips dry; sordes upon the teeth; occasionally spasms, tremblings, and rigidity of the limbs; pulse generally full and quick.

Physical sensations. — Tension and pressure, or sharp, throbbing pains in the head; scalp very painful, especially on pressure; violent heat and burning of the inflamed parts; dryness, smarting, or burning of the eyes; disordered vision; stitching and throbbing pains in the ears, both externally and internally; roaring and humming in the ears; mouth and throat dry, hot, and painful; sticking and burning sensation in the throat when swallowing; aversion to food and drinks, or violent thirst for cold drinks; bad taste in the mouth, bitter eructations, and other signs showing biliary and gastric derangement; short, anxious, and difficult inspirations; great weariness and uneasiness; pains worse in the afternoon and at night, and aggravated by contact or movement.

Mental and moral symptoms.—Vertigo, confusion of ideas, or loss of consciousness, or delirium, violent at night, but moderate during the day; or melancholy, despondent, and apathetic.

Administration.—A drop of the third dilution in water every two or three hours, according to the severity of the symptoms.

Remarks.—It was chiefly from the employment of *belladonna* and *aconite*, that Liston produced the successful results in the North London Hospital, and in private practice, to which we have already alluded. We believe it to be our most valuable remedy in those cases which have been excited by intemperance and violent emotions of the mind. It is applicable also in nearly all cases of erysipelas where there exists prominent cerebral disorder. In these cases, should it not cover all of the important symptoms, we may give some other appropriate medicine in alternation.

Whenever febrile symptoms are strongly pronounced, and there exists a decidedly augmented action of the circulatory vessels, *aconite* will be required, either alone or in alternation with some other remedy. It should be used in the first, second, or third dilutions —a drop in water as often as the exigencies of the case may demand.

Opium is indicated in those cases which supervene during *pneumonia*, typhoid, and other fevers, and present the following signs: profound coma; stertorous respiration; eyes dull and watery; pupils dilated and immovable; general appearance stupid and besotted; spasmodic motions in different parts of the body; pulse slow and feeble, or slow, intermittent, and full; inability to rouse the patient. The second or third dilution may be employed—a drop every half hour until an impression is produced.

When ulcers have formed, and there is a disposition to gangrenous degeneration, we must refer to *ars.*, *carb.*, *veg.*, *sulph.*, *lach.*, *euphorb.*, *sil.*, *clam.*, *acid.*, *nit.* and *acid phos.*

In erysipelas phlegmonodes, when the inflammation is extending into the cellular tissue, our best remedies are *bell.*, *graph.*, *hep-sulph.*, *merc.*, *phos.*, *sil.*, and *sulph.*

If the inflammation exhibits a tendency to shift from place to place, and is attended with gastric or intestinal derangement, and constantly shifting pains, *pulsatilla* will prove specific.

Bryonia has been strongly recommended when the inflammation takes place about the joints, and is accompanied by rheumatic pains.

China will often prove serviceable during convalescence from severe and protracted attacks, when the energies of the system have been exhausted, and there is great irritability of the nervous system. Some of the signs which point to this medicine, are emaciation, œdema of the limbs, deficiency of animal heat, pale countenance, great debility, ringing in the ears, disturbed sleep.

External applications to the affected surfaces, in the form of blisters, and of nit. of silver, have sometimes been employed with success by gentlemen of the old school, and as they are in accordance with our principle of cure, it becomes us to give them all due attention.

Respecting the administration of the remedies above enumerated, we suggest, as a general rule, the employment of the first, second, and third attenuations; but in cases of infants and young children, we may go up to the tenth or twelfth dilution. In acute cases, the dose should be repeated once in two to four hours; but in the chronic varieties, two or three times daily will suffice.

SECTION IX.

THE PLAGUE.

The plague is said to resemble in many respects malignant typhus; the only phenomena which serve to distinguish it from this fever, being the numerous buboes and carbuncles which appear on the body. By many it is supposed to be really nothing more or less than a genuine typhus fever, rendered peculiarly putrid and malignant by the atmospheric and other influences which prevail in Egypt and the other oriental nations in which it has prevailed. As in the worst grades of typhus, maculæ, petechiæ, diarrhœa, hæmorrhages from the bowels, &c., generally supervene in the advanced stages of the disorder, in addition to the buboes and carbuncles.

Our knowledge in relation to this disease is so limited, it being derived solely from the imperfect descriptions we have seen, by other writers, that no attempt will here be made to detail its symptoms. But if we may be allowed to judge of its nature from those phenomena which seem to be characteristic, we suppose the following remedies will correspond with its manifestations, and prove to it homœopathic, namely: *arsen.*, *acid nit.*, *rhus tox.*, *veratrum*, *merc.*, *bell.*, *chin.*, *ipecac.*, *carb. veg.*

CHAPTER XXI.

OF THE CHRONIC CUTANEOUS DISEASES. VESICULAR VARIETIES.

SECTION X.

HERPES.—TETTER.

Diagnosis.—The eruption consists of groups of small vesicles, situated upon red and inflamed bases, and separated from each other by sound portions of skin. As the vesicles increase in size, the colourless fluid which they contained in the first instance, becomes gradually opaque, and in two or three weeks dries up into thin crusts which scale off. When the eruption makes its appearance, there is an unpleasant burning and crawling sensation, which soon settles into a deep-seated, and in some cases, severe pain. It may be confined to a single point, or extend, in clusters of different sizes, over a large surface.

Another variety of tetter, is often observed to commence in the form of broad and irregular clusters of small vesicles, sometimes seated on swollen and inflamed bases, and shortly becoming confluent; or the eruption may appear in distinct groups and unattended with any inflammation or swelling of the surrounding skin. In the first form, when the inflammation is somewhat active, the vesicles often burst and discharge their contents, leaving troublesome ulcers at their bases. This variety is sometimes described under the term *eczema*, or *humid tetter*.

According to Bateman, most kinds of herpes pass through a "regular course of increase, maturation, and decline, and terminate in about ten, twelve, or fourteen days. The eruption is preceded, when it is extensive, by considerable constitutional disorder, and is accompanied by a sensation of heat and tingling, and sometimes by severe pains in the parts affected."

Herpes has been subdivided into many different species, on account of presenting some points of distinction when attacking different parts of the body.

Thus, when the vesicles appear upon the lips during colds, fevers, and inflammations of the mucous membranes of the pulmonary or digestive apparatus, the disease is termed *herpes labialis*. The eruption in this instance, is usually of a more inactive and unhealthy character, than when it occurs in other parts of the body. The matter which escapes from the vesicles is purulent or sanious, and concretes into black crusts.

When the eruption consists of a narrow belt of vesicles, extending partly around the body, or over the shoulder, it receives the appellation of *herpes zoster*, or *shingles*.

Another, and very common form, is thus described by Schroen: "An inflamed red ring, commonly perfectly circular, and upon which numerous small globular vesicles appear, which, though at first perfectly transparent, soon become turbid; these burst, and discharge a thin fluid, which forms a slight lamellated crust that soon becomes detached, leaving a bright red mark. Sometimes the fluid is absorbed, and the vesicles fade and fall off in thin, scurfy exfoliations. The duration of the disease is about seven or eight days for each ring; but as successive rings appear and go through a similar course, it may last between two or three weeks." Schoenlein supposes that a repulsion of this eruption predisposes the patient to *fungus hæmatodes*. This variety is called *herpes circinnatus*, or *ringworm*.

Other subdivisions have been made into *herpes præputialis, herpes iris, herpes phlyctænodes*, &c.; but since the nature of the malady is the same in all these varieties, and as the modifications which occur are dependent in a great measure upon the peculiar structure of the affected parts, we do not deem it necessary to enter into a more minute exposition of the details pertaining to each species.

Causes.—Errors in diet; immoderate use of fat, rich, and indigestible food; a morbid condition of the cutaneous excretion; local irritations from external injuries, and the application of acrid substances. It has been observed that those who have suffered from attacks of syphilis, scrofula, scurvy, or who have taken much mercury, are most prone to the disease. In these cases, a predisposition is established in the skin, so that, from slight causes, herpetic eruptions are excited.

Therapeutics.—When the eruption attacks the face, head, body, or extremities, our best remedies are, *sulphur, calcarea carb., silicea, carbo veg., sepia, rhus tox., belladonna, lycopodium, iodine, graphites, aurum mur.*

Herpes of the lips should be treated with *arsenicum, acid phos., graphites, phosphorus, hepar sulphur.*

If the eruption appears upon the scrotum or prepuce, the appropriate medicines are *mercurius, arsenicum, sulphur, calcarea carb., conium, rhus tox.*

Nearly all cases which occur may be cured by *sulphur, calcarea carb., sepia,* and *mercurius ;* but should these remedies disappoint us, there will be no difficulty in making an appropriate selection from the medicines first enumerated.

Administration.—For the most part, we rely upon the first, second, and third attenuations ; and prescribe drop doses of the dilutions, or grain doses of the triturations, twice daily until a satisfactory amendment is evident.

SECTION XI.

PEMPHIGUS.

Diagnosis—This is also a vesicular affection, characterized by the appearance of single vesicles of large size upon the legs, and occasionally upon other parts of the body. The vesicles are filled with a yellow or straw-coloured fluid, and are seated upon an inflamed, hard, and red base. This disease occurs during the course of fevers, or in old and enfeebled persons, after undue exposure to cold, or improper indulgence in stimulants or indigestible food. "I have frequently seen," writes Mackintosh, "large bullæ take place in the course of slight, as well as severe fevers ; but instead of considering them thereby entitled to any specific character, I have always looked upon their occurrence as an accidental circumstance, and have made no difference in the treatment of the original disease. The appearance of the vesicles is sometimes preceded by slight chills, followed by transient flushes of heat, and other signs indicative of mild constitutional disturbance. In these instances the integuments at the base of the vesicles are hard, swollen, and painful. The ordinary duration of the eruption is from one to two weeks; but in some instances the vesicles continue to appear for months.

Therapeutics.—*Sulphur, rhus, arsenicum, dulcamara, iodine, acid nit.*, and *mercurius.*

Administration.—The medicines may be employed in the same manner as advised in *herpes.*

SECTION XII.

POPULAR VARIETIES.—LICHEN.

Diagnosis.—Many kinds of this malady are described by writers, although the general character of the eruption is in all instances the same. Willan gives us seven different forms; and other authors describe even a greater number. But the propriety of these minute subdivisions is very questionable, since some slight distinctions might be made in almost all cases which occur, and thus lead to a very extensive and inconvenient classification.

The eruption consists of numerous small papillæ upon the breast, arms, and limbs, in the first instance, which afterwards spread over the whole surface of the body, attended with tingling and itching, especially when exposed to heat, or when covered up warmly in bed. The eruption is generally preceded by slight febrile excitement, and symptoms of gastric or intestinal disorder. The bases of the papillæ are red, inflamed, and painful, but they do not often suppurate, or become filled with serum, but continue about eight or nine days, when they dry up, and fall off in the form of scurf.

The eruption which is so often seen in infants during the period of dentition, and known as "*the red gum,*" is a form of lichen. In these cases the colour of the papillæ may be red or white.

Sometimes the eruption appears in the palms of the hands, the arms and legs, when it receives the vulgar appellation of *salt rheum.*

The eruption now and then comes out in a mild form upon the trunk or extremities, attended with heat, and troublesome itching on becoming heated, or from rubbing or scratching, but entirely unattended by febrile excitement. This variety is familiarly known under the designation of *prickly heat.*

Causes.—Irritation of the stomach and intestines from errors in diet, worms, and teething. Also protracted exposure to a hot fire; going into the cool air, after long exertion while in a profuse perspiration; or, sometimes from entering a hot apartment, after having been exposed for a long time to intense cold.

Therapeutics.—The following medicines will suffice for the cure of all forms of this complaint: *sulphur, graphites, calcarea carb., sepia, iodine, antimonium tart., copaibæ bals., acid phos., chamomela, dulcamara, rhus tox., hepar sulphur.*

Administration.—Same as for *herpes.*

PRURIGO.

Diagnosis.—Prurigo is believed by some authors to be a severe form of lichen. The papillæ are, however, larger, "more isolated and distinct, and scattered over larger surfaces" than those of that affection. The eruption is sometimes of a red or pinkish colour, at other times white, like the surrounding skin, and attended with the most intense itching and stinging. The papillæ are most commonly distributed about the labia pudendi, but the disease is not unfrequently observed in other parts of the body.

The causes and treatment are the same as those described under lichen.

SECTION XIII.

PUSTULAR VARIETIES:—SCABIES.—PSORA.—ITCH.

Diagnosis.—The great diversity of appearances which this disease is constantly presenting, renders a complete description almost impossible. It has been regarded by some writers of note, as *papular,* by others as *pustular,* but by the majority as *vesicular.* It consists of a pustular, papular, or vesicular eruption, generally situated between the fingers, on the wrists, near the joints, but sometimes extending over the whole body. The eruption is attended with almost constant itching, which is aggravated by scratching, or by the heat of a fire, or of the bed. The disorder is decidedly contagious in its character, and according to Schroen, "never gets well of itself; but will last for years, and may exist upon the skin a whole life-time, if its cure is neglected." This author recognises four distinct forms:

1. *Scabies sicca*, or *pimply*, or *dry itch*, most common in adults. This form, when repelled, often gives rise to "nervous apoplexy, ascites, or chronic hydrocephalus, and it is best treated by *sulphur*, *mercury*, *causticum*, *carbo veg.*, *psoricum*, *sepia*, *lachesis*, and *veratrum*."

2. *Scabies vesicularis*, or *common itch*, occurring most commonly in highlands,—very rarely in low and swampy districts. When this form is abruptly repelled, it gives rise to serious affections of the cerebral and pulmonary organs, and to the nervous system. *Sulphur* is undoubtedly the appropriate specific, and should be given at the first trituration. In obstinate cases we may employ one or more of the following medicines: *psoricum*, *sepia*, *hepar sulph.*, *arsenicum*, *rhus*, *mercurius*, *iodine*, *copaibæ*, *calcarea carb.*

3. *Scabies purulenta*, appearing in the form of yellow and prominent pustules between the fingers and toes. In this form, Schroen advises *sulphur*, *antimonium tart.*, *sepia*, *cicuta*, *lycopodium*, and *mercurius*.

4. *Crusta serpiginosa*,—"This form resembles crustea lactea, but is marked by the appearance of small vesicles behind the ears, which burst, forming a thin dark-coloured scab, from which an acrid fluid is secreted." The face, neck, arms, and trunk eventually become involved. For the cure of this form Schroen advises *sulphur*, *clematis erec.*, *calcarea carb.*, *lycopodium*, and *arsenicum*.

Causes.—By many the disease is supposed to be owing to the presence in the skin of minute animalcula, of the species *acarus scabei*. It has likewise been attributed to want of cleanliness, and the use of unwholesome food.

Administration.—The remedies should be given at

the first or second attenuation, and repeated two or three times a day until the eruption disappears. In recent cases, Hartmann, Schroen, and Schmid, employ the tinctures and the first dilutions; but in obstinate cases they employ from the third to the sixth attenuations.

SECTION XIV.

ECTHYMA.

Diagnosis.—This disease originates from a morbid condition of the skin, which supervenes during the course of eruptive, and other fevers, venereal diseases, scrofula, scurvy, &c. The pustules are of considerable size, seated upon swollen, bright red, and painful bases, and never running together, but always preserving a distinct character. After a few days the pustules become covered with hard, and dark or greenish scabs, which, in one or two weeks, dry up and disappear. Ecthyma has been subdivided into several distinct varieties, on account of some trifling, and as we believe, unimportant modifications which the eruptions occasionally present, from peculiarities of age, constitution, disease, and habits of life. The most common of these varieties are:

1. *Ecthyma vulgare*, "consisting of a partial eruption of small, hard pustules, on the neck, shoulders, or extremities, which is completed in about three days. They enlarge and inflame, form pus, and then scabs. These eventually dry, fall off, and leave no mark behind. They are chiefly seen in young persons whose health has been impaired."

2. *Ecthyma luridum*, with pustules, "larger, more diffused, more repeated, and fixed upon a hard, elevated base of a peculiar dark red colour."*

3 *Ecthyma infantile*, occurring generally in infants of delicate, or scrofulous constitutions, or in those whose systems have been enfeebled by abuse of drugs.

4. *Ecthyma cachecticum*, peculiar to individuals who are suffering under a venereal, scrofulous, or psoric taint.

* Hall.

RUPIA,

Is another pustular affection, often resembling very closely *ecthyma*. Bateman describes it thus: "an eruption of flat, distinct vesicles, with bases slightly inflamed, containing a sanious fluid, the scabs accumulating, sometimes in a conical form, easily rubbed off, and soon reproduced." Although this author describes the eruption as vesicular, it is now generally conceded that the disease is for the most part pustular. The eruption may be distinguished from that of ecthyma, by the appearance of the scabs, and the ulcerations which frequently occur. Several varieties have been described, but we do not deem it necessary or useful to enter into a particular enumeration of all the minute points of difference in the various cases which present themselves, since the general character of the eruption is sufficiently marked to enable the careful observer to detect its true nature without difficulty.

Therapeutics.—The medicines usually employed in the above complaints are, *sulphur, sepia, mercurius, rhus, antimonium tart., silicea, hepar sulph., aurum mur., arsenicum, iodine, calcarea carb., dulcamara.*

Administration.—Attenuations and repetitions of doses, the same as in scabies.

SECTION XV.

IMPETIGO.

Diagnosis.—The eruption consists of clusters of small pustules, vesicular in the first instance, but soon becoming purulent. After a few days the pustules burst, and thick and dark yellow scabs remain. The skin around the pustules is somewhat swollen, inflamed, and painful, and when the secretion from the ruptured pimples is acrid, the patient is often annoyed with an exceedingly disagreeable burning and itching sensation. Willan, Bateman, Rayer, Schroen, and several other eminent writers on cutaneous affections, recognise five different varieties:

1. *Impetigo figurata*, occurring generally in children during dentition, and in "young men and women of lymphatic or sanguine-lymphatic temperaments." Rayer advises *lycopodium, sepia, sulphur, rhus tox.,*

graphite, *calcarea carb.*, *dulcamara* and *petroleum* in this form of the disease.

2. *Impetigo sparsa.*—In this variety the pustules are isolated, and dispersed over the shoulders, buttocks, face, and scalp, or legs. It generally " appears in the fall and winter, and disappears in spring and summer."—(*Bateman.*) *Mercurius*, *sulphur*, *cicuta*, and *lachesis* will be found specific in this form.

3. *Impetigo erysipelatodes.*—The eruption is usually a disease of the face, and bears some resemblance to erysipelas in the first instance, but soon changes to a pustular character. The scabs which form on the pustules are of a dirty yellow or greenish colour, and are kept soft by the secretion which is under them. Schroen considers *belladonna*, *rhus tox.*, *mercurius*, and *arsenicum*, the proper remedies for this form.

4. *Impetigo scabida.*—This is a severe form, attended with more inflammation and pain in the affected parts, and more extensive ulceration and discharge, than either of the other varieties. We may employ, *hepar sulph.*, *mercurius*, *arsenicum*, and *iodine*.

5. *Impetigo larvalis*, or *crusta lactea*. " Common amongst young sucklings ; characterized by an eruption upon the cheek, of superficial, more or less confluent pustules, united in groups, attended with slight itching, and followed by yellowish and green—generally thin and lamellated, at times, however, with thick and soft crusts, that when loosened, leave a red and inflamed surface, which is quickly covered with new crusts. The best remedies are, *sulphur* and *rhus tox.*," (*Schroen*,) or *dulcamara*, *lycopodium*, and *sepia*, (*Knorre*,) or *graphites* and *mezereum*, (*Lobethal.*)

Administration.—In the same manner as in herpes.

SECTION XVI.

PORRIGO.

This is a contagious disorder, and presents itself in the form of " straw-coloured pustules, sometimes circumscribed, sometimes diffused ; generally, but not always confined to the head ; the pustules break and give issue to a fluid which concretes into yellowish or brownish, thin or thick, crusts or scabs."—(*Hall.*)—It commonly makes its appearance upon the scalp and face, but may occur in any other part of the body. The disease has been subdivided into several different varieties, but the divisions are of no practical utility, and tend directly to create confusion and embarrassment. In some constitutions, the eruption becomes so extensive and severe, as to give rise to troublesome ulcerations, and considerable constitutional disturbance. In cases of this kind, as well indeed as in all others, the utmost care should be taken to ensure cleanliness, so that the secreted fluid shall not accumulate, and thus serve to perpetuate the disorder. The principal remedies are *sulphur*, *rhus toxicodendron*, *calcarea*, *carbo vegetabilis*, *sepia*, *graphite*, and *arsenicum*.

ACNE,

Is another pustular affection, making its appearance generally upon the nose, face, forehead, and shoulders, first in the form of a thickening redness, and induration of the integuments, from which eventually proceed suppurating points or tubercles. The parts affected often acquire a depth of redness and a conspicuousness which much annoy the patient. Plumbe supposes that the malady consists in a diseased condition of the sebaceous follicles, induced by excessive indulgence in the pleasures of the table, sedentary habits, &c. Sometimes it is violent, and extensive inflammation and suppuration occur. The remedies enumerated under porrigo will apply in it.

Administration.—The doses and repetitions of the medicines, the same as in scabies.

SECTION XVII.

SQUAMOUS DISEASES — LEPRA.

Diagnosis.—This disease is characterized by the appearance of spots of various sizes, with red and inflamed borders, slightly raised above the surrounding skin, and covered with scurfy, bran-like flakes or scales, which are constantly falling off, to be reproduced. In some instances, a raw and tender surface remains after the scales have fallen, attended with severe itching and smarting, on rubbing or scratching, or on exposure to a high heat. The eruption is unattended by any febrile disturbance, but is not unfrequently associated with scrofulous or venereal taints, and an impaired condition of the digestive apparatus. The causes which tend to render the eruption severe, extensive, and permanent, are want of cleanliness, constant exposure to a hot sun, and unwholesome food.

PSORIASIS.

Mackintosh regards psoriasis as an aggravated form of lepra. According to Hall, it "differs from lepra chiefly in the irregular form, in the diffusion of the scaly patches, and in the absence of its inflamed borders, depressed centres, and regular oval or circular forms. The subjacent surface is also more tender, more easily denuded, and more prone to become affected by fissures." The disease attacks the scalp, face, the arms, the legs, the palms of the hands, the lips, the prepuce and the scrotum. Occasionally the inflammatory action runs so high that the parts become much swollen and highly painful. In these cases there is usually a considerable secretion from the eruption.

PITYRIASIS.

Simple pityriasis is most commonly confined to the hairy scalp, and displays itself in the form of a superficial bran-like scurf, which may easily be removed by a comb or a brush, but which is speedily reproduced. In mild cases, and with ordinary care, the disease may continue with but slight annoyance for many years, or it may be roused into a more active and troublesome form by general debility, attacks of eruptive fever, and by the relaxing effects of a hot climate.

Therapeutics.—We consider *sulphur*, *iodine*, *conium*, *calcarea*, *carbo vegetabilis* and *sepia*, the best remedies for the above diseases. *Arsenicum*, *graphites*, *acid nit.*, *phosphorus*, *lycopodium*, *natrum mur.*, *copaibæ*, *argenti nit.*, *aurum mur.*, and *hepar sulph.*, have likewise been employed with success.

Administration.—The first, second, and third attenuations should be employed—a dose each day until the morbid action is subdued.

CHAPTER XXII.

DISEASES OF THE ORGANS AND TISSUES CONNECTED WITH THE DIGESTIVE SYSTEM.

SECTION I.

GLOSSITIS.—INFLAMMATION OF THE TONGUE.

Inflammation of the tongue is by no means a common affection, but cases now and then occur in which this organ is so enormously inflamed and swollen, as to place the sufferer in imminent danger of suffocation. It may arise spontaneously, with but few and slight premonitory symptoms of its approach, or it may proceed from derangements of the stomach, sudden changes of temperature, and the application of irritating or poisonous substances. Generally it runs its course rapidly, and if not met by prompt and efficient measures, will so fill the mouth and throat as to suspend respiration.

Diagnosis.—Previous to the pain and swelling of the tongue, the patient is affected with slight chills, loss of appetite, lassitude, indications of disordered stomach, dull pains in the head and back, succeeded with throbbing and aching pains in the tongue, heat of skin, and rapid pulse. The tongue now commences swelling, and often progresses, if the inflammation is not arrested, to an alarming extent. It is usually red and dry, but in some instances continues moist through all the disease.

Causes.—Derangements of the stomach, exposure to strong currents of air, mercurial salivation, smallpox, the application of irritating substances, stings of insects, and certain poisons.

Therapeutics.—The physician is sometimes summoned to cases of this description, where the danger of suffocation is so threatening, as hardly to render it prudent to await the operation of remedies. In these instances free and deep incisions should be made into the substance of the tongue in a parallel direction, which will afford prompt temporary relief, and thus allow us time for the action of our specific remedies.

The medicines which will apply specifically in these cases are, *merc.*, *bell*,. *plumb.*, *aur.*, and *hep.*

Mercurius sol.—External indications.—Expression of countenance, anxious and terrified; tongue inflamed, swollen, red, dry or moist; respiration exceedingly difficult; pulse rapid and full; constant inclination to keep an upright position; skin hot and dry.

Physical sensations.—Febrile symptoms; heat, thirst, pains in the head, back and limbs; throbbing, stinging, or aching pains in the tongue; mouth and throat filled with the swollen organ, giving rise to a dreadful sense of suffocation; symptoms somewhat aggravated during the night; rapid sinking of strength; respiration rather better in the air, and on gentle motion; deglutition partially or entirely suspended.

Mental and moral symptoms.—Excessive anguish, apprehension, and constant and insurmountable dread of immediate suffocation.

Administration.—Divide two grains of the third trituration into six equal parts—one powder dry upon the tongue every half hour in urgent cases, until there is relief or a medicinal aggravation. In less severe cases the medicine may be given once in two, four, or six hours, according to the symptoms.

Belladonna.—External indications.—Face red; eyes bloodshot, or suffused; tongue inflamed, red, dry, and swollen; violent pulsations of the carotid and temporal arteries; pulse rapid and bounding.

Physical sensations.—Congestion of blood to the head; throbbing pain in the head; eyes sensitive to light; skin hot and dry, thirst; throbbing, darting, or drawing pains in the tongue; difficult and anxious respiration; deglutition extremely difficult or entirely suspended; sense of suffocation.

Mental and moral symptoms.—Great agitation; fear of death; anxious and depressed.

Administration.—A drop of the third dilution on two grains of *sugar of milk:* divide into four equal parts, and exhibit one dry upon the tongue once in one, two, or three hours, as the urgency of the case demands.

Plumbum is appropriate in cases of chronic swelling of the tongue, with numbness and *partial paralysis.* Convulsive tremors and general muscular debility are other indications for the employment of this remedy.

In cases of glossitis proceeding from the abuse of mercury, recourse may be had to *aurum muriatic.* and *hepar sulph.* If the inflammation be owing to a wound or injury, *arnica* is the proper remedy.

SECTION II.

TONSILITIS.—QUINSY.

Diagnosis.—Febrile symptoms, succeeded in a few hours by soreness of the throat, painful deglutition, swelling and redness of the tonsils, uvula, and soft palate. As the tonsils continue to enlarge, deglutition and respiration become more difficult, the voice is changed, the pains increase in severity, extending often through the eustachian tubes into the ears, the tongue becomes covered with a thick yellow fur, there is an abundance of viscid saliva on the tongue and tonsils, the breath acquires an exceedingly offensive odour, which, according to Mackintosh, proceeds from sebaceous matter escaping from the mucous follicles.

The disease may terminate in resolution, suppuration, or in permanent induration. When the appropriate remedies are administered at the commencement, the inflammation usually resolves itself without suppuration. If no medicines are given, or those only which are inappropriate, the disorder usually progresses until suppuration ensues, when an artificial opening is made, or the tonsil bursts spontaneously, and the swelling and inflammation gradually subside.

Not unfrequently the tonsils become affected with chronic enlargements and indurations, from frequent and partially subdued acute attacks, which prove exceedingly troublesome by their proneness to take on acute inflammation from the slightest exciting causes.

There is reason to suppose that chronic enlargements of the tonsils often lead to coughs and expectoration of muco-purulent matter, which are confounded with and erroneously attributed to chronic bronchitis, &c.

Causes.—The predisposing causes are: scrofulous dyscrasia, irritability, and chronic enlargement of the tonsils from mercurial salivations, and derangements of the stomach and bowels. The common exciting causes are, cold, atmospheric vicissitudes, wet-feet.

Therapeutics.—The best remedies for acute tonsilitis are, *belladonna, mercurius, aconite, baryta carb., nux, pulsatilla,* and *hepar sulph.*

Belladonna.—External indications.—Cheeks flushed; violent pulsations of the carotids; enlargement of tonsils perceptible on the outside of the throat; tonsils, uvula, and soft palate, inflamed, dark, red, and swollen; tongue dry, or covered with a thick transparent and tenacious mucus; skin hot; pulse full, hard, and frequent; voice hoarse, stifled, or suppressed.

Physical sensations.—Headache; burning and shooting pains in the throat when swallowing; constant inclination to swallow; choking sensation; tonsils painful to the touch; putrid or bitter taste; thirst; eyes sensitive to the light; stitches extending into the ears; deafness from obstruction of the orifice of the eustachian tube; burning fever.

Mental and moral symptoms.—Uneasiness and dejection, worse at night, and occasionally delirium.

Administration.—Two drops of the third dilution to two grains of *sugar of milk.* Divide into six parts and exhibit one dry once in two to four hours as long as necessary.

Mercurius.—External indications.—Offensive, putrid odour from the mouth; tongue covered with a thick yellow fur; mouth dry or filled with viscid saliva; uvula elongated and red; tonsils and soft palate dark red, inflamed and enlarged; roots of the tongue red and swollen; ulcers in the mouth and throat; enlargement of the parotid or submaxillary glands; pulse frequent and moderately full.

Physical sensations.—Heat, alternating with chills; frequent profuse sweats; stinging and shooting pain in the throat, particularly when swallowing; very great difficulty in swallowing, although frequent inclination; glands of the neck painful on motion of the jaws, at sight of savoury food, or on swallowing;

the pains and difficulty of deglutition worse at night; pains darting through the eustachian tube to the ears and parotid glands; loss of appetite and disgust for food; putrid or coppery taste; thirst for cold drinks; symptoms mitigated during repose in bed.

Mental and moral symptoms.—Morose; dejected; uneasy; out of humour.

Administration.—Divide four grains of the third trituration into six powders—give one dry, upon the tongue, once in four to six hours until an impression is apparent.

Aconite is a suitable remedy in cases of tonsilitis attended with a high grade of arterial reaction, painful deglutition, bright redness of the fauces, uvula and tonsils, with pricking or burning pains when swallowing.

Administration.—A drop of the third dilution to two grains of sugar of milk. Divide into four parts and exhibit one dry, once in two hours until the symptoms abate.

Baryta carb. may be given in cases of catarrhal tonsilitis, where there is suppuration of the tonsils, swollen and elongated uvula, raw scraping or shooting pain on swallowing, obstruction, as if by a plug in the throat, bad taste, offensive breath, especially in the morning, and discharge of sebaceous matter from the follicles of the throat.

Administration.—Same as *aconite.*

When derangement of the stomach appears to be the prime predisposing cause of the complaint, and when the symptoms of the acute attack are, scraping pains during deglutition, or when inhaling cold air; obstruction from the enlarged tonsils, choking and spasmodic contractions of the throat when swallowing, *nux vomica* is the specific remedy. It may be administered at the third dilution, by means of sugar, like *aconite.*

Pulsatilla will apply in cases arising from a chill by being wet, wet feet, &c. The signs for this remedy are, burning, scraping, smarting or shooting pains in the throat when swallowing, deglutition obstructed by viscid mucus which adheres to the tonsils and fauces, pains worse in the afternoon and evening, bitter or saltish taste in the mouth, loss of appetite, unnatural taste of food, tongue furred with a thick yellow coat, and breath offensive.

Administration.—A drop of the third dilution on sugar. Divide into four parts, and let one be given dry, once in four hours until the desired effect is produced.

Hep. sulphur has been much employed by our English brethren, in those habitual cases of inflammation and suppuration of the tonsils, which appear to owe their origin to a scrofulous dyscrasia. This medicine occasionally arrests the disease and prevents suppuration, after *belladonna, mercurius*, and *aconite* have entirely failed to produce an impression. It may be given in grain doses, at the third trituration, once in two hours.

SECTION III.

PAROTITIS.—MUMPS.

This affection is classed by writers as an epidemic. It is more prone to attack children than adults, and generally makes its appearance during cold and damp seasons. Its cause is a specific morbific contagion, which may be generated during certain peculiar conditions of the atmosphere, or it may be communicated from the bodies of those having the disorder.

Diagnosis.—Slight febrile disturbance, followed by swelling and pain in one or both parotid glands. Under favourable circumstances the local affection continues to progress until the end of the fourth day, at which time the inflammation and swelling have reached their height: when the tumefaction and pain gradually subside, until at the end of about seven or eight days from the commencement, all traces of the complaint have departed. As soon as the inflammation has fairly declared itself in the glands, the patient experiences much difficulty and pain in moving his jaws, masticating, or even at the sight of savoury food.

It is highly important during its progress, that there be no exposure on the part of the patient, either to cold or dampness, nor from any undue mental or physical excitement. In this manner we may guard against those troublesome metastases to the brain, mamma, and testes, which sometimes supervene from improper exposure, external applications, &c.

Therapeutics.—But little medicinal treatment is required in this malady, provided the precautions just alluded to are heeded; a few doses of the sixth dilution of *mercurius sol.* being all that is necessary to conduct the patient happily through the attack.

Sometimes, however, coma and other alarming symptoms of cerebral disorder, suddenly appear from metastasis of the disease to the brain, which require the prompt administration of *belladonna*, *opium*, or other cerebral specifics. More commonly, however, the metastasis occurs to the mamma or testes, causing inflammation, swelling, induration, and occasionally suppuration in these glands. The remedies in these cases are *merc.*, *sol.*, *bell.*, *nux*, *puls.*, and *acon.* See the particular indications for these medicines under "Inflammation of the mamma and testes."

SECTION IV.

GASTRITIS.—INFLAMMATION OF THE STOMACH.

Diagnosis.—Burning, pricking, or lancinating pains in the stomach, nausea and vomiting, great soreness, tenderness, and pain on motion or pressure, intense thirst for cold drinks, which are ejected almost as soon as swallowed, affording some temporary relief, pricking and soreness in the throat and œsophagus, tongue red at the tip and on the edges, and covered through the centre with a white or yellowish fur, position mostly upon the back or side, with the limbs drawn up and the abdominal muscles relaxed, great depression, anxiety, and fear of death; pulse rapid, sharp, contracted, sometimes almost threadlike; bowels constipated; disgust for food and warm drink, either of which are expelled as soon as received into the stomach; and in severe cases, delirium, and fever of a synochal grade. There is an unusual fulness in the epigastric region, and often of the abdomen. As the disease progresses, the extremities become cold, the features contracted and sunken, the eyes glazed or suffused, and finally diarrhœa, cold sweats, coma, and convulsions supervene.

When death occurs, it is usually caused by ulceration or sphacelation of some portion of the mucous and sub-mucous coats of the stomach.

Causes.—Excessive use of highly seasoned food, stimulating drinks, the introduction of irritating substances into the stomach, poisons, injuries, and the use of emetics, drastics, stimulants, and other medicinal poisons with which the allopathic practice, governed by no scientific method, frequently induces this and other diseases, and destroys the existence it is intended to preserve.

Therapeutics.—The ordinary remedies used in the treatment of gastritis, are, ***arsenicum, veratrum, nux, pulsatilla, aconite, iodium, ipecacuanha.***

Arsenicum. — *External indications.* — Countenance contracted, sunken, and expressive of anguish and anxiety; stomach swollen and hot to the touch; position upon the back: respiration short, rapid, and suppressed; tongue red and clean, or red on the edges with a dirty fur in the centre; pulse contracted, tense, and frequent; voice hoarse, stifled, and suppressed; skin dry and hot, with perhaps cold and clammy extremities.

Physical sensations.—Burning, sharp, or shooting pains in the stomach; aggravation of the sufferings from motion, pressure, coughing, and inspiration; scraping and burning pain in the throat and œsophagus; great prostration; weakness and trembling of the limbs; urgent thirst for cold drinks; persistent nausea and vomiting; all food and drinks speedily and violently rejected; exceeding tenderness in the epigastric region on pressure; respiration suppressed and painful.

Mental and moral symptoms.—Intense anxiety, anguish, depression, and despair; expectation of speedy death; sometimes delirium.

Administration.—Two drops of the sixth dilution in an ounce of water; a dessert spoonful once in two to four hours, until the proper impression is made upon the inflammation.

Veratrum. — *External indications.* — Hippocratic countenance; nose pointed; eyes sunken and glazed; lips bluish and dry; tongue red at the tip and on the edges, with a dark, dry fur running through the centre; pulse quick, weak, and almost imperceptible; stomach and abdomen distended; extremities cold, and covered with a clammy sweat; position on the back, with the knees drawn up; hiccough; and whole appearance indicative of extreme prostration.

Physical sensations.—Feeling of great exhaustion; burning pain in the stomach; rough, dry, and scraping sensation in the throat, rendering deglutition difficult and painful; great soreness in the epigastric region; short, troublesome cough; severe and continued nausea and vomiting; great dread of warm food and drinks; intense thirst for cold drinks; inability to retain anything upon the stomach; spasmodic contractions of the throat, œsophagus, and abdominal muscles; hiccough; painful respiration.

Mental and moral symptoms.—Excessive dejection, discouragement, and sadness; fear of death, complete despair; delirium.

Administration.—In urgent cases we may give a dose of the sixth dilution, in water, once in one hour, until an amendment declares itself, or there occurs a well pronounced medicinal aggravation. We may then await the result, and hold ourselves in readiness to repeat this, or whatever other medicine may be appropriate, as the circumstances of the case may require.

Nux vomica.—*External indications.*—Face bloated; eyelids red, weak, and watery; stomach distended; tongue tremulous, red, and clean, or furred with a whitish coat in the centre; offensive breath; frequent hiccough; pulse frequent, small, and feeble.

Physical sensations.—Burning pain in the stomach, with pulsations and spasmodic contractions in the epigastric region; nausea and vomiting, aggravated after eating or drinking; tenderness and pain in the pit of the stomach when pressed, or during movement; contraction and obstruction in the œsophagus when attempting to swallow; painful sensation of distention of the stomach; dizziness and confusion of the head, on rising from the recumbent position, or in attempting to walk; sour or bitter eructations.

Mental and moral symptoms.—Great uneasiness and

anxiety; morose, peevish, sad, and often disposition to commit suicide.

Administration.—This medicine is peculiarly appropriate in those cases which are induced by abuse of coffee, wine, spirits, condiments, and stimulating food. One drop of the sixth dilution to an ounce of water; a tablespoonful once in two to four hours, so long as the symptoms remain stationary. Occasionally we shall have conjoined with the above symptoms, cerebral disorder, indicated by delirium, optical illusions, and great derangement of the nervous system. In such instances an occasional dose of *belladonna* will prove specific.

Pulsatilla is a valuable remedy when the inflammation is brought on by the use of crude, indigestible, and irritating food. It covers the following symptoms: pressing or shooting pains in the stomach; pulsations in the pit of the stomach; epigastrium sensitive, and painful to the touch, or on pressure; nausea and vomiting after eating or drinking; nausea and disagreeable feeling, extending even to the œsophagus and throat; regurgitation of food; eructations; hiccough; painful distention of the stomach; pulse quick and small; and bitter taste in the mouth.

Aconite, at the third to the sixth dilution, will do good service when the febrile symptoms run high; to be repeated often until amendment ensues, either alone or in alternation with the gastric specifics, as the nature of the case demands.

Iodine, at the third potency, has afforded relief in inflammations of the stomach caused by abuse of mercury and other irritating drugs. The indications for its use are, frequent nausea; vomitings, especially after eating; burning pains and pulsations in the stomach, pyrosis, sour eructations, contraction and burning of the œsophagus; pulse frequent, small and hard. *Colchicum* is an important remedy in cases of metastases of rheumatism to the stomach. It acts specifically as an irritant to the stomach, even when injected into the veins.

A single dose of *ipecacuanha*, at the sixth potency, will sometimes afford prompt relief in cases where vomiting is violent and incessant. It is applicable in inflammation caused by excessive doses of *tartarized antimony, corrosive sublimate, arsenic,* &c., for the purpose of allaying the excessive irritation and vomiting which follow poisonous doses of these articles.

SECTION V.

CHRONIC GASTRITIS. — CHRONIC INFLAMMATION OF THE STOMACH.

Diagnosis.—Many of the symptoms of this malady are similar in character to those which occur in the acute form, but there is a material difference in regard to their grade of violence in the two diseases. Sometimes chronic gastritis is the result of a partially subdued acute attack, which from various causes is kept up for a long period in this state of sub-acute inflammation. At other times it comes on slowly and insidiously, from a combination of causes operating at the same time. Amongst the symptoms which usually attend this complaint, may be enumerated these:—pain and tenderness in some particular part of the stomach, excited by pressure, or by certain kinds of food and drinks; frequent vomiting of food and drink soon after they are swallowed; loss of appetite, putrid taste in the mouth; thirst; fetid breath; acid or bitter eructations; acidity; distention of the stomach with wind, which causes distressing vertigo, and pains in the epigastric and hypochondriac region; tongue red and clean, or furred in the middle with a dirty fur; melancholy; peevishness; irritability; discouragement; and, finally, hectic fever, emaciation, sudden prostration, and death.

Causes.—The most powerful predisposing causes of this malady are, protracted sufferings under the depressing mental emotions and the habitual use of irritating drugs. It often succeeds to acute gastritis which has been but partially subdued; it may also arise from high living, the abuse of wine, liquors, coffee, &c., repelled eruptions, metastases of rheumatism and gout, injuries, and occasionally as a consequence of other diseases which have been badly managed.

Therapeutics.—The medicines to which we have

alluded under acute gastritis, will be the most applicable in the ordinary forms of the chronic variety. The following medicines will likewise cover many symptoms of sub-acute gastritis, namely, *bismuthum*, *baryta muriatis*, *bryonia*, *cuprum met.*, *digitalis purpurea*, *hyoscyamus*, *ignatia*, *mercurius*, *phosphorus*, *arnica*.

SECTION VI.

DYSPEPSIA.—INDIGESTION.

Diagnosis.—This very troublesome malady, regarded for some reason as one of the banes of good society, manifests itself under so many different aspects, and is so entirely irregular in its causes, modes of attack, progress, violence, and duration, that there is a wide difference of opinion amongst physicians in regard to its true nature. While some have referred it to a sub-acute inflammation of the mucous coat of the stomach, others have considered it as in the liver, the cardiac nerves, or the secretory apparatus of the stomach. The nature and precise location of dyspepsia have been, and still are, to a considerable extent, involved in obscurity, and it is a consequence of this that its victims have received so little sympathy or charity either from medical men or from non-professional observers. It is a disease, nevertheless, which in its different phases displays symptoms and sufferings almost innumerable, as is proved from the circumstance of its having been confounded with chronic gastritis, cardialgia, bilious affections, liver complaint, &c. At one time the patient will attribute his sufferings to his head, and entertain the most alarming apprehensions of apoplexy; at another, to his respiratory organs, and imagine he has consumption; again, he describes his malady as in the liver, or the stomach, or the bowels, or the spleen; and thus he continues on from month to month, or from year to year, a martyr to the most distressing chronic affection to which humanity is subject.

Dyspepsia may make its appearance in a gradual and almost imperceptible manner, or it may supervene suddenly in a severe form without previous warning. It may so affect the system as to remind one constantly of its existence, or its symptoms may only manifest themselves after the use of certain indigestible articles of food, or protracted depression of spirits.

Amongst the more common symptoms of this complaint may be mentioned, tenderness and distention of the epigastrium, acidity, flatulency, eructations, sense of weight and fulness in the stomach after eating; also quick breathing, sensitiveness at the pit of the stomach from pressure, tight clothing, &c., pyrosis, vertigo, giddiness, sensation when walking as if the pavement were rising up immediately in front; constipation, pressure in the stomach and epigastrium, hæmorrhoids, sallow or yellow complexion, distention of the abdomen with flatus, loss of ambition and energy, sad, desponding, dread and apprehension respecting the future, frequent inclination to commit suicide, nights restless and disturbed by unpleasant dreams. In the advanced stages of indigestion, there often supervenes a troublesome cough, attended with occasional pains in the chest, and mucous or muco-purulent expectoration, which some writers have termed dyspeptic phthisis. It is probable, in these cases, that the disease is confined to the mucous membranes of the respiratory organs, being a continuation or extension of the gastric disturbance, to the pulmonary mucous tissues.

The character of the gastric sensations is so diverse in different cases, that scarcely a pain or a sensation can be described, which has not been experienced by the dyspeptic. It is often conjoined with cardialgia, chronic gastritis, or chronic hepatitis, and therefore some symptoms of either of these diseases may be present in any given case.

Our own opinion is, that indigestion is not attributable solely to sub-acute gastric irritation, or disease of the cardiac nerves, or of the intestinal canal, or derangement of the gastric secretion, but to a combination of all these maladies. This is satisfactorily evinced from the fact, that in the worst forms of indigestion, many of the principal symptoms of each of these disorders are uniformly present.

Causes.—Protracted depression of spirits, whether occasioned by want of occupation, deprivation of the accustomed mental and physical exercise, pecuniary misfortune, loss of friends, disappointment, or mortification, is a prominent cause of dyspepsia. This cause is very general and extended in its operation, affecting not only the mucous structure of the stomach, but the liver, the bowels, the cardiac nerves, and in some instances the whole nervous system. It is to this variety of indigestion that should be attributed many of those hypochondriacal affections, which are often referred exclusively to disorder of the liver.

Next in importance to the above, may be named, the abuse of rich and highly seasoned food, stimulating drinks, coffee, tea, tobacco, irregular eating hours, and inattention to the daily fæcal evacuations.

When chronic gastritis becomes complicated with cardialgia, chronic hepatitis, &c., the resulting malady will be dyspepsia. Another common cause of this complaint, and one to which we desire to direct particular attention, is the habitual use of cathartics. The belief has so long and so generally obtained, that all of the ills of the organism can be expelled forcibly by inflaming and raking the sensitive and delicate coats of the stomach and bowels with cathartics, that it will be no light task to change opinions which have become (if I may be allowed the expression), *constitutional.* If, however, the intelligent reader will remember that dyspepsia consists in an irritated and weakened state of the nerves, and the mucous coat of the stomach, together with disorder of the liver, he cannot fail to perceive that the effect of purgatives must be injurious rather than beneficial. We are quite aware that some temporary relief is occasionally afforded by cathartics, but innumerable facts warrant the assertion that this slight alleviation is always at the expense of renewed and vastly increased future suffering, and that each new dose communicates an additional impetus to the advancement of the disease towards fatal disorganization.

Another not unfrequent cause of indigestion, is repelled cutaneous diseases, like erysipelas, &c. I have met with a number of well-marked cases of this description, in which alleviation of all the symptoms uniformly occurred when the eruption was upon the surface.

Therapeutics.—An essential condition in the treatment of dyspepsia is the maintenance on the part of the patient, of a healthy, active, and cheerful state of mind. Unless this be accomplished, our remedies will either be of only temporary service, or entirely unavailing. Next in importance, is a course of rigid dietetic regulations. In proposing a bill of fare for the dyspeptic, much must depend upon the circumstances of each particular case. If the patient is of a highly bilious temperament, a much more simple diet will be requisite, than for one who is nervous or sanguine. As a general rule, an intelligent person will be able to select a suitable diet for himself, by observing attentively the effects which different articles exert upon his constitution.

Another equally important condition in the treatment of this complaint, is perfect regularity in all the habits of life, as eating, sleeping, alvine evacuations, exercise, &c. First, sufficient sleep should be allowed, to enable the system to recover entirely from the fatigues of the preceding day; second, moderate and agreeable exercise should be taken for an hour or so, previous to breakfast, bearing in mind that exercise, in order to be beneficial, must not be undertaken and performed as a task, but as a pleasant recreation; third, in partaking of our food, we should never forget, while we are thus repairing the waste of the body, from the exercise of the functions, &c., that this also was intended by our Creator to be a source of pleasure to us. Let the rational man, therefore, and especially the dyspeptic, never eat with disordered rapidity, but slowly, so that, masticated properly, his food may be taken into the stomach in a fit condition for the processes of digestion. This is the true philosophy of eating. Finally, at a certain hour every day, perhaps after breakfast, an evacuation from the bowels should be solicited. It matters not whether the inclination be uniformly present, let the patient never fail in his readiness, and the bowels will soon form the habit of responding. So much are we the creatures of *habit*, that we can train our bodies, our organs, our appetites, tastes, &c., to almost anything we desire, by a steady persistence in our object.

The most approved remedies for the different grades of indigestion, are, *nux, sulph., puls., bry., lycopod., calc. carb., sepia, graph., ignat.*

Nux vomica is well adapted to the cases which occur in sanguine or bilious temperaments, and which have been induced by "high living," sedentary habits, undue mental exertion, irregularity in eating, sleeping, &c. The *external indications* for *nux*, are, florid or pale, sallow or yellow complexion; general expression of countenance, anxious and sad, care-worn; tongue dry, or covered with a whitish coat; occasional fulness in the region of the stomach and bowels.

Physical sensations.—Distress at the stomach after eating; nausea and vomiting of food; eructations; pyrosis; distressing sense of debility; irritability of the nervous system, with constant inclination to roam about; symptoms worse after meals, and in the evening; constipation; hæmorrhoids; tenderness at the pit of the stomach on pressure; vertigo, dizziness, or swimming in the head, particularly when rising in the morning, or on walking about; cramp-like pains at the pit of the stomach, sometimes extending upwards to the diaphragm and œsophagus.

Mental and moral symptoms.—Confirmed *hypochondria;* constant dread of approaching misfortune; inclination to look upon the dark side of everything; trifles exaggerated into matters of importance; *urgent inclination, at times, to commit suicide;* excessive nervous irritability.

When dyspepsia consists simply of impaired activity of the nerves of the stomach, from the causes just named, *nux* is without doubt the appropriate specific; but it is an almost invariable occurrence, that this condition of the stomach is attended with more or less derangement of the nervous system, manifested by loss of animation and energy; depression of spirits; an invincible tendency to look on the dark side of affairs, and an indefinable sense of dissatisfaction, dread, and uneasiness, which impairs the appetite, disturbs the sleep, and almost unfits the individual for the ordinary duties of life. When this condition of the nervous system has existed for a considerable time, it receives the name of *hypochondria*. For this complication, *nux* alone is insufficient, but one or more of the medicines hereafter ennumerated, will be required.

Administration.—In cases of this description, we usually prescribe *nux vomica* from the third to the sixth potency; a dose to be given each night, *as long* as may be necessary.

Sulphur is peculiarly adapted to the treatment of cases occurring in persons of a scrofulous dyscrasia, and to cases which appear to be connected with erysipelatous and other eruptive affections. Dyspeptic symptoms occasionally supervene upon the disappearance of erysipelatous and other eruptions from the surface, also from the sudden suppression of long continued hæmorrhoidal discharges. In many cases of this kind, *sulphur* will be found a valuable remedy.

The *external marks* wich indicate this medicine, are, pale or sallow countenance; light hair; blue eyes; thin skin; white teeth; glandular swellings; eruptions; weak eyes, and the other signs of scrofulous diathesis.

Physical sensations.—Distention and distress of the stomach after eating; nausea; vomiting; pyrosis; frequent eructations, acid or bitter; the symptoms occurring, for the most part, on the disappearance of some eruption or accustomed discharge, and going off on the reappearance of these eruptions or discharges.

Mental and moral symptoms.—Sadness; irritability; moroseness.

Administration.—This medicine may be administered at the third attenuation, in the morning and middle of the afternoon.

Pulsatilla, at the third potency, is a valuable remedy in dyspepsia occurring in females, especially when the malady is complicated with deranged menstruation. If the disorder has arisen from excessive use of greasy and indigestible food, wine, &c., it will also prove a suitable remedy.

Bryonia, at the third attenuation, is well adapted to persons of a bilious temperament, with black hair, dark complexions, and black eyes. The particular indications for its employment, are, yellowness of the skin and eyes; tongue covered with a yellowish fur; bitter taste; vomiting or regurgitation of food soon after eating; sensation of fulness and burning in the stomach after meals; fulness and pains in the region of the liver; urine high-coloured; head confused and giddy; pressure in the head; loss of memory; inability to transact business; great despondency; frequent inclination to commit suicide; constant sighing; sleepless nights, or sleep disturbed by unpleasant dreams.

Lycopodium, calcarea carb., and *sepia*, may be given in mild cases of indigestion, occurring in weakly females and children, and persons of a lymphatic or scrofulous constitution. It may be exhibited at the third attenuation—a dose each day as long as may be necessary. In cases where the above remedies are indicated, a highly nutritious regimen may be enjoined with great advantage, also the constant employment of all those means which tend to invigorate the system, like active exercise, sea air, and bathing; frequent amusement for mind and body, &c.

Graphite is valuable in dyspeptic symptoms which appear to be connected with scrofulous or arthritic affections. It will be found particularly serviceable when they supervene upon the sudden disappearance of eruptions from the skin, or the sudden suppression of old discharges, or the drying up of old sores.

Administration.—Same as *lycopodium.*

Ignatia.—We have witnessed much benefit from the use of this medicine in indigestion afflicting persons of a *nervous* temperament. It covers the following symptoms, viz: countenance pale or sallow; eyes constantly in motion; general expression indicative of anguish and despair; frequent sighing; constant inclination to move about; confusion of ideas; loss of memory; pressure and other bad feelings in the head; distress at the stomach after eating; appetite variable; tongue covered with a thin white fur; entire despair of recovery; feels as if getting worse every day; dread of misfortune, coming want, &c.; frequent inclination to commit suicide; disinclination to see or converse with friends or acquaintances; seeks solitude, and broods over imaginary troubles.

This medicine may be given at the third attenuation, a drop once in twelve hours, until an impression is made upon the malady.

In cases where the nervous system is so much involved that the patient desires to die, and continually contemplates *suicide*, rather than suffer longer from his morbid and unfounded imaginings, and the wretchedness and anguish which tortures him day and night. *aurum muriate* at the first or second trituration, will be found a remedy of the utmost importance. One grain may be given twice daily until an amendment occurs.

The occasional use of mild aperients in certain cases of dyspepsia, as well as in convulsions, diarrhœa, &c., caused by the presence of indigestible food in the stomach and bowels, may be advisable for the same reason that paracentesis is recommended in urgent cases of abdominal or thoracic dropsy. By evacuating the unnatural accumulations, we not only place the disordered parts in a more favourable condition to recover their lost energy, but we also secure a much better state of things for the operation of our remedies. In obstinate constipation, for example, the indurated and impacted fecal matter sometimes induces so great an inactivity of the muscular and nervous structure of the intestinal canal, as to amount almost to paralysis. In these cases, both high and low attenuations now and then prove inefficient; and it is here that mild aperients and injections will sometimes prove serviceable, *not, however as curative agents, but by speedily removing a cause of disease, and thus placing the affected parts in the best possible condition to ensure the proper action of a homœopathic medicine.*

The observations of Dr. Madden, of Brighton, are so just respecting this subject, and so much to the point, that we take pleasure in quoting them in this connection. "But it not unfrequently happens, that the benefit gained by an immediate unloading of the bowels more than compensates for the subsequent increased tendency to constipation. This is acknowledged by all in the case of poisoning. No homœopathist hesitates to give emetics and purges when a person has swallowed a substance which, if not speedily removed, will cause death; but does not the same hold good with an indigestible meal? It is no doubt true that our remedies are often sufficient of themselves to overcome the evil influence of an occasional excess at table; yet I am convinced that it not unfrequently happens, especially in childhood, that a judicious aperient would at once remove a state of things which, if treated otherwise, would entail an illness requiring several days to overcome. There is much unreasonable prejudice among homœopathic practitioners on this point; they will unhesitatingly condemn the use of the mildest medicinal aperient, and yet will order their patients to eat prunes, figs, roasted apples, green vegetables, brown bread, &c., in the hopes of producing the same result. But where is the difference? A dose of castor oil, for example, produces an increased action of the bowels, in virtue of its being an indigestible oil, which passes through the whole intestinal tube unchanged, and perhaps exerting some slight irritating effect on the mucous membrane; whereas the aliments above named produce the same results, in virtue of their having either a large indigestible residuum which irritates by its presence, or by their containing vegetable acids, which directly and specifically irritate the mucous membrane. The result, therefore, is similar in both cases."—*British Jour. of Hom.* No. xxix, p. 311.

In conclusion, we deem it proper to observe, that aperients should never be employed except in very urgent cases, or in those where our attenuations have failed of producing the required effect. In all instances it is to be looked upon as a mere temporary expedient.

SECTION VII.

HÆMATEMESIS.—VOMITING OF BLOOD.

Diagnosis.—Previous to the vomiting there is experienced a sense of weight, fulness, pressure, and disturbance in the stomach, nausea, faintness, debility, general uneasiness, giddiness and confusion in the head, roaring in the ears, anxiety, bitter or saltish taste in the mouth, loss of appetite, occasional chills, and sometimes pains in the stomach, side, or chest. The pulse is for the most part small and contracted, though now and then full and bounding.

"The hæmorrhage no doubt generally occurs from the mucous membrane of the stomach, but it is thought also to proceed in some cases from the liver or spleen. When the blood comes from the former organ, it passes along the common bile duct into the duodenum, and thence regurgitates into the stomach. When the spleen is the source of the hæmorrhage, if this be ever the case, the blood, it is supposed, gains admission into the stomach through the *vassa brevia.*"—(*Dewees*).

The appearance of the blood which is thrown up varies, being in some instances liquid and bright red, at other times black, or coagulated. If the hæmorrhage proceeds directly from the rupture of a blood-vessel in the stomach, it will be red and liquid; but if it has been conveyed from the liver or spleen into this organ, it will be black and perhaps coagulated.

The quantity of blood which is sometimes vomited from the stomach is very great. I have in several instances witnessed the loss of two, three, and even four quarts from this organ without any very serious inconvenience, and that too in persons whose constitutions had been impaired from long-continued intemperance. A not uncommon result of these profuse evacuations is, however, the supervention of dropsy, and I am able to call to mind two instances of this description.

Causes.—Intemperance, suppression of accustomed discharges, as hæmorrhoids, catamenia, &c.: congestions and engorgements of the liver, spleen and pancreas, schirrous and other ulcerations of the gastro-mucous membrane, violent inflammations, whether caused by active drugs or mechanical injuries.

Therapeutics. — The principal medicines for the treatment of this malady are, *aconite*, *nux vomica*, *pulsatilla*, *ipecacuanha*, *arnica*, *veratrum*, *arsenicum*.

SECTION VIII.

CARDALGIA.—GASTRALGIA.

Cardalgia, as we have seen, is usually a symptom of dyspepsia, although writers have classed it as a distinct malady, having no necessary connection with this disorder. The intimate relation between the nerves and membranes of the stomach and the liver, and those which their functions sustain towards each other, incline us to the opinion that derangements of either of these parts of the organism must involve, to a greater or lesser extent, each of the others. The seat of cardalgia is in the nerves of the stomach, and as the healthy tone of the mucous membrane, &c., is dependent upon the normal integrity of the nerves which supply this organ, their mutual dependence will be readily perceived.

Diagnosis. — Pinching, gnawing, and cramp-like pains in the stomach, often extending into the back and loins, relieved on pressure at the epigastrium, or when the abdominal muscles are relaxed, faintness, anxiety, appetite natural, or but slightly impaired, pulse natural; food may be taken into the stomach with impunity; pains of a more severe character than those which occur in chronic gastritis, although there is no feeling of heat or thirst.

Causes.—Highly seasoned or crude and indigestible food, abuse of stimulants, coffee and tobacco, irregularity in eating, and the use of narcotic and other drugs.

Therapeutics.—The following medicines will cover all symptoms which may be present in any case of *cardalgia*, viz., *nux vomica, pulsatilla, acid hydrocyanic, carbo veg., chamomela, cocculus, argentum, sulphur, causticum,* and *bryonia.* For the treatment of other symptoms with which the disease may be complicated, the reader is referred to the chapter on dyspepsia.

Administration.—The remedies may be exhibited from the third to the sixth potency, and at intervals of six to twelve hours, until the desired effect is produced.

SECTION IX.

ENTERITIS.

Under this head we shall proceed to describe two varieties of intestinal inflammation, the peritoneal and muscular, and that of the mucous membrane. The older writers have confounded peritoneal enteritis with ordinary acute peritonitis, but the researches of modern pathologists have pointed out the true location and nature of these different maladies.

PERITONEAL ENTERITIS.

Diagnosis.—Lassitude, rigours, chills, acute pain in some part of the abdomen, swelling and exceeding tenderness in the affected part, nausea, vomiting, *obstinate and persistent constipation*, urgent thirst, bitter taste, loss of appetite, parched mouth, hot skin, inspirations short and painful, position on the back with knees drawn up, and inclination to preserve the recumbent posture, pulse frequent, tense, contracted, and irregular, urine scanty and high coloured.

The above symptoms will be modified according to the particular location of the inflammation. If the small intestines are the principal seat of the disorder, symptoms will obtain which simulate gastritis: if the colon be the part affected, we may expect symptoms resembling hepatitis to be present. This form of enteritis is violent and rapid in its course, and according to most writers is "peculiarly prone to terminate in gangrene. When this termination is about taking place, the pain suddenly subsides, the pulse sinks rapidly, the countenance becomes pale and cadaverous, the extremities cold, the surface covered with a cold clammy sweat, and hiccough, slight delirium, and occasionally convulsions, close the scene. This affection is seldom protracted beyond the seventh or eighth day, without terminating either in resolution or in death."—*Eberle.*

Causes.—The employment of irritating cathartics, like calomel, jalap, croton oil, aloes, scammony, colocynth, colchicum, gamboge, &c., poisons, alcoholic liquors, sudden suppression of accustomed discharges, repelled eruptions, worms, external injuries, persistent constipation, atmospheric changes.

Therapeutics.—*Arsenicum, veratrum, aloes, aconite, nux vom., lycopodium, opium, ipecacuanha, sulphur, plumbum, rhus tox., ac. cuprum.*

Administration.—The principal remedies in the treatment of this malady, are *arsenicum* and *veratrum.*

They may be exhibited at the third potency, at intervals of one to four hours, according to the severity of the symptoms. Should vomiting be very violent and persistent, after the proper administration of *arsenicum* or *veratrum*, recourse should be had to *ipecac.*, third attenuation. When the inflammation attacks the large intestines, *aloes* and *plumbum* may be given in some cases, at the third dilution, after *veratrum* and *arsenicum.* If the disorder has arisen from repelled eruptions, or metastasis of rheumatism, gout, erysipelas, &c., we may resort to *sulphur*, *rhus*, or *ac. cuprum*, as circumstances require. During the course of the disease, *aconite* will occasionally be found useful in controlling the action of the heart and arteries. It may be given at the second potency, either alone or in alternation with *arsenicum* or *veratrum*, according to the symptoms.

Auxiliary to the above remedies, the employment of fomentations, either of warm or cold water, as the case may demand, will prove of eminent service. Cloths should be wrung out, and applied over the affected part, (care being taken to protect the body linen and bed-clothes,) renewing them once in fifteen or twenty minutes, when the inflammation and pain are severe.

SECTION X.

ACUTE MUCOUS ENTERITIS.—DYSENTERY.

Diagnosis.—This disease sometimes commences with *griping pains in the bowels, with frequent discharges of mucus or mucus mixed with blood, attended during the evacuations with more or less straining and burning pain.* After the first two or three evacuations, nothing but mucus, or mucus and blood, are passed. Occasionally the griping and diarrhœa are preceded by lassitude, chills, weakness and pains in the limbs, thirst, bad taste in the mouth, furred tongue, hot and dry skin, frequent and hard pulse, anxiety, and general restlessness. The disease is peculiarly apt to be ushered in with these last-named symptoms, when it has been caused by sudden suppression of perspiration, atmospheric vicissitudes, or miasmatic influences.

The appearance of the fluids discharged, will depend much upon the climate, temperament, the exciting cause, and the particular portion of the intestinal canal affected. If the small intestines are chiefly disordered, the evacuations will consist of dark watery matter, mixed with mucus and blood, while inflammation of the colon and rectum will give rise to discharges of *pure mucus and blood, preceded and attended with distressing tormina, and inclination to remain a good part of the time at stool.* These discharges, which are highly offensive, afford some temporary relief to the patient, only to be renewed with increased severity. There are tenderness of the bowels on pressure, pain and burning in making water, inclination to lie upon the back, with the knees drawn up, great depression of spirits, short and painful inspirations, universal heat and dryness of the skin, more or less derangement in the function of the liver, indicated by an icterode hue of the skin, and the absence of bile in the evacuations, rapid emaciation, loss of strength, and increasing disinclination to physical effort. As the disease advances towards a fatal termination, the countenance assumes a contracted and cadaverous expression, the pulse sinks, the evacuations become more fœtid, and are discharged involuntarily, the pains abate or cease entirely, a cold sweat occurs, hiccough, delirium, cramps, and extreme prostration obtain, and then death.

Causes.—Atmospheric vicissitudes, deranged function of the liver, abrupt checks to perspiration, "*koino miasmata* have frequently an unequivocal agency in the production of this disease," (*Eberle*),—the irritation of teething, worms, and drastic drugs, crude vegetables and unripe or decayed fruits.

Prognosis.—The prognosis of dysentery will vary according to the climate, the location, the season of year, the constitution of the patient, and its complications with typhus, cholera, or other contagious maladies.

Hot and damp regions, abounding in luxuriant vegetation which is constantly undergoing decomposition, and filling the air with miasmatic particles, predispose the system to dysenteric affections, and serve to render them violent and dangerous. Low, marshy, and damp situations favour the formation of the disease, more than elevated and dry locations. It is far more common, severe, and fatal in the months of July and August, in this country, than at any other period of the year; and it is rare that individuals who are strongly predisposed to it, entirely escape during these months. When it is succeeded or accompanied with typhoid symptoms, or when it occurs as a symptom of typhus fever, it may be looked on as a malady of the most dangerous character, and one which will require the most judiciously directed resources of our art. In these instances we have to combat, not only the local intestinal disorder, but also constitutional symptoms of the greatest severity. During the prevalence of Asiatic cholera, dysentery has been observed to assume a more malignant form than in those years when this destructive epidemic has not prevailed. While the cholera was destroying its thousands weekly in our *large* cities, during the last summer, a malignant dysentery prevailed in most of the *smaller* cities and towns, sweeping off numbers entirely unprecedented. In these last examples, the epidemic influence was not sufficiently active to generate the actual cholera asphyxia, but it conduced to aggravate very materially, the type of dysentery.

Therapeutics.—Mercurius, arsenicum, chamomela, pulsatilla, colocynth, aconite, ipecacuanha, nux vomica, carbo veg., sulphur, dulcamara, aloes, acid nit., acid mur.

Mercurius corrosive.—External indications.—Anxious expression of countenance; features distorted by pain; knees drawn up; head and shoulders elevated, or bent forward; fulness of the abdomen; skin hot and dry; tongue dry and dirty; pulse frequent and tense; inspirations short and imperfect, and effected principally with the muscles of the chest; evacuations of pure blood, or mucus mixed with blood, or dark and bilious and fœtid.

Physical sensations.—Sharp, cutting pains in the bowels, accompanied with very frequent and urgent desire to go to stool, and tenesmus; desire to remain long at stool; abdomen excessively painful on pressure, with constant sensation of distention; dryness of the mouth and throat, with intense thirst; involuntary twitchings of the muscles on going to sleep; pain at the neck of the bladder in urinating; cheeks and abdomen hot and flushed, while the extremities are cold; drawings, pinchings, or cramps in the limbs, often deep seated; pains increased at each inspiration; shivering on the least exposure; aggravation of the symptoms at night; sense of pain and fatigue in the joints.

Mental and moral symptoms.—Out of humour; irritable; petulant; desponding; reckless.

Administration.—One grain of the third trituration may be given every hour until the violence of the disease is subdued, when the intervals may be lengthened, or the medicine suspended, according to the exigencies of the case. Some writers advise, an alternation of this remedy with *colocynth,* where the indications point to the latter as well as the former medicine. We have occasionally prescribed these articles in alternation with unequivocal benefit.

Mercurius sol.—This form of mercury is more particularly adapted to the treatment of those cases which are principally located in the upper portion of the intestinal canal, the *external indications* for which are, yellowish colour of the skin; offensive breath; tongue covered with a white, thick, tenacious mucus; distention in the superior part of the abdomen; evacuations of fœtid mucus and bilious matter, of a green or darkish colour, or of bloody mucus; prolapsus of the rectum, which is red and inflamed; urine of a deep red or brown colour and offensive; position, respiration, pulse, temperature, thirst, &c., same as under *merc. cor.*

Physical sensations.—Violent cutting pains in the abdomen, accompanied by shivering, during and after the evacuations; great tenderness on pressure, in the region of the small intestines; frequent desire to evacuate the bowels, accompanied by violent tenesmus; discharges small in quantity; aggravation of pains at night; frequent and urgent desire to urinate; nausea and vomiting, with pain in the stomach; thirst for cold drinks; cramps and contractions in the umbilical region; weakness and rapid sinking of strength; painful sense of distention in the abdomen; sense of fatigue and great weakness in the limbs.

Mental and moral symptoms.—Morose; irritable; great anguish and discouragement; peevish; quarrelsome.

Administration.—Same as *merc. cor.*

Remarks.—In malignant dysentery, *mercurius sol.* and *nitric acid* are unquestionably remedies of the highest importance. In all cases where the symptoms are not covered by one of them, but are entirely so by both, or when either administered singly, does not promptly arrest the disorder, we may use them in alternation with every prospect of success.

The following are the *external indications* of *nitric acid:* countenance pale or flushed, and indicative of anguish and anxiety; evacuations bloody, slimy, and fetid; abdomen distended; urine red, or dark and turbid; body hot, while the extremities are perhaps cold; pulse hard and frequent.

Physical sensations.—Frequent evacuations with severe tenesmus, and urging to urinate; headache; fever; thirst; sweat during the night and occasionally in the day time; sense of fulness and pain in the abdomen; general character of the disease typhoid.

Mental and moral symptoms.—Sometimes delirium; or anxiety, fear, apprehension, depression, and sleeplesness.

Administration.—We may give a drop of the second or third dilution in water, after each evacuation: or when used in alternation with *mercurius*, after every other discharge from the bowels.

Mercurius viv.—This medicine covers the same range of symptoms as the *merc. sol.*, and may be substituted for it, if desired, in the treatment of dysentery. Its mode of administration is also the same.

Arsenicum alb.—Where dysentery has arisen from the abuse of drastic and other debilitating medicines, after excessive loss of blood, or after the organism has been enfeebled from previous disease, *arsenicum* will often prove an efficient remedy. It is also peculiarly useful in dysenteric affections, occurring in individuals of a nervous, dropsical, or lymphatic constitution, and when the disease is attended with typhoid complications.

External indications.—General appearance of debility and prostration; trembling or stiffness of the limbs; face pale or yellowish, hollow and cadaverous; position on the back, with tendency to sink to the foot of the bed; eyes dull and sunken; lips dry and dark-coloured; tongue dry and brownish; abdomen swollen and hard, or tympanitic; fæces offensive, putrid, and variable in colour, but generally slimy and streaked with blood, or greenish or darkish; skin cold and bluish, or dry and shrivelled; breathing short and oppressed; pulse frequent, small, thready, sometimes irregular.

Physical sensations.—Violent, sharp and cramp-like pains in the abdomen, accompanied with nausea and vomiting; sensation of fulness and burning in the bowels; frequent eructations; flatulency; frequent evacuations with some tenesmus, burning pain at the anus, and nausea; retention of urine, or burning pain in making water; pain increased by the slightest motion; faintness upon the least exertion; great tenderness of the abdomen; colliquative sweats; entire inability to sit up, or make any effort; puffiness of the eyes or cheeks; disturbed sleep, with constant jerking of the limbs, and tossing.

Mental and moral symptoms.—Sad; desponding; anxious; discouraged; irritability, impatience; delirium; loss of consciousness.

Administration.—One grain of the first trituration to two ounces of distilled water—a teaspoonful once in two or three hours until the required effect is produced.

Chamomela.—A useful remedy in dysenteric affections arising from a sudden chill, from difficult and protracted dentition, from violent grief or passion. It applies especially to affections of this nature which occur in women and children, and when judiciously prescribed, will often act promptly and efficiently. Laurie has found it of service after *aconite* in cases attended with inflammatory symptoms, which have been partially subdued by this medicine. It may be given at the third potency, as circumstances require.

Pulsatilla.—This remedy has been highly recommended in *fall dysenteries,* and in some cases of *chronic dysentery.* The indicatlons for its use are, nausea, vomiting, bad feeling in the head; bruised sensation in the integuments of the abdomen; cutting pains in the bowels, with discharges of sanguineous mucus; pain in the small of the back; chilliness, especially towards night; bad taste in the mouth; eructations, acid or bitter; prickling or numbnesss of the skin; constant inclination to sleep during the day; yellow tinge of the skin.

Administration.—Four drops of the third dilution to an ounce of distilled water—a dessert spoonful every two, four or six hours in acute cases. One dose every afternoon in chronic dysentery.

Colocynth should be exhibited in cramp-like, colicky pains in the bowels, with inflammation of the whole abdomen; slimy or bilious evacuations, with pains and contractions at the rectum; bitter taste, with urgent desire for cold drinks; nausea and vomiting of bilious fluids; shooting and cramp-like pains on one side of the body; pains in the head, and throbbing of the temporal arteries.

Administration.—Same as *chamomela.*

Nux vom. sometimes effects speedy cures in protracted dysenteric discharges, which appear to be kept up from relaxation and loss of tone in the abdominal mucous membrane rather than from actual inflammation. By imparting tone and vigour to the enfeebled nerves of the stomach and intestines, it cures the disease, and enables these organs to resume their healthy functions. The indications for its employment are, fulness and distention of the abdomen; contractive or cramp-like pains in the umbilical, epigastric, or hypochondriac region; frequent small evacuations of mucous and bloody matters; contractive pain in the rectum during the discharges; bowels and cheeks hot; thirst; fæces putrid and offensive.

Administration.—A drop of the third potency may be given every two to six hours, as the urgency of the symptoms demand, until an impression upon the disease is apparent.

Another medicine which has proved highly serviceable in my hands, is *aloes soc.* The indications for its use are similar to those of *colocynth;* and in some cases where *colocynth* has failed to afford the desired relief, this medicine has succeeded promptly.

Rau has also used *aloes* with distinguished success in purely *inflammatory dysentery*. The *external indications* are: abdomen distended and tender to the touch; stools slimy and mixed with blood, or thin and watery; urine scanty and high-coloured; tongue red and dry; pulse full and rapid; skin hot and dry, &c.

Physical sensations.—Severe pressing, cutting and burning pains in the lower part of the abdomen; violent tenesmus and smarting in the rectum, during the evacuations, with sharp pains extending to the sacrum and abdomen; high fever; pain in urinating, &c.

Mental and moral symptoms.—Anxiety and general indications of nervous excitement.

Administration.—Same as *chamomela.*

Dulcamara may be used in dysentery arising from cold, and attended with cutting pains in the intestines, bloody discharges, burning and itching at the rectum, heat of skin and thirst. It may be prescribed at the third potency—a dose once in two to six hours, according to circumstances.

Carbo veg. may succeed or alternate with *arsenicum* in certain low forms of dysentery, when the former does not act with sufficient efficiency. It may be given for the same train of symptoms, and at the same potency as *arsenicum.*

Sulphur is a remedy which deserves consideration in instances where the more ordinary remedies fail in affording prompt relief, and especially, if any latent miasm is suspected to have conduced to the disease, or prevented the usual action of the medicines administered. It is also often serviceable in the dysenteries of hæmorrhoidal patients.

Sulphuric acid has been highly commended in *putrid dysentery*. The *external indications* are: thin, bloody, and very fœtid stools; red, or darkish urine, turbid, or depositing a dirty sediment; burning hot skin; apthæ; petechiæ; blood-blisters; vomiting of water and food.

Physical sensations.—Frequent inclination to go to stool, with severe tenesmus, nausea, and vomiting; desire for acids, fresh fruit, &c.

Mental and moral symptoms.—Indifferent, or irritable; irascible and peevish. It may be given in the same manner as *nitric acid.*

Belladonna is indicated in *inflammatory dysentery,* with *determination of blood to the head, and delirium.* There is constant tenesmus, but nothing is evacuated, with violent fever, vomiting, tympanitic distention of the abdomen, &c.

In *bilious, catarrhal, erethistic,* and *rheumatic* forms of dysentery, examine *colocy., puls., nux vom., cup., cham., chin., rhus,, sulph., ip., dulc., euph., canth., ant. crud., rheum.*

When the malady degenerates into a chronic form, our best remedies are, *phos., acid nit., sulph., china, lach., acid phos., calc. carb., verat., merc., ferr.,* and *colocynth.*

We have often observed the most decided benefit follow the employment of enemata of cold water, in dysenteric inflammations. They may be administered after each evacuation, in suitable cases, and when they afford evident relief.

SECTION XI.

ACUTE PERITONITIS.

Diagnosis.—Three varieties of this disease have been recognised, viz.: first, natural peritonitis; second, puerperal peritonitis; third, chronic peritonitis. We shall, however, include under the present head, each variety, detailing, as we proceed, the characteristic symptoms pertaining to all of the different forms of the malady.

Acute peritonitis is usually ushered in with more or less of the ordinary symptoms of fever, as lassitude, irregular chills, succeeded by flushes of heat, headache, frequent pulse, uneasiness, or pressure in the region of the stomach, nausea, and loss of appetite. These symptoms are speedily succeeded, and occasionally accompanied, by a pain and tenderness in the abdomen, either confined to circumscribed points, or universally diffused over its whole extent. Generally the abdomen is excessively tender and painful upon pressure, often rendering the weight of the bedclothes intolerable; but in some instances, the pain is slight from the commencement to the fatal termination of the malady. The tongue is moist and covered with a white fur, in the first instance, which soon becomes dark and dry in the centre, with red edges. The bowels are constipated, but may be readily acted upon by appropriate remedies. The pulse is commonly frequent, tense, corded, and wiry, though in some instances it varies but little from the natural standard. This, like most other inflammations of the abdominal viscera, imparts to the countenance a contracted, sharp, and anxious expression, indicative of both acute physical and mental suffering. The patient inclines to relax those muscles which operate upon the abdominal parietes, and on this account we find him with his legs drawn up, his head and shoulders elevated, and his respiration short, imperfect, and exercised almost entirely by the muscles of the chest.

Puerperal peritonitis is that form of the disease which occurs in females after confinement, and is known as puerperal fever. It differs from ordinary peritonitis, in being more sudden and violent in its attack, and in having a tendency to run its course with greater rapidity. Among the first symptoms are pain and tenderness in the hypogastric region, occurring soon after delivery, and succeeded by chills, &c. Some authors assert that the lochia are almost invariably suppressed, while others of equal eminence, assure us that this discharge is often but little affected, and never entirely suspended. The secretion of milk is also either partially or entirely suppressed; and if the secretion has not yet taken place, it does not occur at all. In many cases of both forms of this disease, the brain is affected at an early period, and demands special attention.

In regard to the precise character which this malady may be likely to assume, much will depend upon the peculiar constitution and circumstances of the individual, the season of year, the prevalence of epidemic or contagious influences, &c. "There is also an entire extinction of the maternal feeling," (*Dewees*,)* and

* Dr. Dewees considers this one of the most remarkable circumstances attending this disease.

frequent inclination to pass water, which is often attended with pain. The duration of this malady is from twenty-four hours to two or three weeks.

Chronic peritonitis, although often consequent upon a partially subdued acute attack, may also arise independently from sudden changes of temperature, insufficient clothing, irritating food, external injuries, surgical operations, and chronic bowel complaints. Many of the symptoms of this disease are like those of dyspepsia, as sensation of fulness, distention, weight, and occasional pains in the region of the stomach and bowels, constipation, loss of appetite, depression of spirits, restlessness at night, distress and pains, aggravated after eating, emaciation, thirst, frequent pulse, foul tongue, &c. This form of peritonitis may terminate in a few weeks, or it may run on for a year or more, and then result in ulcerations opening into the intestines.

Causes.—Certain occult conditions of the atmosphere, undue exposure to cold, excessive physical exertion, injuries, labour, miscarriage, over-exertion when the organism is weakened by previous disease, atmospheric vicissitudes, metastases of rheumatism, and gout, suppressed discharges, &c.

Therapeutics.—The most approved remedies in the treatment of peritonitis are, *aconite, belladonna, bryonia, arnica, bismuth., chamomela, coffea, colocynth, ipecacuanha, mercurius, nux vom., pulsatilla, rhus tox., sulphuris, veratrum.*

Administration.—We advise the employment of the three first attenuations—and a repetition of the dose every one, two, or three hours, according to the urgency of the case.

SECTION XII.

COLIC.

Under this head, we shall describe three varieties: first, *bilious colic*; second, *flatulent colic*; third, *painter's colic.*

1.—BILIOUS COLIC.

Diagnosis.—The first symptoms of this disease, are

headache; nausea; bitter taste; bilious vomiting; foul tongue; loss of appetite; thirst, and uneasiness in the bowels. These symptoms are speedily followed by severe griping, twisting, or shooting pains in the umbilical region; hot skin; painful distention of the stomach and abdomen; obstinate constipation, and finally, tenderness of the abdomen; yellow cast of the skin and eyes; coldness and torpor of the extremities; cold sweats; feeble or extinct pulse, and other signs indicative of a fatal termination of the disorder. During the first stage of the malady, the patient involuntarily makes firm pressure over the navel, which affords temporary relief, and it is by this symptom that we may distinguish the disease from inflammation of the bowels, in which pressure is attended with an aggravation of the pain.

Causes.—Deranged function of the liver, is supposed to be the chief cause of this complaint, but what the precise nature of this derangement consists in, we know not. Dewees supposes that the liver is in a state of morbid activity, and secretes bile of an acrid quality, which serves to irritate the stomach and intestines, and thus induce the disease. Gregory, Eberle, Johnson, &c., assert that this organ is in a torpid condition, and consequently secreting only a small amount of bile, thus leaving the ingesta to be only partially acted upon by one of its natural solvents, and thereby rendering the half digested food an irritant to the digestive organs. From the fact of its occurring only at particular periods of the year, it is reasonable to conclude that atmospheric causes exert some influence in its production.

It is quite evident, however, that derangement of the liver is intimately connected with genuine bilious colic, and it therefore behooves those who have been afflicted, to take every precaution to ensure a healthy condition of this organ.

2.—FLATULENT COLIC.

Diagnosis.—Flatulent colic may be distinguished from the variety last described, by the greater distention of the stomach and bowels with flatus; frequent eructations; borborygmus; the pain, although as severe as in bilious colic, yet coming on more in paroxysms, absence of nausea and bilious vomiting, and from the fact that it usually occurs an hour or two after eating something indigestible.

Causes.—Indigestible food, unripe or decayed fruits; beer; mental emotions, or any other cause capable of morbidly altering or suspending for a time, the healthy action of the stomach and bowels, in such a manner as to cause them to generate an unusual quantity of gas.

3.—COLICA PICTONUM.—PAINTER'S COLIC.

Diagnosis.—Lead colic commences with feelings of lassitude; dull pains in the head; loss of appetite; bad taste in the mouth; wandering pains in the bowels and limbs; transient chills, and depression of spirits. After these symptoms have existed for some time, the pain in the region of the umbilicus becomes exceedingly severe, obliging the patient to make firm pressure against the abdomen, with the body in a bent position; indeed, so intolerable is the pain, that the patient is unable to remain quiet in any position. He is now in a state of great agitation and excitement, and feels confident that he must die unless speedily relieved. It is important to observe, that in all the varieties of colic, the skin is cool or not above the natural standard, and sometimes covered with a cold sweat. The pulse, also, exhibits but little arterial excitement. These last symptoms, together with the relief which firm pressure upon the abdomen affords, in the early stages of the malady, indicates its spasmodic character, and will serve to distinguish it from enteritis and other inflammatory conditions of the abdominal viscera.

Therapeutics.—The specifics for the different kinds of colic, are, *colocynth, plumbum, nux vomica, arsenicum, chamomela, hyoscyamus, stramonium, veratrum, cocculus, senna, colchicum, phosphorus, pulsatilla.*

Auxiliary to the above remedies, we beg leave to impress upon the practitioner the importance of *fomentations and enemata of warm water*. These measures, conjoined in certain cases with the tepid bath, are worthy of high consideration, and should never be lost sight of in the treatment of this, as well as other maladies of a spasmodic character. The fomentations should not only be applied to the abdomen, but to the extremities, more especially if these parts are cold and inclined to cramp. In moderate cases, fomentations, together with an ordinary enema, and the proper specific, will suffice to effect a speedy cure; but if the case has been very violent and obstinate from neglect or mismanagement, by *calomel* and *opium*, a *general bath*, with *very copious injections* of warm water while immersed in the water, cannot be too highly recommended. Indeed, we have in several instances, observed the abdominal spasms to relax, the pains to cease, and free evacuations of fæcal matter and of wind to occur, while the patient was yet in the bath. By adopting this course, we secure the advantage of *internal*, as well as *external* fomentations, and thus bring a safe, yet efficient remedy, to bear directly upon the parts affected. All who have practically tested the soothing influence of warm water applications upon the nervous system, when in a state of unnatural erethism, will appreciate the truth of our remarks.

The medicine which is most generally applicable in the treatment of colic, is *colocynth*. It is particularly appropriate when the complaint has been caused by a chill, by mental emotions, as grief, indigestion, mortification, &c., also when biliary derangement has been the exciting cause.

The *external indications* are, inflation of the abdomen; position of the body bent forward, so as to relax the abdominal muscles; cramps in the calves of the legs; general agitation; temperature of the skin, about the natural standard, or cold and covered with sweat; pulse natural, or but slightly increased in frequency; tongue covered with a yellowish fur, or natural; face pale and indicative of intense suffering; rigidity and contraction of the abdominal muscles, as well as of the tendons in other parts of the body.

Physical sensations.—Violent cramp-like contraction or cutting pains in the abdomen, generally in the region of the umbilicus; painful cramps in the calves of the legs; sensation of faintness, with coldness and shuddering; bitter or insipid taste in the mouth; nausea; loss of appetite; disgust for drinks; constant inclination to move about, to grasp objects violently, and to make pressure against the abdomen; empty eructations; pains in the back and loins, especially semilateral; obstinate constipation, or small and loose evacuations.

Mental and moral symptoms.—Most intense anguish and agitation; dejection; extreme restlessness and desire to move about; fear of speedy death.

Administration.—From the first to the sixth dilution may be employed according to the age, sex, constitution, temperament, and severity of the disease. A dose may be given every half hour in urgent cases, until amendment or medicinal aggravation occurs, to be resumed and repeated as the exigencies of the case may require.

Plumbum.—On account of the very marked and decided specific action of *lead* upon the colon and ileum, whether introduced into the blood through the stomach, rectum, lungs, or skin, this drug is peculiarly appropriate for the treatment of some of the varieties of colic. The practitioner will, of course, avoid exhibiting it in that variety of colic which has been caused by the absorption of *lead*. The following are its

External indications.—Rigidity and contraction of the abdominal muscles; hard ridges, or elevations in the abdomen; borborygmus; frequent expulsion of offensive flatus; eructations; tremblings, jerkings, or cramps of the limbs; face and skin pale, bluish, or yellow; surface cold, and covered with clammy sweat; mouth dry or moist, and clammy; pulse weak, and somewhat frequent; body bent double.

Physical sensations.—Violent constrictive, shooting, or pinching pains in the umbilical region; constant and urgent desire to eructate and expel flatus; chilliness or shuddering during the paroxysms; sensation of faintness; torpor, numbness, stiffness, and weakness in the limbs; desire to press the abdomen against something hard; extremities cold; dizziness; sweetish or bitter taste; thirst; vomiting of bilious or fæcal matters; pressure and cramps in the stomach; obstinate constipation; evacuations, scybalous and difficult to expel; shooting pains in the loins, and back, and limbs; cramps in the feet, excessive agitation and restlessness.

Mental and moral symptoms.—Very great anguish and uneasiness; melancholy; discouragement; impatience.

Administration.—Same as *Colocynth.*

Nux vomica is very useful in colic, arising from torpor of the liver, indicated by deficient secretion of bile, indigestion, flatulence, &c. It is also useful in *flatulent colic,* occurring in dyspeptic subjects after the use of improper articles of food. In cases where *nux* is indicated, the face is pale or yellowish, the stools, previous to the attack, light and clay-coloured, the abdomen distended, there are frequent eructations, hiccough, sharp and cramp-like pains in the stomach and bowels, rumbling in the bowels, giddiness, sensitiveness of the stomach and abdomen when pressed upon.

Administration.—This medicine may be used at the second or third attenuation; a dose once in half an hour to two hours until relief is obtained.

Arsenicum is specific in colic pains coming on in *regular paroxysms,* and attended with decided remissions. In extreme cases, it may also be resorted to with advantage, where the powers of the system have been exhausted, and other remedies seem to be incapable of arresting the disease. The first to the third potency may be used, and repeated as circumstances appear to require.

Chamomela is advised by Hahnemann in the colics of pregnant and parturient women, of new-born infants, and of children during dentition. It is also recommended for the colics of nervous and hysterical females. If this medicine does not afford the desired relief, resort may be had to *hyoscyamus, stramonium,* or *senna.*

Administration.—A dose of the third to the sixth dilution every hour or two as long as necessary.

Veratrum, cocculus, and *colchicum,* will often prove valuable in spasmodic and flatulent colic occurring in nervous and hysterical females, and in persons of a mild and phlegmatic temperament. In instances where the above described remedies do not correspond, let the indications of these articles be considered.

Pulsatilla is principally useful in colics arising from

the abuse of crude, esculent vegetables, unripe fruits, and abuse of fat and greasy articles of food. The pains are very severe, and usually occur a few hours after eating, attended with borborygmus, and the expulsion of large quantities of flatus. We have often seen the most prompt relief follow a single drop of the tincture, and we have rarely been obliged to repeat the dose more than two or three times.

Phosphorus will apply to cases occurring in persons of a feeble organization, who have been weakened by long-continued gastric affections, and especially for those who are afflicted with disease of the *mesenteric glands.* A dose of the third trituration may be administered every two hours until relief ensues.

SECTION XIII.

ASIATIC CHOLERA.

When the Asiatic cholera first pursued its destructive course amongst the millions of Europe and America, the disciples of the ancient school of medicine stood aghast and almost powerless before the awful scourge, their best resources often hastening rather than retarding the work of the destroying angel. Destitute of an accurate or reasonable system of practice, without any definite rules of action, or any true knowledge of the operation of medicines, the allopath brought to the treatment of the malady his vague, indefinite, and uncertain remedial theories; and in contemplating the numerous and contradictory modes of treatment advised and adopted by different eminent persons of this description,—the ridiculous, and often fatal *experiments,* by means of which they hoped to *guess out* and blunder on to some actual remedy—we are forcibly reminded of the entire worthlessness and unsoundness of their system. Here was a violent and relentless enemy, seizing its victim with unwonted energy, and pursuing its deathly course with rapid strides—one requiring active, prompt, and decided processes to stay its fatal ravages,—and what course did the allopath adopt in the fearful crisis? Did he attack symptom after symptom with medicines which possessed specific, uniform, and decided effects, and thus repel the invader step by step? Did he administer his stimulants, opiates, mercurials, and counter-irritants with that confidence which an exact and correct system of medicine must naturally inspire? Let their results and confessions everywhere answer.

It is universally conceded, at the present time, that homœopathy is far more efficient in the treatment of cholera than any other mode of practice. During its prevalence in Europe, from 1831 until its disappearance, the average mortality of cases under this treatment was about one in twelve, while under allopathic treatment, the average was one in three. In Germany, Russia, France, and other European kingdoms where our system had become known, even distinguished gentlemen of the old school were forced to admit its vast superiority over their own system; and it was undoubtedly this superior efficacy and success which caused so many distinguished men of Europe to investigate the claims of the doctrine of "*similia similibus*," renounce the fallacies of Hippocrates and Galen, and throw their influence on the side of truth.

Being a disease of extreme violence, and having a tendency to run its course with great rapidity, there was no time to apply remedies according to the principle *contraria contrariis*, nor would its severity permit the additional waste of strength and nervous energy which ever follow opiates, stimulants, and counter-irritants. A positive *specific*, a real *antidote*, could alone reach the seat of the disease, and arrest its progress; and to the disciples of Hahnemann is due the credit of bringing forward these *specifics*, and demonstrating to the world their tremendous power and efficiency over this world-wide scourge.

Diagnosis.—Asiatic cholera varies much in its mode of attack, violence, and duration. It may seize its victim in such a manner as to produce an immediate prostration of strength, together with most of those symptoms which indicate an almost total loss of vitality, as a sunken and cadaverous expression of countenance, small and almost imperceptible pulse, surface of a bluish tinge, and cold, cramps in the calves of the legs and fingers, burning in the stomach and throat, extreme anguish or stupidity, vomiting, diarrhœa, and an almost entire loss of power over the voluntary muscles. Other cases set in with vertigo, humming in the ears, oppression and burning pain at the pit of the stomach, nausea, vomiting, griping, and purging of a liquid resembling "rice water," which are soon succeeded by oppression of the chest, difficulty of breathing, cramp-like pains in the extremities and abdominal muscles, intense thirst, great loss of strength, bluish colour of the lips, nails, and skin, pulse almost imperceptible, hippocratic countenance, delirium, cold, icy skin, profuse sweats, weak, hoarse voice, and sometimes sopor, with eyes half open and fixed, with partial or total loss of consciousness. A few or the whole of these symptoms may be present in any given case, according to the constitutional, predisposing, and exciting causes which may exist.

Causes.—A peculiar subtle poison, capable of being conveyed by currents of wind from place to place, either dissolved in aqueous vapour, or in some other manner, and possibly, by attaching itself to articles of clothing, &c., capable of communication in this way. Whether this infinitesimal, imponderable morbific agent is generated during the prevalence of some peculiar conditions of the atmosphere, from vegetable or animal matters in a state of partial or total decomposition, or from some other source, is as yet a matter of speculation. Like most other of the more potent agents in nature, the particles of the poison are in so minute a state of subdivision, and so subtilely diffused in the air, that in the present imperfect condition of the sciences, we are entirely unable to investigate or appreciate their nature. That the cause or agent is *material*, however, no one can for a moment doubt; for it must be *something* or *nothing;* if it is the former, it must be composed of minute particles or atoms of matter, which, by being absorbed, produce those specific effects which constitute cholera. If it is contended that the cause is not material, but simply a *property of matter;* something spiritual, unreal, intangible, and yet capable of producing powerful impressions; we say proofs of this view are wanting, and we reason upon fallacious, if not absurd data. We hear much said respecting the "*properties of matter*," when abstruse subjects are the topics under consideration, and this unmeaning phrase serves the purpose of explaining everything which is obscure, and cannot be explained by the existing knowledge concerning the nature of certain imponderable substances. *Properties of matter* are merely *effects* produced upon the organism by actual contact of *material* atoms, and must never be substituted or confounded with the agent—the morbific cause itself. Let medical men, therefore, confess their ignorance respecting the causes and physical character of those imponderable atoms, which so often contaminate the atmosphere, and by being absorbed into the blood, induce those baneful specific diseases which so sorely afflict mankind.

Therapeutics.—Dr. Lobethal, of Germany, who had charge of a large cholera hospital (*allopathic*) during the prevalence of the epidemic in 1831, and who treated an immense number of cholera patients *homœopathically* in the summer of 1847, and again in 1849, observes: "It has been reserved to the 'specific' healing art, generally known under the name of homœopathy, to stand the test of practical observation, and to demonstrate its superiority in combatting this fearful disease, (cholera,) the appearance of which, followed by an immense number of well substantiated cures, has tended in the highest degree to the spread of the new healing art. In 1831, I learned from experience that the various methods of treatment pursued in the old school, in spite of all the science on which it was based, led, on the average, to very unfavourable results; whereas in 1848 and 1849, by adopting the homœopathic treatment, *I lost but few out of a very great number of patients.*"

When the cholera is preceded by nausea; loss of appetite; constant borborygmus; violent thirst; slight febrile symptoms; frequent thin watery discharges; *absence of pain in the bowels,* and other symptoms, generally known under the term "*cholerine,*" Dr. Lobethal has derived marked benefit from the use of *phosphoric acid,* repeated every two or three hours until the symptoms are better. If the above symptoms are attended with coated tongue, vomiting, debility, and indigestion, *ipecac.*, of the third dilution, is required.

When cholera has actually made its appearance, a remedy which covers the exact symptoms of the case, ought to be immediately exhibited. Our best remedies are *verat.*, *ars.*, *cup.*, *camph.*, *canth.*, *carb. v.*

In the *forming stage* of cholera, and in *cholerine*, with cramps in the calves of the legs, give tincture of *camphor*; "and for aching or burning in the epigastrium, *ac. phos.*, *ars.*, *cup.*, *phos.*, *ver.*; for rumbling in the belly, *ac. phos.*, *ver.*, *phos.*; for diarrhœa, *ac. phos.*, *ars.*, *ip.*, *phos.*, *sec.*, *sulph.*, *ver.*"—(*Nusser*).

In the third stage, or collapse, *ars.*, *phos.*, *verat.*, *carb. v.*, *laurocer.*, &c., are to be used.

During the prevalence of the epidemic in England and France in 1848-9, and in America in 1849, almost every individual experienced unusual intestinal irritation and disposition to *diarrhœa*. In the large cities, especially, very few exceptions to this rule could be found. Even the most strict regard to diet, and avoidance of all exposure, was no security against this weakness and rumbling of the bowels, and a certain lassitude and uneasiness which constantly attended it. Most of these cases subsided without any serious disturbance; others passed into *cholerine*, which could generally be controlled when promptly taken in hand; while those cases which were neglected, or improperly managed, usually terminated in *cholera*. In rare instances, individuals would be attacked suddenly and violently, without any *apparent premonitory symptoms*, but cases of this description have almost invariably occurred in those whose constitutions were impaired from intemperance, disease, or who had been deprived of proper repose, by mental application, excitement, fear, &c.

Dr. Hencke found *camphor* a positive specific in the *spasmodic form* of cholera, "when the patients were suddenly taken with rigor, and even cold in the back, which was soon followed by faintness and weakness, sinking sensation in the stomach, *vertigo*, nausea, *aching*, *contracting pain in the epigastrium*, gagging, vomiting, *spasms in the calves*, general *tonic* spasms, disappearance of the natural warmth, therefore coldness of the hands and the whole body, *depression of the pulse*, which could hardly be felt, lividity of the lips, *anxious expression of the countenance*, &c., sometimes diarrhœa." Dr. H. advises that the patient be well covered, and dry heat applied to his body and limbs, and that strong spirits of camphor be given in drop doses every five minutes, until reaction occurs, warmth returns, and perspiration sets in. Dry frictions may at the same time be employed. As soon as we observe signs of reaction, we must either omit the remedy, or if the urgency of the case demands further remedial means, give the *camphor* at the first or second dilution until reaction is fully established. It was a very common occurrence for patients to be taken in the night, generally after midnight, with cramps in the stomach, nausea, vomiting and purging of a watery fluid, without pain or effort on the part of the patient; sense of exhaustion and debility, and great anxiety. If these symptoms were not speedily arrested, there soon succeeded extreme prostration, almost constant vomiting and purging of rice-coloured fluid; contractive or burning pains in the stomach; coldness of the surface; spasms or cramps in the calves and other parts of the body; countenance sunken, altered in expression, and indicative of extreme anxiety; voice feeble or hoarse; marbled appearance of the skin; skin shrunken and shrivelled; cold breath; cold and pasty sweat; burning thirst; marked loss of power in the circulatory and respiratory organs.

Camphor, *veratrum*, *arsenicum*, *cuprum*, *acid hydrocianic*, *secale*, *laurocerasus*, and *carbo veg.*, have been most successful in the epidemic of 1848 and 1849, both in Europe and America.

Dr. Griesselich, of St. Petersburgh, considers *veratrum* by far the most important remedy in cholera. In Russia, this remedy was so notoriously efficacious, "*that the homœopathic drug shops were overrun by allopathic physicians and druggists to procure it.*"

Dr. G. found *acid phos.* exceedingly efficacious in *cholerine.*

In fully developed cholera asphyxia, as it occurred at Breslau in 1848 and 1849, Dr. Schweikert, of Breslau, found *ver.* first, and *secale* first, a drop every five minutes, *in alternation*, more commonly indicated than any other remedies. When asphyxia took place, Dr. S. relied upon *ac. phos.*, either alone or in alternation with *secale;* but in a few cases he used *tinct. phos.*, first or second dilution, with success.

Probably in no part of America did the cholera rage with more violence in 1849, than at Cincinnati, Ohio. Two physicians, Drs. Pulte and Ehrmann, treated 1,116 genuine cholera patients, in all stages of the disease, *and with a loss of only thirty-five*—two Americans and thirty-three Germans. These gentlemen also treated 1,350 cases of *cholerine*, and many cases of malignant dysentery, after the subsidence of the cholera, without the loss of a single patient. Of the cases of genuine cholera asphyxia, 538 had *vomiting, diarrhœa*, and *cramps*—70 of these being in a state of collapse, and the balance, 578, presented with *vomiting* and *rice-water* discharges. These last being subjected to prompt treatment, were speedily restored without the supervention of more serious symptoms.

The treatment adopted by Drs. P. and E. was as follows: in the *first stage* of the malady, *tinct. camphor*, one or two drops every five minutes for one to two hours, or until profuse perspiration ensued, which should be kept up for several hours, care being taken to keep the patient well covered. This remedy was perfectly effectual in almost every case during the early part of the disease. In the *second stage*, when cramps, general prostration, and rapid sinking of the physical energies appeared, *veratrum* when the cramps were in the lower extremities; *cuprum*, if in the bowels and breast, and *secale cornutum*, were relied on. The latter medicine was found of eminent service in elderly people. In cases of *decided collapse, arsenicum* and *carbo veg.* were the remedies employed. Mild frictions of the extremities with the hands alone, were the only external means made use of.

In St. Louis, New Orleans, and other cities of the west and south, a similar plan of treatment was adopted by homœopathic physicians, and with results which, for the most part, compare favourably with those detailed by Drs. Pulte and Ehrmann.

During the prevalence of cholera, much may be done towards warding off its attacks, and thus disarming it of a portion of its terrors. The most important rule which we would inculcate, is the cultivation of presence of mind under all circumstances, cheerfulness, contempt of danger, and strict temperance and regularity in all the habits of life. Other precautions are, frequent ablutions, so as to ensure perfect cleanliness, and a healthy action of skin, careful ventilation, frequent changes of body linen, moderate and agreeable exercise, good company, and a clear conscience.

As a prophylactic, many European authors have highly recommended camphor in tincture, in doses of a drop or two once or twice in twenty-four hours. From its extensive application as a medicinal antidote, we are disposed to believe that it may possess virtues of a high order, as an antidote against the poison of cholera.

The medicines which have been found, upon the whole, most serviceable in the treatment of this malady, as it occurs in different localities, and in its various forms, are, *veratrum*, *cuprum*, *arsenicum*, and *camphor*. Symptoms often supervene, also, which call for the exhibition of *secale cornutum*, *nux vomica*, *phosphorus*, *phosphoric acid*, *ipecacuanha*, and *carbo veg.*

Veratrum.—External indications.—General coldness of the surface of the body; cold perspiration on the face, and sometimes over the whole surface; skin white, or of a bluish tinge; bluish colour around the nails, and of the lips; contraction of the muscles of the extremities; nausea, vomiting, and purging; face pale, sunken, and hippocratic; nose cold and pointed; breath cold; pulse almost imperceptible; general appearance of prostration.

Physical sensations.—Painful cramps in the limbs; sensation of extreme debility and faintness; nausea; vomiting and purging; vertigo and confusion in the head; constrictive pain in the throat; oppressive and burning pain at the pit of the stomach; painful contraction of the abdomen; oppression in the chest;

fulness and pressure in the region of the heart; obstructed respiration; rumbling and griping in the bowels; thirst; great restlessness.

Mental and moral symptoms.—Excessive dejection, anguish and despair; constant disposition to turn from side to side, or otherwise to change position; sometimes loss of memory and stupidity.

Administration.—The first to the sixth dilution should be employed, a dose every ten, fifteen, or twenty minutes in urgent cases, and extending the intervals as the symptoms demand.

Arsenicum alb.—External indications.—Skin of a pale or bluish colour, and cold; face wan and cadaverous; eyes sunken; nose pointed; general expression of countenance unnatural and indicative of pain; lips bluish, or black and dry; trembling or stiffness in the limbs; skin cold and covered with a clammy sweat, or dry and shrivelled; pulse very weak, irregular, and trembling; watery discharges by vomiting and purging.

Physical sensations.—Burning pain in the stomach, worse after vomiting; cramps in the calves of the legs, toes and fingers; dizziness; nausea; frequent inclination to vomit and purge; rumbling in the bowels; ringing in the ears; feeling of extreme debility; very great restlessness and agitation; intense thirst, which affords but slight relief; spasmodic contraction and burning in the throat and œsophagus; cramp-like pains in the stomach and abdomen; frequent desire to pass water, or retention of urine; difficulty of respiration, with hoarseness; general sensation of coldness and loss of vitality.

Mental and moral symptoms.—Intense anguish, anxiety and discouragement; dread of death; constant uneasiness; confusion of ideas; delirium.

Administration.—The lower potencies of this medicine should be used, and in urgent cases, the doses may be repeated once in fifteen or twenty minutes until the symptoms yield. Some writers extol it highly in alternation with *veratrum*, and where either of these remedies does not afford prompt relief by itself, by all means let them be given in alternation.

Camphor.—It is not alone as a prophylactic that this

medicine has been advised. Hahnemann made use of it in all stages of cholera, but he found it particularly successful in the *first* stages of the malady, when vertigo, extreme weakness, cramps in the calves of the legs and muscles of the abdomen, burning and heat in the stomach, convulsive distortion of the features, eyes sunken, face and hands bluish and cold, anguish, dulness, loss of consciousness, and hoarseness, were present. It has been found most useful in those cases which have been almost entirely unattended with nausea, vomiting, and diarrhœa. It has in some instances restored patients who were apparently in *articulo mortis.*

Secale corn. and *cuprum* are appropriate remedies when there are distortion of the limbs; jerking and convulsive movements in the limbs ; great desire to sleep ; great coldness in the back, abdomen, and limbs ; cold clammy perspiration ; suppression of urine, and pains in the extremities.

Nux vomica may be used when the principal sufferings seem to be in the stomach, as anguish and oppression at the pit of the stomach, and severe spasms in the stomach, also tenesmus with an increase of the spasms at each discharge.

In some severe cases where the previous remedies have failed to afford relief, the practitioner should take into consideration, *phos.*, *phos. acid*, *ipecac.*, *carb. veg.* *canth.*, *sulph. ether*, *chloric ether*, *&c.*

SECTION XIV.

SPORADIC CHOLERA.—CHOLERA MORBUS.

Diagnosis.—Distressing nausea and vomiting, with great fulness and oppression at the stomach ; severe griping or colic pains in the umbilical region ; frequent watery discharges ; twisting and cramps in the abdominal muscles and calves of the legs ; tongue slightly furred ; pulse quick and weak ; countenance expressive of suffering and anxiety.

Causes.—Torpor of the liver ; obstruction of the biliary ducts ; unripe or decayed fruits ; crude esculent vegetables ; constant exposure to a cold and damp atmosphere.

Therapeutics.—The most efficacious medicines in the

treatment of this complaint, are, *veratrum, arsenicum, colocynth, chamomela, pulsatilla, ipecacuanha.*

Veratrum alb.—External indications.—Countenance pale or bluish, cold and disfigured; eyes sunken; nose pointed; mouth parched, lips dry or cracked, and of a dark colour; surface cold, or hot and dry; contraction of the muscles of the abdomen and extremities; pulse frequent and very weak; cold sweats; evacuations watery, light, greenish, or brownish.

Physical sensations.—Severe cutting pain in the umbilical region; violent nausea and vomiting, with diarrhœa; burning sensation in the stomach; speedy rejection of food or drinks; stomach and abdomen tender on pressure; cramps in the abdomen and in the extremities; extreme prostration; great oppression and distress at the stomach; intense thirst; general uneasiness.

Mental and moral symptoms.—Excessive anguish; fear of death; despair of recovery; delirium.

Administration.—This medicine may be used at from the first to the third dilution—a dose every half hour, in urgent cases, until the requisite impression is produced. In slight cases, two or three doses of the third dilution, at intervals of two to four hours, will suffice for the cure.

Arsenicum alb.—The indications for this remedy are somewhat similar to those of *veratrum*, but it is especially useful when the disease is violent from the commencement, attended with an almost immediate prostration of strength; trembling of the limbs; severe burning pain in the stomach; constant nausea and vomiting; diarrhœa; ringing in the ears; vertigo; giddiness; great anguish and restlessness; skin dry or cold, and bluish; hippocratic countenance; eyes sunken, dim, and suffused; thirst; distress from swallowing the blandest liquids; tongue and lips dry, dark, and cracked; breath cold; excessive anguish, anxiety and despair.

Administration.—Same as *veratrum.*

Colocynth will occasionally serve us in cases attended with moderate nausea, vomiting and purging; violent cramp-like pains in the region of the navel; cramps in the extremities; tongue loaded with a yellow fur; bitter taste in the mouth; great dejection and anxiety, and general restlessness. It may be given at the third potency every two hours, gradually lengthening the intervals as the pains subside.

Chamomela has been highly recommended when the disease has been "excited by a *fit of passion.*" The symptoms which point to this remedy, are, frequent vomiting of food, or of mucous, sour, or bitter substances; great anguish and pressure at the pit of the stomach; cramps in the calves of the legs when lying down; tearing and cutting pains in the abdomen.

Administration.—Same as *colocynth.*

Pulsatilla is chiefly useful in cholera which has been induced by the abuse of fat, crude, and indigestible food. In cases of this description, it is often promptly serviceable, administered at the first or second dilution, as circumstances require.

Ipecacuanha is the remedy when vomiting is the most prominent and troublesome symptom. It may be given at the third potency every half hour, until the symptoms abate—afterwards, as the exigences of the case demand.

SECTION XV.

DIARRHŒA.

Diagnosis.—Looseness of the bowels, with or without griping pains; discharges feculent, or thin and watery; respiration, circulation, skin, and the organs generally in a natural condition.

Causes.—Dentition, worms, irritating articles of food, cold, mental emotions, hectic fever, repelled eruptions, epidemic influences, &c.

Therapeutics.—For the diarrhœas which supervene during dentition, suitable remedies will be found in *chamomela, ipecacuanha, dulcamara, mercurius, sulphur, calcarea carb., rheum, coffea,* and *aconite.*

When the disease has been caused by the use of fat and indigestible food, and the discharges are pultaceous, mucous, liquid, or fœtid, attended with burning or excoriation of the anus, nausea, regurgitation, colic, and aggravation of the symptoms in the night, *pulsasatilla* is appropriate.

Dulcamara is a remedy of the very highest value,

in diarrhœas, and it covers a much wider range of symptoms than has generally been attributed to it. It has been employed principally in *watery* diarrhœas, which have arisen from cold; but we have used it with distinguished success in bowel complaints which have been caused by teething, worms, repelled eruptions, errors in diet, &c., and in which there were mucous, slimy, bilious, greenish and sanguineous evacuations. Dr. Rummel expresses the opinion that nine-tenths of all cases of diarrhœa may be cured with *dulcamara*, and we are satisfied that he is not very wide of the mark. It may be employed in the first or second dilution, and given in drop doses, with water, after each evacuation.

If the complaint appears to be characterized by prominent biliary derangement, specific medicines will be found in *mercurius, chamomela, pulsatilla, nux vom., arsenicum,* and *bryonia.*

If the discharges are mucous, slimy, or sanguineous, and preceded and accompanied by griping and tenesmus, our best remedies are, *acid nit.*, and *mercurius sol.*, in alternation. We may use the third attenuations,—a dose after each evacuation. Other remedies are, *arsenicum, ipecacuanha, sulphur, acid phos., acid sulph., petroleum, colocynth, veratrum, phosphorus,* and *dulcamara.*

For the diarrhœas which supervene during dentition, suitable remedies will be found in *chamomela, calcarea carb., ipecacuanha, rheum, magnesia carb., coffea, dulcamara, mercurius, sulphur.*

When bowel complaints arise in consequence of violent mental emotions, we employ *chamomela, ignatia, colocynth, veratrum, antimonium crud., coffea, nux vom., phosphorus, arsenicum, pulsatilla,* and *ferrum.*

If the discharges can be traced to the presence of worms, we give *sulphur, cina, spigelia, aloes, mercurius, nux vom., carbo veg., ferrum.*

For the diarrhœas which occur during hectic fevers, especially if connected with a scrofulous dyscrasia, the appropriate medicines are, *sulphur, calcarea carb., acid nit., acid phos., iodine, ferrum, mercurius, sepia, kalmia.*

For painless chronic diarrhœa, we suggest *phosphorus, ferrum, veratrum, china, natrum mur., acid nit., sulphur, lachesis, lycopodium, graphite, arsenicum.*

When the diarrhœa occurs during dentition and is connected with some chronic cutaneous affection, it will be necessary to exhibit *sulphur*, either alone, or in alternation with *dulcamara*, *chamomela*, or *mercurius*. It has not unfrequently occurred to us, that after *mercurius*, *chamomela*, and other apparently appropriate medicines have failed in arresting the relax, a few doses of *sulphur* has either put a stop to the malady, or placed the system in such a condition that it will respond readily to the remedies first employed.

Administration.—Our attenuations may range from the first to the sixth—one drop, if a dilution, or a grain, if a trituration, after each evacuation.

SECTION XVI.

HÆMORRHOIDS.—PILES.

Diagnosis.—This very common and troublesome complaint will probably demand the attention of the physician more frequently than any other single malady; nor, when we consider the causes which originate it, and their almost constant and universal prevalence, shall we be surprised at this. Any cause which operates upon the rectum in such a manner as to impair the integrity of its vascular and muscular structures, may induce the disease. The effects in these cases are, a permanent dilatation of the veins, and a relaxation of the mucous membrane of the part, causing tumours of various sizes, at the verge of the anus, and within the rectum, and in some instances, a protrusion of a portion of the rectum itself. When this last result obtains, we are presented with the disease known as *prolapsus ani*.

Hæmorrhoidal tumours may be *external* or *internal*—hard or soft—sensible or insensible. Their general appearance, in regard to colour, size, &c., will depend much upon the amount of inflammation present, the causes which have been in operation, and the length of time which has elapsed since the commencement of the malady. During a "fit of the piles," the tumours are usually red, or purple, inflamed, and painful, the pain is of a severe kind, aggravated to an almost intolerable degree when at stool, and accompanied by tenesmus and frequent discharges of blood. The location and character of the pains vary much in different cases, being sometimes confined to the tumours themselves, and at others extending upwards into the intestines, or into the perineum, down the thighs, &c. The pains may be itching, burning, aching, throbbing, darting, or shooting—constant, or only when at stool, or on sitting down.

When the mucous membrane of the rectum is much relaxed, we almost always have as a complication, *prolapsus ani.* Although this complaint sometimes originates independently of any hæmorrhoidal enlargements, in the majority of cases the two diseases are conjoined; and this is explicable from the circumstance that the causes of both are generally the same. The most common of these causes is habitual *constipation,* induced for the most part, by the reprehensible practice of inattention to daily alvine evacuations. We have before observed that the protracted presence of indurated fæcal matters in the rectum gives rise to a semi-paralytic condition, which impairs the tone of the parts, and thus induces *constipation, piles,* and *prolapsus ani.* The evils, then, to which this condition of the lower bowels give rise, may be summed up as follows: first, *constipation,* and the numerous and grave consequences which often result from it, in the form of determinations of blood to the brain, lungs, and intestinal canal; also mania, hypochondria, neuralgia, dyspepsia, bowel affections, colic, fistula in ano, &c.; second, *piles,* and its train of unpleasant symptoms; third, *prolapsus ani.*

Causes.—Other causes of these affections, in addition to the one already mentioned, are abuse of cathartics which operate specifically upon the lower portion of the intestinal tube, excessive exercise on horseback, long continuance in the standing posture, or in certain other constrained positions, protracted bowel complaints, general debility, dyscrasias, sedentary habits, indulgence in highly seasoned food, wines and liquors.

Therapeutics.—The first object with the physician in the treatment of hæmorrhoids, should be to ascertain the cause or causes upon which the malady depends, so that immediate and efficient measures may be taken to remove them. In a majority of instances the disease is unquestionably connected with *constipation;* which should therefore receive a due share of attention. Nothing can remove the torpid condition of the bowel, upon which the constipation depends, unless all indurated fæcal matters be removed daily, in order that sufficient time may elapse to enable the debilitated parts to recover their impaired tone. The first step necessary to secure this result, is to adopt suitable dietetic regulations. In many instances this alone will suffice to regulate the bowels, and thus to remove all traces of the hæmorrhoidal affection. Amongst the articles of food which we particularly commend in these cases, is bread made from unbolted wheat. A liberal and daily use of this highly nutritious substance, and of other articles of a similar character, with an occasional indulgence in ripe and wholesome fruits, will often surpass our most sanguine expectations in abolishing diseases of the rectum. Should these simple means alone prove ineffectual after a thorough trial, we may then call in the aid of enemeta of cold water. This last resource will rarely disappoint us, provided the case is recent, and the cause has not been very long in operation. When the hæmorrhoidal tumours are much inflamed and very painful, great service will frequently be derived from external applications of cold water, and in some instances, of ice enclosed in a linen cloth, and applied to the parts as long as may be deemed expedient. In troublesome cases of prolapsus ani, also, these applications and injections will sometimes afford prompt relief.

The medicines which are entitled to the highest consideration in the complaints under consideration are, *nux vomica, sulphur, rhus toxicod., sepia, bryonia, lycopodium, opium, pulsatilla, aloes, carbo vegetabilis,* and *calcarea carb.*

Nux vomica is appropriate when the disease has been caused by inactive and sedentary habits, high living, or the depressing mental emotions, and is attended by constipation, prolapsus, and general loss of power over the muscular structure of the rectum.

The second or third trituration may be employed—one grain every night as long as is deemed expedient.

Sulphur is well adapted to cases occurring in individuals tainted with syphilis, scrofula, psora, or mercury. If the piles bleed frequently and profusely, and there exists considerable inflammation of the surrounding mucous membrane, with darting pains up the bowel, tenesmus, discharges of mucus or of fæcal matters mixed with blood and mucus, this medicine will generally prove effective. It should be given at the third attenuation—one grain morning and evening until the desired effect is produced.

Rhus tox., in alternation with *sulphur* or *nux*, has been eminently useful in piles and prolapsus conjoined, which appeared to be connected with some latent impurity of the blood. We are accustomed to use the first or second attenuations in these cases—giving a dose daily, and changing the medicine every other week.

When the hæmorrhoidal tumours protrude, and are inflamed, red and painful, with profuse hæmorrhage during each evacuation, we may consider *acid nit.*, *acid mur.*, *aloes*, *calcarea carb.*, and *sepia*.

If the disease arises during pregnancy, and constipation is unusually obstinate, we advise *pulsatilla*, *opium*, *bryonia* and *platina*.

Administration.—This malady responds most satisfactorily to the first, second, and third attenuations—given in grain or drop doses once or twice in twenty-four hours.

SECTION XVII.

ACUTE HEPATITIS.—INFLAMMATION OF THE LIVER.

Diagnosis.—When the disease occupies the *convex* surface of the liver, we shall have fulness and severe pain in the region of the liver, increased on pressure, either of a sharp, aching, or burning character; pains extending into the chest, under the clavicle, between the shoulder blades, into the top of the right shoulder, and sometimes down the arm; short, dry cough; dyspnœa; difficulty in lying upon the left side; hot and dry skin; thirst; scanty and high-coloured urine; constipation; clay-coloured evacuations; full, hard, and frequent pulse; headache, and more or less mental disorder. If the inflammation is in the *concave* portion of the liver, we shall have, in addition to the symptoms already enumerated, distressing nausea and vomiting; tongue covered with a white or yellow fur; bitter taste; urgent thirst; an aggravation of the pain in the hypochondrium on pressure; urine scanty, and of a dark yellow or saffron colour; eyes and skin tinged with yellow; bowels constipated or relaxed; pains in the back and limbs; ideas confused; mind clouded or delirious.

In most instances of acute hepatitis, it is highly probable that the peritoneal covering of the liver is implicated to a greater or less extent, and this may serve to render the pains more severe, and the accompanying symptoms more violent.

CHRONIC HEPATITIS.

Diagnosis.—The symptoms of chronic liver complaint are somewhat similar to those of the acute form, but much more mild in their character. For example, the pain in the right hypochondrium is dull, heavy, and dragging, that in the shoulder and arm of a vague and heavy kind; the skin is somewhat hot and dry; the tongue furred; the countenance and albuginea yellow; the urine and perspiration of a dark or yellowish colour; the bowels costive, sometimes alternating with relax; evacuations light; occasional cramp-like pains in the stomach; great weakness and loss of energy throughout the entire system; inclination to sleep a good part of the time; trembling of the knees on the slightest exercise; dejection and indifference to life; enlargement and induration of the liver.

Causes.—This is a disease of hot rather than of temperate latitudes, and may arise from a too free use of animal food, stimulating drinks, and other articles abounding in carbon. As the blood passes through the liver, its office is to separate the carbon, &c., which is not wanted in the system. We can, therefore, readily perceive how prone this important organ must be to be overtasked, in so rarefied a temperature, unless the utmost care is taken to retain the organs in a healthy state, as well as to avoid highly seasoned animal food, stimulants, &c.

The chronic form of hepatitis often follows, and is a consequence of dyspepsia. Indeed, there are but few, if any, cases of the latter disorder, which are entirely unattended with derangement of the liver.

Want of exercise, depression of spirits, misfortune, sudden suppression of perspiration, accustomed discharges, &c., may often exercise a powerful influence in inducing this disease.

Therapeutics.—Aconite, mercurius, china, eupatorium, perfoliatum, nux vomica, bryonia, sulphur, conium, taraxacum, pulsatilla, lachesis.

Administration.—The medicines may be used from the first to the sixth attenuations, and repeated, in acute cases, every two, four, or six hours according to circumstances. In chronic hepatitis, a dose of the appropriate specific should be given once or twice in the twenty-four hours, at the same time inculcating the importance of rigid dietetic regulations.

In chronic hepatitis, there is a peculiarly dry and harsh state of the skin, and on this account we strongly advise the daily use of *cold sponging, or bathing*, to be followed by vigorous exercise, in order that the pores may be opened, and the cutaneous functions thus restored.

CHAPTER XXIII.

DISEASES OF THE RESPIRATORY ORGANS.

GENERAL OBSERVATIONS.

In all of our investigations touching affections of the lungs and their appendages, whether acute or chronic, a few preliminary inquiries are essential, in order that we may be able to arrive at accurate opinions respecting the seat, nature, treatment, and probable termination of each particular case. Although we are to be governed, as a general rule, by *symptoms*, yet certain constitutional or accidental peculiarities, connected with a given train of symptoms, might induce us to select one specific in preference to another, which was equally homœopathic to the disease. Thus, cough, copious expectoration, pains in the chest, and tickling in the throat, &c., which had followed immediately upon the suppression of some chronic eruption, might be completely covered by *bryonia, ipecacuanha, phosphorus, phosphoric acid, staphysagria, silicea*, &c., so far as the mere *symptoms* are concerned; but who would not prefer, in cases of this description, *sulphur*, or some other specific which would have a tendency to reproduce the eruption, while, at the same time, it would be perfectly homœopathic to these indications? So in regard to temperament, habits of life, occupation, medicinal symptoms, age, sex, climate, &c., our remedies should always be selected in such a manner as to bear upon any occult miasm, or other latent cause which may be operating upon the organism, and thus either directly or indirectly aggravating and complicating the apparent symptoms.

When called to treat lung diseases, therefore, let the physician inquire, first, Is there any hereditary predisposition on the part of the patient to scrofula, consumption, dropsy, erysipelas, nettle-rash, syphilis, &c.? Second, Is the chest well developed and symmetrical, so that the lungs can have ample room to perform their functions? Third, Is the subject, during health, put out of breath by slight exertion? Fourth, Has the malady supervened on, or shortly after the disappearance of an eruption? Fifth, Do all parts of the chest dilate equally and properly during inspiration, and is the respiration natural during health?

Respecting this last question, it is proper to observe that a difference of opinion exists amongst authors, Laennec considering respiration natural "when the anterior and lateral parts of the chest dilate equally, distinctly, yet moderately, during inspiration, and when the number of inspirations, in a state of repose, is from twelve to fifteen in the minute;" while Andral, Broussais, Müller, Forbes, and others, suppose that Laennec has placed the mean number of inspirations too low. These gentlemen assure us that the "mean average of respirations is more than sixteen or eighteen in the minute, in the healthy adult, and that most persons in health breathe from eighteen to twenty-four times in a minute." From much observation in reference to this subject, we are disposed to adopt the opinion of Laennec, rather than that of Andral, &c., and therefore estimate the mean number of respirations in a healthy adult at fifteen or sixteen in a minute.

We beg leave in this place to recommend, in strong terms, the use of *auscultation* and *percussion* in the investigation of chest diseases, if for no other reason than to form an accurate diagnosis and prognosis. In order to acquire skill in the use of the stethoscope, percussion, &c., a patient and careful course of study and practice upon both healthy and diseased subjects, is indispensable. By this means, the physician will be able to pronounce with certainty the seat and nature of the malady, and its probable termination. As we advance in our descriptions of the different affections of the respiratory organs, we shall point out the peculiar sounds elicited by percussion and auscultation, in the several varieties of disease.

SECTION I.

CATARRH, CORYZA, OR COLD.

Diagnosis.—This disease consists of an inflammation of the mucous membrane lining the frontal sinuses and the nostrils. It usually commences with lassitude, a sense of coldness, slight shiverings, sneezing; dull and heavy feeling in the head, succeeded in a short time by lachrymation; more or less obstruction in the nose; sense of fulness, or pain in the region of the frontal cavities; swelling or inflammation of the nostrils; nose dry and tender, or constant discharge of mucus, of a mild, burning, or corrosive character; eyes inflamed, watery, and sensitive to light; buzzing, or roaring in the ears; drowsiness, heaviness, and dull pains in the head; chills, alternating with flushes of heat; pains and soreness in the limbs and bones; thirst, worse in the night; cold sores upon the lips; stupid, languid, and indifferent, or irritable and ill-humoured.

When the inflammation extends to the mucous membrane of the throat, larynx, and trachea, it has received the name of

INFLUENZA, (INFLUENZE DELL ARIA,) OR, INFLUENCE OF THE COLD.

In addition to the symptoms just enumerated, we have, febrile symptoms; hoarseness; severe cough, either dry and racking, or hollow and loose; wheezing, or difficult respiration; impaired appetite; soreness, oppression, or stitches in the throat and chest on coughing; incapacity for mental or physical exertion; bowels constipated or relaxed.

Sometimes the inflammation appears to extend to the membrane of the thorax and of the bronchial tubes, giving rise to sharp, stitching pains, or a sensation of rawness in these parts, severe and painful chest cough, thick, tenacious, and semi-purulent expectoration, oppression of the chest, and difficult respiration. In these instances, the inflammation is of a lower grade than obtains in acute bronchitis, pleuritis, or laryngitis, and, consequently, the symptoms are more slight and less dangerous. In some cases, the disease commences with soreness and burning in the scorbiculus cordis, which gradually extends to the chest and throat, nose and head, when coryza, obstruction of the nose, and other signs of influenza, manifest themselves.

Therapeutics.—The chief remedies are, *nux, arsenicum, mercurius, dulcamara, ammonium, carbon, ipecacuanha, causticum, belladonna, bryonia, pulsatilla, chamomela.* When the complaint is attended with marked febrile excitement from the first, our treatment should always commence with *aconite;* but when the local symptoms manifest themselves without much constitutional disturbance, we may commence with the appropriate local specific immediately.

For common cold, with evening chills, sneezing, free discharge of thick, yellow, green, or offensive matter, loss of smell, taste, and appetite, pain and fulness in the region of the frontal sinuses, *pulsatilla* is specific.

Drs. Shue and Taft have found *tartar emetic*, at the first or second attenuation, the most efficient remedy in the early part of the influenzas which usually prevail in this region.

Nux vomica, ipecacuanha, and *arsenicum*, will also be found appropriate in many instances of the complaint, as it occurs in this latitude.

My friend, Dr. Shue, has employed *sabina* with excellent success in several cases of *chronic catarrh* occurring in females. The cases which have responded the most promptly to this remedy, have been those in which the catarrhal discharge appeared to alternate with *leucorrhœa*, disappearing when the *fluor albus* was profuse, and returning again at every suppression or material diminution of the discharge.

If *hoarseness* be an attendant symptom, and proceeds from an inflammation of the mucous membrane of the larynx, *causticum, bryonia, capsicum, carbo veg., mercurius, rhus tox.* and *belladonna* are our best remedies.

When the hoarseness has arisen from loss of tone of the nerves of the throat, an alternation of *carbo veg.* with *nux vom.*, will usually prove curative. *Belladonna, causticum*, and *mercurius* will also occasionally demand our attention.

"Hoarseness, with bruised and pricking sensation in the larynx, coryza, moist cough, pain in the chest, and complete loss of voice, responds to *pulsatilla*."—*Croserio.*

Administration.—We usually prescribe from the first to the third attenuations; the doses to be repeated, in severe cases, once in two to four hours, according to circumstances, and in chronic cases, once or twice daily.

SECTION II.

CYNANCHE TRACHEALIS.—CROUP.

Until the present century this disease was confounded with hooping cough, asthma, and bronchitis, and the fatal cases were supposed to be violent forms of one of these maladies.

In the hands of the allopath, croup has ever proved

a most formidable and fatal disease. Acting, in the application of their remedial measures, only indirectly upon the part affected, by venesection, leeches, blisters, emetics, mercurial cathartics, expectorants, &c., it is not a matter of surprise that they are so often baffled in subduing a malady of so violent a character as the one under consideration.

It is especially in diseases of this nature, that the truth and value of a system of practice may be satisfactorily tested; for it is here that a prompt, efficient, and specific remedy is imperatively demanded, in order that the progressing inflammation may be at once arrested, and the patient saved. These are the cases which try the truth and soundness of a theory: which convince the *public*,—who appreciate *facts*, if they do not comprehend abstruse theories—which school possess the knowledge and skill that should command approbation and support. On the result of these tests we are willing to rest the claims of homœopathy. Indeed, the records of the homœopathic practice show conclusively a large balance in its favour, over the other systems, in all maladies of an acute as well as chronic character.

Croup rarely occurs after the age of seven years, and may therefore be accounted a disease almost peculiar to childhood. Its seat is the mucous membrane of the larynx, trachea and bronchia, and sometimes of the fauces and palate.

Diagnosis.—Croup may with propriety be divided into two principal varieties, viz.: first, the *false*, *pseudo*, or *non-membranous;* comprising, however, under this head, the *spasmodic*, *catarrhal*, and *slightly inflammatory* kinds; and second, the *true*, or *membranous* croup.

Some recent writers have distinguished *four* distinct varieties, each one forming a distinct and independent disease, and not liable to run into either of the other forms.

It is doubtless true that these several varieties do often exist as distinct and clearly defined maladies, and that the remedies homœopathic to these varieties are also entirely distinct, but we are by no means certain that the different forms do not run into each other.

Be this as it may, it is of importance that an accurate knowledge should be acquired respecting the seat, nature and symptoms of the malady in all its forms, so that we can exhibit without delay a remedy which shall be truly specific and homœopathic. First, *False or non-membranous croup.*

Spasmodic croup usually makes its appearance suddenly, with considerable difficulty of breathing, noisy and wheezing inspirations, a short, *dry*, hoarse cough, occurring but rarely, and an entire absence of febrile symptoms.

Catarrhal croup also commences suddenly, with a "croupy cough, hoarse voice, shrill, wheezing, and sonorous inspirations, oppression and tightness at the chest, and sudden attacks of dyspnœa; *but in a few days the croupy character will wear off of itself, leaving simple catarrhal symptoms only.*"—(*Watson.*)

In the *simple inflammatory* croup, in addition to the loud, harsh, and wheezing respiration, and hoarse, croupy cough, we have usually sore throat, some thirst, and nightly febrile exacerbations. This, like the preceding variety, will often wear off spontaneously, leaving only some slight symptoms behind.

An important peculiarity of all the varieties of false croup, consists in the *suddenness* of their attacks. Children may retire to their beds in the most perfect health, and yet in an hour or two be disturbed from a sound sleep with an apparently alarming attack of croup. It is important, however, that all should be aware that these seemingly dangerous cases are much less to be dreaded than those which make their appearance in a more slow and insidious manner, as will be seen by the following description of the *true* croup. In all of the varieties above described, although there may be very difficult, laboured, anxious, and wheezing respiration, hoarse, harsh, and croupy cough, hoarse voice, and the patient may seem to be in imminent danger of suffocation, yet the fact that the attack has occurred *suddenly*, and that the cough bears no resemblance to the dreadful *metallic* cough of real croup, will afford us sure indications of its nature, and enable us to assure those interested that the attack will speedily be subdued.

Second, *True* or *membranous croup* is usually ushered in with the ordinary symptoms of catarrh, as chilliness, sneezing, some soreness of the throat, hot skin, thirst, slightly accelerated pulse, hoarse voice, and some little impediment in respiration. At this period a whistling or "buzzing sound may be heard at the rima glottidis, by placing the ear upon the back of the neck, or over the larynx."—(*Ware.*) Even at this early period the commencement of the false membrane may be observed upon the tonsils, and sometimes upon the uvula and pharynx, which gradually increases in thickness and strength unless the peculiar inflammation be arrested.

As the disease advances, the febrile symptoms increase, the respiration gradually becomes more laboured and difficult, the inspirations, particularly after coughing, being slow, sawing, sonorous or ringing, while the expirations are quick, the cough is dry and gives forth a *metallic* sound, the voice becomes more shrill, the pulse is frequent and small, the expression of countenance swollen and anxious, the head is thrown back, the extremities are cold, while the rest of the body retains its exalted temperature, there is often a profuse perspiration, until finally the respiration is so much impeded that the blood is but slightly oxygenated, the cheeks and lips become livid, the eyes red and sunken, the pulse extremely small and frequent, the whole organism prostrated, and the child expires in a state of asphyxia or suffocation.

In membranous croup the inflammation is of a peculiar character ; for from the very commencement of the attack, the mucous membrane continues to pour out coagulable lymph, which becomes adherent to the parts affected, forming the tough artificial tube known as the false membrane. We believe that the progress of this fictitious formation is never entirely arrested until a healthy medicinal inflammation is made to supersede the peculiar morbid action.

"The false membrane which so frequently forms on blisters, is, of itself, sufficient to prove that it is much less to the *degree* than to the *nature* of the inflammation, that we are to attribute this concretion or coagulation of pus in certain cases."—(*Laennec.*)

Causes.—A cold and damp atmosphere, wet feet, and exposure to the air which blows from seas and lakes. It appears to be necessary also that there should be a certain predisposition on the part of the patient, in order to contract the disease, since all of the children of some families are constantly liable to its attacks, while those of other families, constantly exposed to precisely the same influences, are exempted. This predisposition may frequently be traced back through several generations, while in other families the reverse is true, no instances of the malady having ever been known to exist in them. Croup sometimes follows as a sequence of scarlatina, measles, &c., and has by some writers been confounded with the former disease, and from this circumstance has originated the idea of its contagious nature.

Therapeutics:

Spasmodic croup.—Aconite, spongia, hyoscyamus, belladonna, nux, musk, cuprum, ipecacuanha, camphor and *lobelia inflat.*

Catarrhal croup.—Aconite, tartar emetic, spongia, hepar sulph, drosera, lachesis, sambucus, chamomile, and *nux.*

Simple inflammatory croup.—Aconite, spongia, hepar, tartar emetic, phosphorus, iodine, and *belladonna.*

True or membraneous croup.—Kali, bichrom, bromine, ammonia caustic, hepar sulph., argentum nit., sambucus, spongia and iodine, senega, tartar emetic.

We introduce the following excellent indications for the employment of *spongia, hep. sulph., bromine, caustic ammon., bichrom,* and *potash,* arranged by several homœopathic physicians in Pressburgh, and translated by Ch. J. Hempel, M. D., for the Homoœopathic Examiner.

SPONGIA—CROUP.

"Hollow cough; with expectoration; with pain in the chest and trachea; roughness in the throat; (night-cough with weeping expression); breathing aggravated, as from a plug in the throat, slow or quick; panting; larynx painful, as if from pressure—worse when touched; scratching, burning, and constrictive sensation in the larynx; painful feeling of swelling in the cervical glands near the larynx and trachea; stinging in the throat and sensation in the outer parts of the neck, as if something were pressing out, morning and evening; painful tension, on the left side of and near the apple of Adam, when turning the head to the right side; the eyes are sunken; the urine deposits a thick, grayish-white sediment; general morning sweat; pulse quick and hard; drowsiness; lassitude of the whole body; out of humour; everything puts him out of humour, even talking and answering questions."

HEPAR CROUP.

"Violent fits of cough, as if one would suffocate or vomit; deep; occasioned by tightness of breathing; husky, accompanied with painful soreness of the chest at every turn of cough; violent; the air rushing violently against the larynx, which causes a pain in that part; scraping; scratching; with mucous expectoration; the cough being occasioned by titillation in the throat, or by a scraping in the trachea; increased unto vomiting by a deep inspiration; weakness of the organs of speech and chest, preventing her from talking aloud; short breathing; pressure in the throat, occasioning a constrictive feeling, as if he should be suffocated; urine pale, clear while being emitted, afterwards becoming turbid and thick, depositing a white sediment: or flocculent, turbid while being emitted: dark-yellow: burning during emission; great, unconquerable drowsiness; profuse sweat day and night; viscid, profuse night sweat; sweat before midnight; sad; apprehensive; inclined to weep."

BROMINE CROUP.

"Formation of pseudo membrane in the larynx and trachea; spasm in the larynx occasioning suffocation; cough with croup-sound, hoarse, wheezing, fatiguing, not permitting one to utter a word; accompanied with sneezing; with violent suffocative fits; respiration characterized by mucous rattling; wheezing; alternately slow and suffocative, and hurried and superficial; laboured; painful; oppressed; gasping for air;

heat in the face; increased secretion of urine; pulse rather hard; slow at first, afterwards accelerated."

CAUSTIC AMMONIA CROUP.

"Deep, weak voice; fatiguing, interrupted speech; increased secretion of mucus in the bronchi; violent cough, with copious expectoration of mucus, especially after drinking; difficult, rattling, laboured breathing; stertorous breathing; suffocative fits; spasm of the chest."

BICHROMATE OF POTASH CROUP.

"Symptoms approach gradually and insidiously; at first, slight difficulty of breathing when the mouth is closed; slight elevation of temperature; pulse irregular and intermittent, or frequent and small; as the disease progresses, the difficulty of breathing increases; the sound of the air as it passes through the trachea is shrill, whistling, as if it passed through a metallic tube; voice hoarse; cough not frequent, but hoarse, dry, barking, and *metallic*; deglutition painful; tonsils and larynx red, swollen, and covered with an appearance of false membrane; after a time, breathing affected in part by the action of the abdominal muscles, and those of the neck and shoulder-blades; head inclined backwards; breath offensive; finally, diminished temperature of the skin; prostration; stupor."

The medicines, of which the pathogenetic symptoms we have here detailed, are those which are most completely specific against croup. It is true that the other articles alluded to, as *aconite*, *iodine*, *belladonna*, *nux*, *hyoscyamus*, *sambucus*, *tartar emetic*, *lachesis*, *phosphorus*, *drosera*, *arsenicum*, &c., cover many of the symptoms usually present, especially in non-membraneous croup, but they cannot be considered positive and reliable specifics against the disease fully developed. So far, however, as certain special indications are concerned, these medicines may often be employed with very great advantage.

The following is Dr. Bosh's method of treating croup: "If the disease begins, as it frequently does, with an inflammatory fever, then I give first, according to circumstances, every quarter to half hour, one to two drops of *aconite* (the dilution second or third, depending upon the age), and then I let the child rest from one to two hours, when I give the remedy, which I found in my practice to be the main remedy, *spongia*, first, second, or third dilutions, according to the severity of the disease; eight drops in four ounces of water, of this every quarter to half hour, or, in less intense cases only every hour, half a table spoonful. If the disease has proceeded further, and paralytic signs are perceptible (by continued obstruction of the respiration, congestions to the brain, &c.), then I give *spongia* alternately with *phosphorus*. If, notwithstanding these means, the disease increases, I give *spongia* in alternation with *tartar stibiatus*."

Tartar emetic is not only useful in the early stage of croup, but it is also indicated when there are signs indicative of partial paralysis of the pneumo-gastric nerve, viz., face livid and cold; cold sweat on the forehead or body; respiration exceedingly difficult, short, hoarse, shrill, or whistling; head thrown back; pulse small and rapid, or feeble and slow; great weakness, anxiety, and uneasiness; difficulty in swallowing; short, hoarse, and barking cough; disposition to sleep. The remedy should be given in the first attenuation, and the dose repeated every twenty or thirty minutes, until relief is obtained.

In *spasmodic* croup, Dr. Dunsford relies upon *aconite*, *hyoscyamus* and *belladonna*.

When, in addition to high febrile excitement, the local croupy symptoms are urgent, we must alternate the proper local specific with *aconite*. In this way we may often give *spongia*, or *hepar sulph.* and *aconite* advantageously in the first instance, or *tartar emetic* and *aconite*. When the disease obstinately resists *aconite*, *spongia*, *hepar sulph.*, *tartar emetic*, both alone and in alternation, we may consult *phosphorus*, *lachesis*, *sambucus*, *senega pol.*, &c.

As we progress in the knowledge of medicinal substances, a still greater number of pure specifics will undoubtedly be added to our Materia Medica.

Before taking leave of this subject, we ask attention particularly to the employment of one remedy previously named, for the cure of membraneous croup. We refer to the *nitrate of silver* as a direct application to the affected membrane. For some years, we have been in the habit of employing a strong solution of this salt, by means of a sponge moistened with it and introduced into the larynx; and in several instances the most satisfactory results have followed. This remedy has been used to a considerable extent by French allopathists, and within the last few years by a number of American physicians, and in many cases they have saved life when every other means had failed. The principle on which it cures, however, is strictly homœopathic, for it is due solely to the *medicinal*, or *artificial action of the remedy*, that the morbid croupy inflammation is superseded, and the false membrane gradually destroyed and expelled.

It may be used in any stage of true croup, and will sometimes succeed in effecting a cure when every internal remedy has failed.

A little tact will enable the physician to apply the solution to the larynx, or trachea, in an efficient manner, and with perfect safety. For minute directions upon the subject, the reader may consult "Trousseau and Belloc," and Dr. Green's work upon Bronchitis, &c., published in New York.

Administration.—In the treatment of croup, we generally employ the lower potencies. In regard to the repetition of doses, no definite rules can be given, but the practitioner must be guided by the variety of the disease, the severity of the symptoms, and the effects of his remedies.

SECTION III.

ACUTE BRONCHITIS.

This complaint is of most frequent occurrence in old age and in childhood. Its seat is in the mucous membrane of the bronchia, but authors assure us that the bronchial inflammation is always accompanied with considerable "sanguineous congestion of the lungs." Effusion into the substance of the lungs, is peculiarly apt to occur in this disease, and it is to this circumstance that its danger is to be attributed.

Diagnosis.—Constriction and aching sensation, extending over the whole chest; breathing very much oppressed, quick, anxious, irregular, laboured; the voluntary muscles of respiration often called into play; expectoration at first dry, soon becomes viscid and frothy, and sometimes streaked with blood; more or less cough, hoarse and painful in children; throbbing pain in the forehead and aching pain in the eyes, aggravated on coughing; face red or pallid; tongue moist, and covered with a white fur; bowels costive; temperature of the skin nearly natural, but sometimes hot and dry; pulse at first but little increased in frequency, becoming, as the disease advances, very rapid; urine scanty and high coloured; vertigo; rattling in the throat and chest; wheezing respiration. As the malady approaches towards a fatal termination, the skin becomes suffused with a cold perspiration; the cheeks and lips pale and livid; the extremities cold; rattling and sense of suffocation in the throat; extreme prostration and complete insensibility.

The peculiar respiration (the mucous rale or rattle of Laennec) which is so apparent in bronchitis, is owing to the "passage of air through the diseased secretion of the air-passages, and may be heard by placing the ear to the chest, long before it becomes so severe as to be distinguished by any other means."—*McIntosh.*

The inflammation in bronchitis is of a much more intense character than that which is present in *catarrh* or *influenza*, and there is always more or less sanguineous congestion of the lungs. Many of the more urgent symptoms of the complaint are due to this last circumstance, like the great difficulty of breathing; the painful sense of tightness; stricture and oppression in the chest; wheezing respiration; severe cough; pallid countenance; vertigo; pain in the head, &c. During the progress of this disease, the substance of the lungs often becomes hepatized.

CHRONIC BRONCHITIS.

Chronic bronchitis is at the present time an exceedingly common and fashionable disease. From the fact of its occurring for the most part in clergymen, lawyers, and other public speakers, it has acquired "*caste*," and therefore, it may be that every slight affection of the respiratory apparatus is now denominated *bronchitis*. It occurs at all periods of life, and in general, is insidious in its approach, though it occasionally succeeds to acute bronchitis.

When the disease follows an acute attack, the patient will be left with some cough; expectoration of viscid or puriform sputa; dyspnœa on the slightest exertion; nocturnal exacerbations of fever; emaciation, and in some instances hectic symptoms.

The stethoscope usually gives us the sound of the crepitous ronchus at certain points, and now and then over the whole chest, while at the same time the respiratory murmur may often be heard.

Those cases which come on more insidiously, will be often found complicated with chronic laryngitis, indicated by *hoarseness* of the voice; raw or scraping sensation in the larynx, and extending over the chest; copious expectoration of opaque or purulent sputa, which affords relief to the patient; hoarse, hollow, and painful cough; increased susceptibility to changes of temperature; night sweats, and general debility.

When the expectoration is copious, we shall have the crepitous ronchus, either at isolated points or over the whole chest; but if there is no expectoration, then the sound which will be elicited by auscultation, resembles snoring, and has been termed "*dry sonorous rattle*;" or in some instances, the "*sibilous rattle*," like the chirping of birds. Laennec also mentions a "clicking" sound, which he compares to the action of a valve.

Percussion affords us no aid in our investigations of bronchitis, but pressure with the hand upon the chest, will often enable us to detect the mucous rattle without difficulty.

Causes.—Protracted exposure to cold; alternations from heat to cold; inhalations of dust and other irritative substances; insufficient clothing, and improper exposure of the throat and neck, after much talking, public speaking, or singing.

We believe that one great cause of the very frequent occurrence of chronic bronchitis, may be found in the reprehensible fashion of shaving the beard. That this ornament was given by the Creator for some useful purpose, there can be no doubt, for in fashioning the human body, he gave nothing unbecoming a perfect man, nothing useless, nothing superfluous. Hair being an imperfect conductor of caloric, is admirably calculated to retain the animal warmth of that part of the body which is so constantly and necessarily exposed to the weather, and thus to protect this important portion of the respiratory passage from the injurious effects of sudden checks of perspiration.

When one exercises for hours his vocal organs, with the unremitted activity of a public declamation, the pores of the skin, in the vicinity of the throat and chest, become relaxed, so that when he enters the open air, the whole force of the atmosphere bears upon these parts, and he sooner or later contracts a bronchitis; while, had he the flowing beard with which his Maker has endowed him, uncut, to protect these important parts, he would escape any degree of exposure unharmed.

The fact that Jews and other people who wear the beard long, are but rarely afflicted with bronchitis and analogous disorders, suggests a powerful argument in support of these views.

Therapeutics.—The medicines most worthy of consideration in the treatment of acute and chronic bronchitis, are, *aconite, tartar emetic, belladonna, bryonia, hepar sulphur, carbo vegetabilis, spongia, ammonium carb., rhus tox., mercurius, sulphur, sambucus, arsenicum, digitalis, hyoscyamus, pulsatilla.*

As in other inflammatory diseases, *aconite* is also indicated in acute bronchitis, whenever there is a rapid and full pulse, hot skin, and other symptoms indicative of a high state of febrile excitement. It may be given at the second or third potency, and repeated every hour until a decided amendment ensues.

Tartar emetic is indicated when there are severe paroxysms of coughing, with suffocating obstruction of respiration; wheezing respiration; mucous ronchus; very great shortness of breath, with anxious oppression at the chest; great anxiety and agitation; palpitation of the heart; pain in the back and loins; pressure on the eyes; pains in the head; thirst.

Administration.—A grain of the first trituration of

tartar emetic, to four ounces of water—a teaspoonful every one, two, three, or four hours, as the urgency of the symptoms may demand.

In cases of acute bronchitis in which the predominant symptoms are, oppression and weight at the chest; short, anxious and rapid respiration; shaking, spasmodic cough, and decided cerebral disturbance from the commencement, *belladonna* is our most valuable remedy.

Administration.—Like that of *aconite.*

The indications which point to *bryonia*, are, headache aggravated by movement; pressure in the eyes; dryness in the throat; respiration difficult, short, and anxious; pressure on the chest as if from a weight; stingings in the chest; cough with stingings in the chest, or with severe aching pains in the head. In the acute attacks of children, with suffocative cough, very great oppression at the chest, exceedingly difficult, rapid, and anxious or sighing respiration, loud mucous ronchus, rapid pulse, hot skin, thirst, great agitation and anxiety, this remedy is also especially called for.

It may be exhibited at the first to the sixth potency, and frequently repeated until the disease subsides. The practitioner may sometimes alternate it with *aconite*, with benefit. *Pulsatilla* is indicated in bronchitis when the cough is dry in the first part of the complaint, but soon becomes moist, "with easy expectoration of abundant yellow and bitter, or saline and disgusting matter; sometimes with nausea or retching, or a sensation of reversion in the stomach, as if about to vomit. The cough occurs principally at night, on lying down; proceeds from a tickling or itching in the larynx, or by scraping and dryness in the trachea, accompanied with fatiguing pains in the abdomen, and stitches in the back, shoulders, sides, or chest, and relieved on rising up in bed."—(*Croserio*). It may be given in the same manner as *bryonia.*

In *chronic bronchitis,* characterized by anxious, hoarse, and wheezing respiration, much aggravated on lying down; attacks of suffocation, which force the patient to throw the head back, in order to take breath; dyspnœa; dry, rough, and hollow cough;

cough, with expectoration of mucus; hoarseness of voice; exacerbations of fever in the after part of the day, succeeded by night sweats, *hepar sulph.* is an important specific. In cases which seem to have been connected with suppression of salt rheum, or other eruptive disease, or metastases of arthritic inflammations, this remedy should always be borne in mind. It is also useful in those cases which threaten to terminate in tubercular consumption.

The third trituration may be used: a dose from two to four times in twenty-four hours.

When bronchitis is complicated with *angina trachealis*, we may resort to *spongia tosta* with confidence, either alone or in alternation with *hepar sulph.* If febrile symptoms run high, these remedies should be preceded by *aconite.*

When suffocation is threatened from loss of tone and power of the respiratory organs, rendering them incapable of expelling the morbid secretions which obstruct the free entrance of air into the pulmonary structure, *ammonium carb.*, *rhus tox.*, *sambucus*, *arsenicum*, *digitalis*, *hyoscyamus*, and *stannum*, are worthy of careful examination. In making our selection from these medicines, regard should not only be had to the actual symptoms present, but to the temperament, hereditary predisposition, and the remote cause of the malady. For example, if in any given case the indications actually present, point equally to *hepar sulph.* and *rhus tox.*, but the attack was found to be connected with a repelled eruption, our choice would evidently rest upon the former medicine; while if the disease was found to be dependent upon an arthritic habit, *rhus* would be the appropriate remedy.

In the last stages of acute bronchitis, when there is danger that the malady will run into the chronic form, *sulphur* has been highly lauded by many eminent practitioners. If the disease occurs in persons of lymphatic constitutions, and subject to eruptions, swelling of the glands, &c., this remedy can scarcely be dispensed with during the progress of the attack.

For the profuse and debilitating sweats which now and then occur during the continuance of the symptoms, valuable specifics will be found in *mercurius*, *acid nit.*, and *acid phos.* Many physicians have commended *carbo veg.* in the strongest terms, in *chronic bronchitis*, and it has doubtless effected many excellent cures. It may be used at the third attenuation, one grain once or twice daily.

SECTION IV.

PNEUMONIA.—LUNG FEVER.

Diagnosis.—The symptoms of lung fever vary so much in different cases, that an exact portrait, which shall be recognisable in all instances, can hardly be given. The signs, however, which are more particularly characteristic, may be enumerated as follows: dull or deep-seated pain, or a tightness in the chest; frequent short cough, with expectoration of a viscid, tenacious matter, of a yellow, green, or pale colour, sometimes tinged with blood; rapid and difficult respiration; inclination for the most part to lie upon the affected side, or the back; great heat of the skin; headache; thirst; rapid and full pulse (though this last symptom is by no means uniformly present, as the disease sometimes runs on to a fatal termination without any material change in the pulse); general restlessness; urine scanty, very red, and sometimes scalding. The character of the expectoration during the first stage of the malady is supposed by many to afford a characteristic mark of the malady; and it is from this circumstance that Laennec has denominated the sputa expectorated, *pneumonic*, or *glutinous*. During the stage of hepatization, the sputa diminish in quantity, become lighter in colour, and less transparent, until finally, when the third stage supervenes, expectoration of almost a mucous character occurs.

Sometimes pneumonia is complicated by more or less derangement of the biliary organs, when we shall have superadded to the lung affection the symptoms indicative of such derangement. This variety of the complaint is termed *bilious pneumonia*.

M. Saucerotte recognises a kind of latent pneumonia, depending upon a certain peculiarity of constitution, entirely unlike ordinary pneumonia, and which seems to commence by the second stage, or that of hepatization. His description of the disease is as follows: First, "*Premonitory symptoms*, either entirely absent, or of slight importance, consisting of lassitude, with shivering, loss of appetite, and but little fever."

Second, "*Symptoms*. The temperature of the skin is not sensibly augmented; the pungent heat of ordinary pneumonia seldom present; pulse usually but little affected; respiration natural, and no pain in the chest. Percussion always elicits a dull sound over a considerable extent, and bronchial respiration is audible over the same locality. In some cases, slight crepitation may be heard around the hepatized spot."

Third. "*Progress* and *duration* variable. In some cases we have seen the disease linger for six or seven weeks. When the case terminates favourably, the dulness gradually disappears, and the bronchial souffle is replaced by crepitation; respiration becomes more free, and the general aspect of the patient improves.

Fourth. "*Diagnosis*.—Pleurisy is the affection with which latent pneumonia is apt to be confounded. In chronic pleurisy, however, there is more constantly a pain in the side, and the region of the dulness varies with the position of the patient. Apoplexy, and the bulging of the intercostal spaces, shortly clear up the diagnosis. The history of the case distinguishes it from phthisis.

Fifth. "*Causes*.—For the most part, exposure to cold."

Although Dr. Saucerotte is a practitioner of the old school, his sole internal remedy in this affection is *tartar emetic*, our own specific in similar cases.

Viewed anatomically, inflammation of the substance of the lungs presents, according to Laennec, three different degrees, or stages, which he designates, first, *engorgement*, or *congestion*; second, *hepatization*; third, *purulent infiltration*.

In the first degree, the lung loses in a measure its crepitous feel, is of a livid colour, and more solid than natural.

In the second degree, the lung presents the appearance of liver; it is not crepitous, is heavier than in the first degree, and shows a granular appearance when cut into, or torn asunder. Laennec, Andral, and Louis, suppose this hepatization to be owing to the conversion of the air-cells into solid grains, by the hardening of a concrete fluid, which is poured out during the inflammation; while Dr. Williams supposes that "these granulations contain no viscid mucus, but consist of little bunches of vesicles, which have been obliterated by the swelling of their membranous tunics, and the enlargement of their blood vessels."

In the third degree, the external appearance of the lung is similar to that of the second degree, but of a lighter colour. The same heavy, hard, and granular character obtains, but when the lung is cut into, a yellowish and purulent matter makes its appearance. As the disease advances, the granular condition disappears, and purulent abscesses take its place.

The phenomena elicited by auscultation and percussion, during the stage of engorgement, are the *crepitous rhonchus*, the respiratory sound being yet audible, and the ordinary healthy sound on percussion.

As soon as hepatization has occurred, percussion over the affected part yields a dull sound, and neither the respiratory murmur nor the crepitous rhonchus can longer be heard. There are certain other sounds, like bronchophony, a kind of blowing, &c., which may exist in certain cases of hepatization, but these signs are so vague and uncertain. that immense practice is requisite to enable the physician to form an accurate judgment respecting them.

After the third stage has existed a little time, and the pus begins to soften, the mucous rhonchus may be heard in the bronchi. In some instances the pus is not expectorated or absorbed. but forms an abscess in some part of the pulmonary tissue. We shall then have a mucous rhonchus over the seat of the abscess, also pectoriloquy, and what is termed a "bronchial or cavernous cough."

When the disease terminates favourably, and resolution takes place. it will be found that the lungs gradually and by successive degrees, return to their original state, as is indicated by the diminution of the crepitous rhonchus, and the return of the natural respiratory sound, when the inflammation had ceased at the first stage; also by the reappearance of the crepitous rhonchus, &c., when the malady had progressed to the second and third stages.

Causes.—Lung fever is a disease peculiar to temperate and cold latitudes, and usually occurs during the winter months. The usual causes are, undue exposure to intense cold, sudden suppression of perspiration, epidemic influences, and the inhalation of noxious vapours or gases. Laennec and Forbes assert that pneumonia is sometimes induced by the bite of the rattle snake, (*crotalus horridus,*) and of other venomous serpents; and that it may also arise from the "injection of various medicinal substances into the veins." These assertions go far to prove a specific operation of these substances upon the respiratory organs, and may afford a valuable hint respecting their homœopathic application in pneumonia.

Therapeutics.—The prominent medicines for the treatment of pneumonia, are. *aconite, bryonia, belladonna, tartar emetic, phosphorus, ipecacuanha, sambucus, sulphur, lachesis, rhus tox., arsenicum, mercurius, acid phosphoric, arnica.*

In the first stage of the disease, when symptoms indicative of a high grade of febrile excitement are present, as hot and dry skin, great thirst, rapid and hard pulse, scanty and high coloured urine, &c., *aconite* and *belladonna* may be given in alternation, until the inflammatory symptoms subside. These remedies are often alone sufficient to break up the disease in this stage; and even when they fail of effecting a complete cure, they generally moderate most essentially the fever, and mitigate all the other symptoms.

If, after the subsidence of these symptoms, stitches in the side, difficult and anxious respiration, and troublesome cough continue to harass the patient, recourse must be had to *bryonia.*

When, however, the second stage, or *hepatization* has occurred, indicated by dull sound on percussion, bronchial respiration, &c., we should at once have recourse to *tartar emetic* or *phosphorus.*

The *external indications* which point to the use of *emetic tartar,* are, dull sound on percussion; absence of the respiratory murmur, or bronchophony ; skin cold, and covered with a clammy sweat ; considerable expectoration of a yellowish or brownish colour, and mixed with blood ; pulse small, soft and frequent ; tongue covered with a dry and dark fur, and perhaps red at the edges.

Physical sensations.—" Great oppression and difficulty of breathing ; cough loose, and accompanied with rattling of mucus ;"—(*Müller*)—burning under the sternum, and sometimes as high up as the throat ; sensation as if the chest were lined with velvet ; want of air and want of breath previous to the paroxysms of coughing ; also *pneumonia biliosa*, with gastric and bilious symptoms, as yellow tinge of skin ; yellow or brownish fur upon the tongue ; bitter taste ; nausea and bilious vomiting ; yellow or dark urine ; headache ; general sensation of lassitude and debility.

Mental and moral symptoms.—Anxiety ; restlessness ; confusion of ideas ; sometimes furious delirium.

Administration.—A grain of *tartar emetic* to six ounces of pure water—a teaspoonful every one, two, three or four hours as required.

Phosphorus has been highly extolled also in the second stage of pneumonia, and in certain cases of pleuro-pneumonia, where *aconite* and *bryonia* have failed in effecting a cure. Dr. Fleischmann has used it successfully in all stages of lung fever.

Buchner, Griesselich, Horner, Bosch, and Shellhammer, have employed it with advantage when the third stage had set in with great prostration, livid or hippocratic countenance, sunken eyes, cold, viscid sweats, tremulous and feeble pulse, dry and dark lips and tongue, difficult expectoration of a brown or rust colour, extreme anguish, subsultus tendinum, muttering or furious delirium, with grasping at flocks, sense of suffocation, and involuntary stools.

Müller describes the special pathogenetic symptoms of *phosphorus*, having reference to pneumonia, as follows : " Sticking and violent stitches in various parts of the chest, left and right side, sometimes accompanied with burning, in rest and during motion, especially when sitting and taking an inspiration ; pain in the chest, especially during an inspiration ;

itching in the interior of the chest, with dry cough; feeling of heaviness in the chest; anxiety in the chest, with arrest of breathing, and beating in the right side of the chest; great oppression of breathing; great shortness of breath; oppressive tightness, and tensive sensation in the chest, as if a band were encircling it; tension and dryness in the chest; constrictive clawing and pressing in the upper part of the chest; loud, rattling breathing; dry, hollow cough, without expectoration; a sort of hacking cough, with huskiness of the chest, and expectoration of some mucus; cough, with expectoration of transparent mucus, accompanied with tensive pain, and afterwards with sticking pain in the chest; fatiguing cough, with white, tenacious expectoration; the expectorated mucus is streaked with blood; bloody expectoration, with mucus, accompanied with short, slight cough; coughing up small clots of pus, with smarting burning behind the sternum; sticking pain in the pit of the stomach when coughing, compelling one to lay the hand upon the pit; short breath after every turn of cough."

From the above it will be seen that *phosphorus* includes a greater range of symptoms than *tartar emetic.* In typhoid pneumonia, especially, it is often of distinguished service where hepatization has occurred, and the symptoms point to the third stage.

Administration.—It may be employed at the first, second, or third attenuation, and the dose repeated according to circumstances.

In *typhoid pneumonia,* as well as in cases attended from the first with great debility and prostration of the energies of the system, *rhus tox.* will be found a remedy of much efficiency, either alone, or in alternation with some other specific. Should the case be complicated with pains in the chest or side, of a rheumatic character, *rhus rad.* may occasionally be employed with advantage. This medicine is usually given after *aconite* and *bryonia.*

Sulphur is an important remedy in certain protracted cases of pneumonia occurring in psoric or scrofulous subjects, and which threaten to terminate in phthisis. Indeed, in most of those cases of chronic pneumonia which seem to have arrived at a fixed point, the patient neither improving nor apparently retrograding, we should always bear in mind this powerful antipsoric.

When the disease has reduced the patient, notwithstanding our remedies, to a state of extreme prostration, with very short breath on the slightest exertion, dry and dark tongue and lips, extreme anguish, stitches in the side, great thirst, diarrhœa, ringing and buzzing in the ears, *arsenicum* is the proper remedy. In examples of this description, the remedy should be frequently repeated until a decided impression is produced.

If the pulmonary inflammation threatens to run into gangrene, as will be indicated by fetid and greenish, or dark expectoration, *arsenicum* is appropriate, as are also sometimes *carbo veg.* and *china.*

Pneumonia occurring in old and feeble persons, and attended with symptoms showing a low grade of inflammatory action, will require the use of *phosphorus, ipecacuanha, sambucus, veratrum, nux vom., china, belladonna, lachesis, lycopodium,* and *cantharis.*

Arnica is applicable in pulmonary inflammations proceeding from mechanical injuries.

The symptoms of pneumonia and bronchitis combined, will be covered by *tartar emetic, aconite, mercurius, phosphorus, capsicum, bryonia, carbo veg., pulsatilla, senega,* and *nux vom.*

We usually select one of the low attenuations, and repeat the dose once in two, three, or four hours, until a marked impression is produced upon the symptoms.

SECTION V.

PLEURITIS.—PLEURISY.

Diagnosis.—This malady commences with lassitude, chills, and other febrile symptoms, succeeded in a short time by the following local phenomena: "The stitch, dyspnœa, cough, and recumbency on the affected side."—*Laennec.* Dr. Wurm, of Vienna, maintains, however, that "the posture of the patient is usually upon the *back.*" The inspirations are short, rapid, and attended with severe sharp stitches, unless the inflammation be very slight, in which case, but little alteration will be observed in the breathing; there is often experienced a sense of tightness and oppression at the chest; there is generally little or no cough unless the lungs or the bronchia are involved, when there occurs a short and dry cough, with but a small quantity of glairy expectoration, and very painful; the pulse is rapid and full; skin hot and dry; urine scanty, and of a deep red or dark colour; the pain is almost invariably confined to one side of the chest, and increased by inspiration, coughing, and movement; urgent thirst; great dyspnœa; constant inclination to lie upon the affected side or back; abdominal respiration, and pain in the intercostal spaces on pressure. These symptoms are speedily succeeded by others, which indicate that *effusion* has taken place. Laennec, Johnson, and Mackintosh believe that effusion commences as soon as the inflammation is established; while others, equally eminent, contend that a considerable period elapses before it occurs. But the weight of testimony seems to be in favour of the opinion of the former gentlemen. Amongst the signs which are characteristic of pleurisy with effusion, are, increased size of the affected part of the chest, apparent to the eye, or by mensuration; also ægophony, perceptible by the stethoscope from the commencement of the inflammation, or after a moderate quantity of fluid has been effused, disappearing when the effusion becomes very large in quantity, and re-appearing as absorption takes place, and the liquid diminishes; dull sound on percussion, and failure of the respiratory murmur in the affected side.

Should the lungs happen to be involved, the sputa will be tinged or streaked with blood, and more copious than in simple pleuritis. Other symptoms will also obtain which characterize pleuro-pneumonia.

The effusion in pleurisy may be either of a plastic, serous, or hæmorrhagic character. The severity of the febrile, and other symptoms, will depend upon the rapidity of the effusion, and its quality and quantity.

Causes.—Atmospheric vicissitudes, sudden checking of the perspiration, metastases of rheumatism, erysipelas, gout, &c., mechanical injuries, surgical operations upon cancerous and scrofulous parts. We have witnessed two cases of pleurisy which supervened as a consequence of surgical operations. One of these cases occurred after amputation of the thigh for a malignant disease of the leg, and proved speedily fatal. The other case came on about two weeks after excising a large fungous tumour from the breast of a female, which also proved fatal. Both of these cases were unusually violent, and ran their course with very great rapidity. It is worthy of remark, that in both, the wounds by the operation were progressing as favourably as usual. Whether pleurisy, in these instances, is attributable, as some writers suppose, to the absorption of pus into the system, or to some other cause, we are at a loss to determine; but that the disease is peculiarly violent and fatal, has been observed by all who have witnessed its occurrence.

Therapeutics.—The most valuable remedies in the treatment of pleurisy, are, *aconite*, *bryonia*, *tartar emetic*, *phosphorus*, *arsenicum*, *rhus tox.*, and *arnica.* During the progress of the disorder, we should also bear in mind *sulphur*, *scillae*, *rhus rad.*, *lachesis*, *silicea*, and *china.*

Aconite is eminently appropriate, either alone or in alternation with other specifics, whenever the inflammatory action runs high, accompanied with hot skin, quick and full pulse, urgent thirst, and general suspension of the secretory functions. Wurm and Trinks commend it in the highest terms in that variety of pleuritis which is characterized by the plastic nature of the effusion, and the severity of its inflammatory fever. It should be exhibited at the very commencement of the disease, and in the lowest potencies, and repeated, in urgent cases, every hour until the fever subsides.

Bryonia is a specific of great value in the malady under consideration, and the power which it possesses of promptly controlling and subduing the most violent cases of pleurisy, is a matter of astonishment to us, who formerly believed copious and repeated venesections to be the only safe means of effecting a cure. We have treated a great number of cases, in which *bryonia* has been our chief remedy, and we have not failed in a single case, but our cures have been far more prompt, pleasant, and satisfactory, than we ever effected under the old treatment. The effusion has invariably been more speedily absorbed, and the pleura and lungs, as well as the system at large, have more perfectly recovered their original tone and vigour, than in cases which have been treated by the old method. Nor will this appear at all strange, when it is remembered, that by one method, the structure actually diseased is *alone* acted upon, while by the other, the *whole organism* is subjected to the influence of the most powerful medicines, impairing the integrity and vigour of almost every part, without producing any certain or decided effect upon the pleura, or any other pulmonary tissue.

Let the sceptical allopath prove upon his own person in health, the pure effects of *bryonia, tartar emetic, phosphorus, lachesis, scillæ,* &c., upon the respiratory organs, and then test them judiciously in cases of disease after the homœopathic principle, *similia similibus,* and he will forever abandon the uncertainties and dangers of the lancet, mercurials, counter-irritations, &c.

Bryonia may follow or alternate with *aconite,* advantageously. The *external indications* are, cheeks flushed and hot, dry or moist ; respirations short and rapid, and performed principally with the abdominal muscles ; position upon the affected side ; pulse quick and full ; tongue dry ; breath hot ; urine scanty, and red or dark ; dull sound on percussion of the affected side ; respiratory murmur indistinct or entirely wanting.

Physical sensations.—Stinging, shooting, or burning pains in the side, aggravated on inspiration, coughing, on movement ; respiration difficult, short, anxious, and rapid ; sense of tightness ; a weight or oppression at the chest ; painful cough, dry or with expectoration of a glairy sputa, sometimes tinged with blood ; great heat of skin, alternating with frequent coldness and shivering ; urgent thirst ; pain in the intercostal spaces on pressure ; weariness and inclination to retain the recumbent position.

Mental and moral symptoms.—Anxious, apprehensive, desponding; fear; irritability; peevishness; restlessness.

Administration.—A dose of the first dilution every hour, alone or in alternation with *aconite*, until the pain, difficulty of breathing, &c., are relieved.

Tartar emetic.—According to Majendie, this medicine possesses the specific power of causing engorgement and inflammation of the lungs when given in large doses. There can be no doubt that it is an absolute and decided specific over the respiratory organs as well as the gastro-intestinal membrane. This has been demonstrated by Cloquit, Müller, Majendie, Gross, and others, by autopsical examinations, and by numerous provings upon persons in health.

It is a common remedy with the old school, in affections of the respiratory organs; yet they are entirely ignorant of its curative action. It is only necessary to refer to the unsatisfactory and contradictory opinions of Laennec, Rasori, Broussais, Eberle, Payne, Blake, and Barbier, upon this subject, to be convinced of the utter want of accurate knowledge and uncertainty of principle amongst allopathists in the administration of medicines.

The homœopathist, on the contrary, demonstrates by numerous provings in health, that it exerts a specific force upon the lungs and their appendages, and he therefore gives it in inflammations of these organs with confidence and success. With him there is no random and crude speculation—no breaking down of the organism by violence, hoping in the general ruin to crush the malady, but having a definite object, and seeing his goal, he quietly, safely, and surely attains it.

The *external indications* for *tartar emetic*, are: face flushed, hot and dry, or pale, wan and anxious, and covered with sweat; respirations short and obstructed; surface burning hot and dry, or cold and bathed with cold perspiration; pulse quick, weak, or full; tongue moist and clean, or loaded with a white or brown fur; urine scalding hot, red or brown; mucous or bloody expectoration; general appearance indicative of great anxiety and physical prostration.

Physical sensations.—Respiration short, difficult, obstructed, and attended with stinging or shooting pains; cough with expectoration of mucus, sometimes tinged with blood; violent throbbing of the heart; coldness and shivering whenever the bed clothes are raised, or on motion; fever with adypsia, or moderate thirst; lassitude, debility, and disposition to syncope; trembling of the limbs, from the slightest exertion; sense of suffocation.

Mental and moral symptoms.—Agitation; apprehension; discouragement; despair.

Administration.—From half a grain to a grain of the *tartar emetic*, may be dissolved in a tumblerful of pure water, and given in teaspoonful doses, every one, two, three, or four hours, as the urgency of the case demands.

Phosphorus.—*External indications.*—Countenance pale, alternating with redness; eyes hollow and surrounded by a blue circle; respiration short, difficult, and noisy; tongue dry; pulse quick and hard; expectoration slimy or bloody.

Physical sensations.—Respiration rapid, short, and difficult; lancinating pains in the chest, mostly on the left side; sharp pains on pressing the intercostal spaces; anguish, fulness and tension of the chest; palpitation of the heart; dry, shaking cough, or cough with expectoration of bloody mucus; weakness, pain and trembling of the limbs; mouth and throat dry; thirst.

Mental and moral symptoms.—Uneasiness; melancholy; anguish; dread of the future; indifference to everything; passionate and irritable.

Administration.—Same as *bryonia.*

After the more violent febrile symptoms have subsided, and those of effusion into the cavity of the pleura remain,—as enlargement of the affected side, dull sound on percussion, absence of the respiratory murmur, oppression and constriction of the chest, difficult and short breathing, with occasional attacks of suffocation, dry cough, coldness of the body, clammy sweats, anxiety and general sense of prostration, *arsenicum* is our remedy. It may be given in these cases, at the third potency, a dose once in two to four hours, lengthening the intervals as improvement occurs.

Rhus tox. is sometimes useful after the febrile symptoms have subsided, and there yet remain wandering pains in the chest, shortness of breath, and general debility. In cases also which have arisen from metastases of rheumatism or gout, this remedy is peculiarly appropriate. It may be administered in the same manner as *bryonia.*

When inflammation of the pleura has arisen from a contusion, bruise, or other injury, *arnica,* both internally and externally, is our best specific. For internal exhibition, we may use one of the lower dilutions; externally, a lotion made of a drachm of the tincture to twelve ounces of water.

The other medicines to which we desire to call attention, and which will often be found highly serviceable in some of the sequela of pleuritis, are, *sulphur. scillae, mar., rhus rad., lachesis, silicea,* and *china. Sulphur* especially, is recommended by Wurm, in plastic pleurisy, and in cases complicated with pneumonia and hepatization, after *aconite* has moderated the more active symptoms. He uses the tincture.

SECTION VI.

PERTUSSIS.—WHOOPING COUGH.

Diagnosis.—Most writers recognise three distinct stages in whooping cough, viz.: first, the *forming stage,* presenting symptoms like ordinary catarrh, as sneezing, watery eyes, dry cough, headache, constriction and oppression at the chest, feverish nights, &c., which continue for two or three weeks, when the *second* or *convulsive stage* sets in. At this period of the malady, there are violent paroxyms of cough of a convulsive and suffocative character. This cough is distinguished from others by a peculiar stridulous or whooping sound, which occurs during inspiration, while the expirations are interrupted by frequent fits of coughing. This whooping sound is owing to a spasmodic contraction of the glottis, which renders respiration very difficult, and gives rise to a sense of obstruction and impending suffocation. This spasm and contraction, together with a tickling in the throat, come on previous to the paroxysms, and subside somewhat after the coughing has ceased. The duration of the paroxysms varies from one to five minutes, at the termination of which there is often vomiting or expectoration of mucus. This stage usually acquires its greatest degree of violence in from one to two weeks, and its continuance is from five to six weeks, when the third, or *stage of declension*, commences. At this period all of the symptoms gradually become milder; the paroxyms are less frequent,—the cough less urgent; the contraction and obstruction less strongly marked, until at the end of two to four weeks, under favourable circumstances, all of the symptoms have disappeared.

Causes.—Pertussis is unquestionably attributable to the absorption into the organism of a *miasm* of a specific nature. We know nothing of its chemical or physical character, but in this, like other maladies, the system must be rendered susceptible by previous preparation, or predisposition, to enable the miasm to exercise its specific effects and induce the phenomena of whooping cough.

Whether this specific miasm operates primarily upon the mucous membrane of the air passages, the stomach, the diaphragm, the lungs, or the eighth pair of nerves, we are unable to decide in a satisfactory manner. It would seem that the advocates of each particular opinion in regard to its primary location, have found in their autopsical examinations, appearances which indicated that there had been inflammation in each of the structures alluded to. That the pneumo gastric and other nerves, as well as the membrane of the glottis, larynx, &c., are involved, either as a primary or secondary effect of the contagion, there can be no question.

The causes which act upon the organism in such a manner as to render it susceptible to the action of the miasm, are, atmospheric vicissitudes, colds, debility and chronic diseases of the respiratory organs, inhalation of irritating substances, fatigue and exhaustion of the physical or nervous system.

Therapeutics.—In the first stage of the malady the ordinary remedies for catarrh are appropriate, as *nux vom., chamomela, belladonna, ipecacuanha, mercurius, aconite, dulcamara, pulsatilla, arnica, bryonia, &c.*

In the second, or *convulsive stage*, the best remedies are, *tartar emetic, veratrum alb., carbo veg., chamomela, cuprum acetat., sambucus nig., conium mac., drosera, hyoscyamus, ipecacuanha, nux vom.*

In the third stage, we may consult, in addition to the medicines already enumerated, *pulsatilla, hepar sulph., sulphur, lachesis, arsenicum, sepia, acid phos.*, and *china.*

Dr. Bosh speaks very strongly in favour of *cuprum metallicum* in firmly developed whooping cough.

"In simple whooping cough of children under one year of age, I give in the morning and evening, *cuprum* third, one grain ; in older children, *cuprum* second, one grain twice a day, and in this way the disease was generally removed under gradually decreasing coughing turns." When the cough is complicated with symptoms arising from dentition, or other affections disconnected with the cough, these symptoms should be met by appropriate remedies, either alone, or in alternation with *cuprum.*

Administration.—Our attenuations may range from the first to the sixth, in this disease, according to the age, temperament, and impressibility of the patient. The doses should be repeated at intervals of six or eight hours.

SECTION VII.

ASTHMA.

Diagnosis.—For a week or two previous to an attack of asthma, the patient will often be troubled with sneezing every morning, itching at the inner canthi of the eyes, irritation of the throat, with constant disposition to hem or hack, lassitude, dull pains in the head, back, and limbs, loss of appetite, dry hacking cough, and great depression of spirits.

The attack most commonly commences during the night, with tightness and constriction about the chest; urgent and distressing dyspnœa, aggravated by the slightest movement; inspirations short and strong, while the expirations are long, laboured, and wheezing ; great and rapid movement of the nostrils ; countenance bloated and livid, and indicative of intense distress and anxiety ; inclination to retain the erect position ; even during the forming symptoms, inability to lie upon the right side or back ; more or less prickling or burning heat after the attack commences, aggravated by scratching ; symptoms aggravated by eating even bread ; respiration very difficult, as if from want of air, yet the wind from a fan or the draft from a door or window, stops the breath, and cannot be borne ; face and forehead livid, or pale ; sharp pain through the temples ; inability to lie upon a feather bed from the first ; during the paroxysm must constantly retain the erect posture ; the dyspnœa, &c., worse in the night, and remitting during the day ; dry cough in the first instance, sometimes but not always, followed in a few hours by expectoration of a viscid mucus; perfume of flowers, hay, &c., increases the symptoms, and almost puts a stop to the breath during the paroxysm ; extremities cold ; respiration through the mouth ; attacks brought on from excitement, particularly grief and fear ; also certain odours or irritating substances inhaled ; palpitation during the attack ; the asthma occurs for the most part during the season of flowers; tongue foul ; breath offensive ; eructations ; flatulency ; urgent desire for cool, fresh air ; pulse variable.

Causes.—It has been often observed that asthma almost always occurs in individuals who are suffering from some chronic miasm. In numerous instances we have been able to trace a direct connection between an attack of urticaria, but partially developed, and then suddenly suppressed, and asthma. Indeed, it may be safely asserted, that a majority of the cases of true asthma, are attributable to this or some other miasm, which has been thrown, from some exciting cause, upon some portion of the respiratory apparatus. We are confirmed in this opinion, from the fact that in several instances where an attack of asthma has been seriously threatened, and even commenced, we have been able to cut it short by administering a remedy like *puls.*, *bry.*, and *cup. acet.*, which had the effect to develop the nettle rash, and thus relieve the air passages.

Other causes, which are, properly speaking, exciting causes, may be enumerated, as humid easterly winds, atmospheric vicissitudes, inhalation of certain medicinal and other irritating substances, like *ipecac.*, the odours of certain plants, and electricity in the air, the inhalation of the imponderable particles of which often causes severe paroxysms of the malady; also indigestible food, anger, fear, the irritation of pregnancy, spinal disease, sedentary habits, &c.

Therapeutics.—*Pulsatilla, ipecacuanha, arsenicum, bryonia, nux vomica, belladonna, china, sulphur, lobelia inflata, coffea, digitalis,* and *acid hydrocyanic,* are the principal remedies in this complaint.

Pulsatilla.—This remedy is indicated in cases occurring in persons of a mild temper, light complexion, hair and eyes, from suppressed or confined rash, cessation or other derangement of the menses, and inhalation of the vapour of *sulphur.* The *external indications* are: short, suffocating, and extremely difficult respiration, as if from want of sufficient air, or choked by some irritating substance; the patient is obliged to retain the erect posture; his movements are rapid, and his whole appearance indicates great distress and anxiety; tongue loaded with a thick coating; breath offensive; frequent eructations; hiccough; countenance pale, sometimes alternating with redness; attacks usually coming on in the night during sleep.

Physical sensations.—Cramp-like and constrictive tension of the chest or larynx; respiration impeded and distressing, increased by motion, walking in the open air, or by eating; short spasmodic cough; nausea; palpitation of the heart; sensation of fulness and distention in the stomach; throbbing pain in the forehead; bad taste in the mouth; cramp-like pains in the abdomen; itching, burning, or prickling sensation in the skin, in the evening or during the night; pains in the limbs; nausea and vomiting; smarting or burning pain in the canthi, and pressure in the eyeballs.

Mental and moral symptoms.—Very great depression of spirits, and melancholy from the onset of the symptoms; intense anxiety, agitation and dread of suffocation during the paroxysms.

Administration.—From the third to the sixth dilution may be used—a dose every half hour in urgent cases—until aggravation or amendment occurs.

Ipecacuanha.—In asthma caused by the suppression of miliaria, urticaria, and by the inhalation of irritating vapours, *ipecacuanha* at the first to the third attenuation, may be exhibited. The signs which particularly indicate this medicine, are, spasmodic contraction of the larynx and chest; anxious, sighing, or panting respiration; palpitation of the heart; air seems full of dust; face pale; extremities cold; nausea; vomiting; coated tongue; insipid or bitter taste; dry, spasmodic cough; irritability, impatience and fear of death.

Arsenicum alb., is a valuable remedy in bad cases occurring from suppressed eruptions or catarrh, also in persons of feeble or impaired constitutions, whether from excesses, previous sickness, or old age. The following symptoms point especially to this medicine, viz.: feeling of extreme lassitude and debility; difficult, stifling dyspnœa, with attacks of suffocation; spasmodic constriction of the larynx and chest; respiration short, anxious, and wheezing; irregular throbbings of the heart; sufferings aggravated at night by lying down, movement, eating, mental excitements, or exposure to the cool fresh air; distention and cramp-like pains in the abdomen; frequent eructations; nausea; vomiting; burning sensation at the stomach; fœtid breath; smarting or burning sensation in the throat; pressive burning pains in the eyes; face pale or bluish; anxious and desponding. The first to the third trituration may be employed, regulating the repetition according to the urgency of the symptoms.

Bryonia is applicable in cases arising from suppressed eruptions, or rashes but partially developed. It is also appropriate in cases complicated with catarrhal and pulmonary disorder.

The paroxysm usually occurs in the night; the respiration is difficult, short, sighing, impeded by stingings in the chest, and aggravated by exercise; there are oppressive, tensive or contractive pain in the chest;

cramp-like pains, cuttings or shootings in the abdomen; bitter or acid eructations; throbbing or pressive pains in the head, increased by movement; pressure and burning pain in the eyes on motion. It may be exhibited in the same manner as *pulsatilla.*

Asthma which has been caused by derangement of the digestive functions, excessive study and watching, sedentary habits, and abuse of drugs, liquors, coffee, &c., may often be cured by the use of *nux.*

The *nux* symptoms are, weight and constriction at the chest; great difficulty of breathing, aggravation of the symptoms in the night, on walking, eating, or lying down in the evening; heat and burning in the chest; bitter and acid eructations; pressure and contractive pains in the stomach and epigastrium; palpitation of the heart; short, dry, spasmodic cough, sometimes attended with a scraping in the throat; fœtid breath; loaded tongue; heartburn; distention of the abdomen after eating; heaviness, or tearing, throbbing, drawing or jerking pains in the head; frequent sneezing, with coryza; hypochondria, anxiety and irritability. It may be employed like *pulsatilla.*

Belladonna has been especially recommended in cases occurring in females of an irritable constitution, also in cases where there exists a tendency to spasms, or any organic lesion. Hartmann asserts that "it often proves radically curative after the exhibition of some intercurrent remedy, particularly in cases which have not become too chronic by repeated relapses, under which circumstances we must have recourse to *sulphur, calcarea,* or some other proper antipsoric."

It is particularly called for when the paroxysms come on in fits of short, difficult, irregular, and suffocating respiration, accompanied by dry cough; pressure on the chest; violent beatings of the heart; vertigo, swimming or darting pains in the head; pains in the small of the back and limbs; cramps in different parts of the body; anxiety, irritability, and fretfulness.

A dose of the second or third dilution every hour or two until an impression is produced.

Chamomela is an important remedy in the flatulent asthma of children, also that following a suppressed catarrh. It is likewise specific in those attacks which are caused by anger, grief, fear, &c., in adults. Among the symptoms which point to it, may be mentioned, distention and sense of fulness of the stomach and bowels; pressure, anxiety, and fulness in the region of the heart; short, wheezing respiration; great restlessness; dry irritating cough; bad taste; tainted breath.

Administration.—Same as of *belladonna.*

Lobelia inflata is a remedy of great value in cases of spasmodic asthma induced by humidity, and certain other conditions of the atmosphere. It is indicated when the attack is preceded or accompanied by a kind of "prickly sensation through the whole system, even to the extremities of the fingers and toes;" constriction across the chest; short, anxious and wheezing respiration; nausea; vomiting; sense of prostration; trembling of the limbs; giddiness and headache; spasmodic cough; burning sensation in passing urine; intermittent pulse; cramp-like pains in the abdomen; cold sweats.

Administration.—Potencies from the third to the sixth,—a dose every two to four hours, as the symptoms require.

In cases of asthma of long standing, and which appear to be connected with some chronic miasm lurking in the organism, *sulphur, digitalis, acid hydrocyanic, calcarea,* &c., are worthy of consideration, and will sometimes effect cures when the other medicines enumerated have disappointed our expectations.

There are other remedies, like *coffea, ignatia, stramonium, china, arsenic, arnica,* &c., which should always be borne in mind by the practitioner, for instances may occur in certain complicated cases, where one or more of them will be required.

SECTION VIII.

PHTHISIS PULMONALIS.—CONSUMPTION.

We come now to the consideration of that disease which has proved the most destructive of human life of all that claim the attention of the profession. Slow, insidious, and gentle in its progress, from causes which have been in operation for years, it steadily draws its victims to the brink of the grave, before they have an apprehension of danger, or are conscious of even serious indisposition. We are accustomed to regard with terror the yellow fever, because its subjects are seized suddenly, and destroyed by a single blow. But if this fearful agent of death possesses, in the torrid climates to which it is almost always confined, a nearly indiscriminate and unlimited dominion, during two or three of the sultriest months of summer, consumption, with its deliberate and almost invisible step, traverses all the world, destroying in its treacherous and fatal embrace innumerable numbers, of every age, and sex, and condition. The yellow fever indeed strikes suddenly and violently, and leaves the patient no hope or consolation; but consumption quietly and gently fastens its chains upon its victims, while brightening the intellect, charming the spirit, and tinting the cheeks with the colours of the lily and the rose, distracting their attention with songs of hope and security; and the poison pervades its subject organs, and the deluded patient sooner or later awakes, from his fancied safety, scarcely in time to realize his peril ere he yields his life.

How few physicians are there, of extensive practice, whose diaries might not furnish histories of the most touching pathos, in connection with the treatment of this disease, which (it may be by a perversity of the judgment) seems to fulfil its mission in disappointing the fondest expectations, and in blighting the fairest creations of human loveliness! A maiden, perhaps, becomes the belle of the season, in which she makes her entrance into the gay world. To an assured position of the highest elevation in society, she brings the most exquisite physical beauty, and grace and elegance of manner, and the finest and rarest moral and mental endowments, subtlest intelligence and quickest wit, and a sweetness of disposition which crowns a sudden admiration with the dearest and most permanent affection. When Hope comes to her with the most enchanting promises, the Angel of Ill approaches also, in the guise of consumption, and the two contend until the last is victor, and his triumph is celebrated with all the displays of unaffected wo. Or it is a young man, who has scaled the difficult heights that obstructed an ambitious vision, and is about to grasp the prize upon which his eagle eye has been steadily fixed through years of varying toils and storms. The moment he dares to dream of rest, the enemy that has dogged his steps, unseen, through half his career, is disclosed, and leads him from the presence of Hope into that of Despair. With what a profound interest must the physician contemplate a disease of which the path is constantly thus marked!

True tubercular phthisis, when once fully developed, is beyond question incurable by medical means. The physician may palliate symptoms, and often protract for a considerable period the fatal termination of the malady, but he cannot remove those foreign accumulations which constitute tubercles, either by a gradual absorption or in any other manner, so as to prevent the formation of ulcerous excavations, nor can he heal these ulcerous cavities when once formed, since they are constantly being disturbed and irritated by the incessant motions of the lungs. The few instances of spontaneous cures of ulcerated lungs, reported by Laennec and others, are only exceptions to the general principle which we have advanced. Much, however, may be done in the early stages of phthisis, while the tubercles are yet small, and but slightly irritated, to retain them in a latent condition for an indefinite number of years. We are aware that in some instances there will be great difficulty, even on the part of the physician, in detecting the insidious advances of the disease at this early period, but by watching with great care every slight indication of disturbance connected with the respiratory organs, by ascertaining whether any hereditary predisposition exists in the family, by examining the physical conformation of the chest, the respirations, as relates to their strength, freedom, number per minute, and whether unduly increased by exercise; and finally, by investigating minutely the previous history of the individual, in order to be able to judge whether any cause may have been in operation which might originate the disorder, we may be able to advise such measures as shall retain the tubercles in a latent and undeveloped condition, and thus for years prolong life.

The most common period for the occurrence of phthisis is between the ages of eighteen and thirty; and it is probable that more deaths occur in persons under the age of eighteen, than after thirty. It is calculated by Drs. Forbes and Clark, "that above one quarter part of the individuals who die before the age of puberty, die with tubercles!" It is also estimated by the latter gentleman, "that the maximum of mortality in this disease is at thirty, and that from this point it gradually diminishes." No age, however, is exempt from it; for infancy, childhood, youth, manhood, and extreme old age, are all more or less subject to its withering attacks.

Females also suffer more from the malady than males, as is shown by the statistical facts which have been published by Louis, Forbes, Skoda, Laennec, Andral, Clark, Young, and others. Nor is this at all surprising, when we reflect upon the education, and the habits of life of the women of civilized countries. Born and reared during infancy in hot-houses, where the invigorating breath of heaven rarely penetrates; their childish intellects crammed with ideas which they are unable to understand, while their physical frames are permitted to wither in crowded schoolrooms, without that free and abundant exercise and indulgence in childish sports, which are so absolutely essential to their growth and well being; submitted at the period of puberty to those instruments of torture and distortion, stays, in order that the symmetrical figures which God in his wisdom has given them, may be contracted sufficiently to meet the ideas of an abominable *fashion;* rejecting constant and vigorous exercise in the open air, early hours, regular habits, and all of those means which tend to promote physical strength and vigour: is it strange, in view of these things, that the seeds of phthisis are so often and so early planted?

There are habits also prevalent among the youth of the male sex, which conduce in an alarming degree to generate and develope phthisical affections. The vice to which we allude, from false delicacy, from its solitary nature, and from the very gradual manner in which it impairs the nervous system and undermines the constitution, has either been entirely overlooked, or but slightly touched upon by writers. But unless we are much deceived, a very large number of consumptive cases, especially in young men, are attributable to onanism, as their remote cause; and we are sure that those who have minutely investigated the previous histories of consumptive patients, will fully coincide with us.

It is quite true that there are many other habits and customs which pertain to refined society, that also have their effect in engendering phthisis, but we believe that the cause just touched upon has been productive of more evil amongst the youth of the male sex, than any two other causes combined. This cause applies, to some slight extent, to females, but, compared with the male sex, it is trivial and unimportant, for the reason that women are, *by nature*, purer, less sensual, and less addicted to gross, carnal, and beastly thoughts, than a vast majority of the other sex.

Let parents, then, banish all mawkish delicacy upon this subject, and caution their children against this dreadful evil. Let them talk plainly, and display before their minds the inevitable consequences, in the form of consumption, idiocy, lumbar abscess, &c., to which an indulgence in this degrading and pernicious vice so surely leads.

There are many other causes of phthisis which we might here dilate upon, but we shall allude to them under the head of "*causes of phthisis.*"

The appearance of the tuberculous formations vary in different subjects, some being small as millet seeds, and irregular in shape, either distinct or running into each other, of the consistence of cheese, and of a light yellowish colour. This variety, which is by far the most common, has been termed the *miliary tubercle.*

Another variety is called the *granular tubercle*, which, according to Laennec, is only the ordinary tubercle in its first stage. Bayle and McIntosh entertain different opinions, the former believing the miliary granulations to be distinct from tubercles, while the latter supposes them to be genuine tubercles, but *sui generis*.

Bayle, Laennec, and others, also assert that they have met with a few cases which they term *encysted tubercle*. Other writers speak of the occasional occurrence of this variety of tubercle, it being semi-transparent, whitish, and in consistence like hard cheese.

Laennec describes, likewise, three kinds of *tuberculous infiltration*, viz., the *irregular*, the *gray*, and the *yellow*. This infiltration is generally formed around tuberculous excavations, but it may exist where there are no tubercles. It is sometimes found in large masses, "occupying the whole lobe of the lung, and having no connection with the miliary tubercle."—*Mc Intosh.*

Respecting the nature and cause of these tuberculous formations, there is a wide difference of opinion. Broussais supposed that *irritation*, or *inflammation*, were only "degrees of the same affection, and that they may produce, indifferently, tubercles, encephaloid cancer, melanosis, fibrous, bony, cartilaginous growths, &c."

Laennec and Andral maintain that they are "*accidental productions*, foreign to the natural organization of the lungs," and caused by an aberration in the nutrition of the organ.

Others are of opinion that tubercles are primitively hydatids.

In the first stage of development, tuberculous matter is "a gray, semi-transparent substance, which gradually becomes yellow, opaque, and very dense. Afterwards it softens, and gradually acquires a fluidity nearly equal to that of pus; it being then expelled through the bronchi, cavities are left, vulgarly known by the name of *ulcers of the lungs*, but which I shall designate *tuberculous excavations*."—*Laennec.*

Whether these accidental formations are inorganic substances deposited in the pulmonary structure, like pus or calculous concretions, by a kind of exudation, or whether they are organized, and possess life and vitality, cannot easily be determined. We incline, however, to the latter opinion.

For a more particular description of the morbid appearances found on dissection, the reader is referred to the writings of Louis, Laennec, Skoda, Bayle, Forbes, and Clarke.

Diagnosis.—One of the first symptoms which announces the approach of phthisis, is an undue *shortness of breath* after exercise. If, in addition to this, there are hæmoptysis, wandering pains, constriction and tightness at the chest, great sensitiveness of the lungs to cold air, a dry morning cough, a dull sound in the clavicular region on percussion, and a partial or total absence of the respiratory murmur, the most serious apprehensions may be entertained.

Let all remember, also, that it is only at this early stage of the malady, that our preventive and remedial measures can be brought to bear with any assurance of success, and on this account, we shall dwell particularly upon these primary indications, trusting that we may in this way impress upon the minds of all their vital importance.

In all of our investigations of diseases of the chest, it is a matter of importance, in the first instance, to ascertain whether any hereditary predisposition exists on the part of the patient to tuberculous affections. Secondly, whether from occupation, previous habits, excesses, protracted mental anxiety and depression, and frequent exposure, without a sufficient supply of wholesome, nutritious food, the patient has not acquired those peculiarities of constitution which render him susceptible to attacks of phthisis; and, thirdly, whether the physical development of the chest is such that the lungs can have ample room to exercise their functions.

In making up our diagnosis in the early stage of any given case, much will depend upon the presence or absence of these remote causes, for most of the symptoms enumerated may exist in a man with a large and well formed chest, and with no hereditary or acquired predisposition to the malady, and yet excite no serious apprehensions, while the same symptoms in an individual with a narrow, flat, and ill-shaped thorax, with a predisposition to the disease, would induce us to form a diagnosis of an entirely different character. Commencing, then, with the primitive symptoms of consumption, we shall notice first—

The respiration. "Healthy respiration," according to Marshall Hall, "is performed with ease and freedom, and without the aid of the auxiliary muscles, in any of the usual positions of the body. It is effected by a nearly equal elevation of the ribs, and depression of the diaphragm, except in females, in whom the thorax is observed to move more than in men; each side of the thorax moves also in an equal degree, and inspiration and expiration occupy nearly equal spaces of time."

Laennec considers the respiration natural "when the anterior and lateral parts of the chest dilate equally, distinctly, yet moderately, during inspiration, and when the number of inspirations in a state of repose is from *twelve* to *fifteen* in the minute."

Andral puts the mean average of respirations in a healthy adult, at more than sixteen or eighteen in the minute, Majendie at twenty, and some writers even as high as twenty-six.

Taking, then, the mean number of respirations of a healthy adult to be eighteen per minute, and bearing in mind the natural movements of the healthy thorax during inspiration and expiration, we shall be enabled to form a pretty satisfactory opinion respecting the condition of the respiratory organs, by judicious comparisons of different stages of disease with the supposed natural standard.

We are convinced, from much observation, that Laennec, Andral, and Louis, have laid quite too little stress upon this important indication; for, although individuals may now and then be short breathed who have no tendency towards diseases of the lungs, yet, when taken in conjunction with an hereditary predisposition, unusual susceptibility of the lungs to cold, slight, dry, hacking cough, narrow or flat chest, or occasional wandering pains in the chest, we may be certain that mischief is threatened.

A very fleshy person, or one afflicted with disease of the heart, and certain other maladies, may be short breathed after slight exercise, but these cases can never be mistaken by the observing physician as phthisical, since the history of the case, as well as the general aspect of the patient, sufficiently mark the distinction in all instances.

Whenever, therefore, an individual has more than the usual number of respirations during repose, the expirations and inspirations being unequal in point of time, and is put out of breath after the slightest exercise, it is the duty of the physician to ascertain the cause of this unusual action, and whether consumption is not insidiously approaching. Is his chest large, full, and well developed,—are its movements natural during inspiration and expiration,—is scrofula hereditary in his family,—is he troubled with tightness or pains in the thorax,—is he subject to cough upon the slightest exposure,—is he inclined to stoop when sitting or walking,—is his respiration sighing,—has he a slight morning cough,—finally, is the sound in the clavicular region, or in any other part of the chest, dull on percussion, and is the natural respiratory murmur absent at this, or any other point? Upon the presence or absence of these symptoms will depend our diagnosis. Taken as a whole, they indicate clearly the existence of phthisis pulmonalis; and where there is a family tendency to phthisis, even dull sound on percussion, and absence of the respiratory murmur, with dyspnœa after ascending a stairs, or other moderate exercise, will warrant the opinion that tubercles exist in the lungs. If, furthermore, one or more of the other signs enumerated obtain, our opinion must be still more decided and unfavourable.

Physical conformation of the thorax.—One of the causes which especially favours the formation and development of tubercles, is a small, flat, and contracted chest. This want of symmetry and proportion may be owing to natural organization, or it may be acquired from indulgence in sedentary habits, stooping, a neglect to keep the body in the erect posture, and to breathe in that full, free, and vigorous manner which is so essential to the development and well-being of the lungs.

If the thorax is *naturally* contracted and ill-shaped, a suitable course of physical culture should be promptly adopted and persisted in until it has acquired sufficient size and symmetry. This result is practicable in all cases by steady perseverance and energy on the part of the patient.

The means of accomplishing this desirable end, are gymnastic and other exercises which particularly bring into action the muscles of the chest, constant exercise with the body erect, in the open air, the habit of taking long, free and full inspirations in order that all portions of the lungs may constantly receive a due proportion of air, and thus execute their functions properly, and lastly, the use of tubes for the purpose of exercising more efficiently the pulmonary organs. By a regular and systematic employment of these means, the size of the chest may be increased to a surprising extent, and the lungs made to acquire a degree of strength and vigour which could have been attained by no other method.

There are other instances where well-formed chests are contracted, distorted, and weakened, by the wearing of *tight clothing*, *stays*, *&c.*, and by sedentary occupations and habits, with the body constantly inclined forward and bent over. These pernicious habits are so commonly indulged in, and have become so much a part of our social system, that their important influences,—their baneful consequences upon the most vital part of the organism, are almost entirely overlooked. Yet no one who reasons at all, can be unaware of the dangerous and undermining effects of these things; and to those whose pride, or indolence, or imbecility, still prompts them to persist in such habits, we would say, and without much sympathy for their sufferings, "you have sown the wind, and you shall reap the whirlwind."

Hereditary and acquired predisposition to phthisis.—An alarming circumstance connected with the history of any individual, even when no symptoms point to an approaching consumption, is an hereditary predisposition to tuberculous disease of the lungs. To know that the seeds of a dreadful malady are implanted in the system, liable at any moment to be roused into activity by the numerous exciting causes which prevail, is enough, one would naturally suppose, to call forth all of the energies of the individual in order that he may escape the threatened evil;—yet how few under such circumstances use proper means of prevention, and exercise that care and attention towards themselves which these cases require!

But the root of the evil must be traced farther back to those injudicious marriage connections, where one or both of the parties are labouring under a *scrofulous taint.* It appears singular that intelligent persons of this description should be willing to enter the matrimonial state, when they are so certain of entailing upon their offspsring, disease, misery, and an early death; yet how often do we see the desire for temporary self-gratification, for riches, display, or pride, outweigh the potent reason named, and induce the unfortunate victim of the malady, to plunge herself and her children into almost certain future suffering!

A predisposition to phthisical affections is often *acquired* by constant exposure in small, damp, and ill-ventilated habitations, insufficient clothing, scanty and unwholesome food, free use of pork, incessant occupation in close rooms and constrained positions, onanism, protracted depression of spirits, and certain occupations, like the stone-cutter, scythe-grinder, &c.

All of these causes exert a powerful influence in bringing the system into that condition which renders it peculiarly susceptible to tuberculous formations in the lungs, and for this reason, should be avoided as much as possible by individuals, and should receive the attention of all benevolent men.

Amongst the first signs which should lead us to suspect latent phthisis, are, an ill-formed thorax, respirations above the natural standard, and greatly accelerated on slight exercise, and the existence of an hereditary taint. Whenever these signs obtain, the chest should be at once explored by auscultation, and percussion, so that if tubercles are discovered, immediate measures may be taken to keep back or prevent their development. Sometimes a slight dry cough, with tightness and pains in the lungs, are the first symptoms which announce the affection: at other times the disease supervenes suddenly, after a pleurisy, or an influenza, or some other acute malady. In the majority of instances, however, the symptoms occur in the order enumerated, viz., habitual shortness of breath, especially after exertion, short and dry cough, burning in the palms of the hands and soles of the feet, constriction and pains in the chest on inspiration, sensitiveness of the lungs to cold. These symptoms may remain stationary for months or years, when from some exciting cause the pulse becomes unnaturally frequent, there are febrile exacerbations in the evening, and generally about noon, the respiration becomes more rapid and laborious, being often executed by the diaphragm, the anterior and lateral parts of the chest dilate unequally during inspiration and expiration, particularly in the recumbent posture, the catemenia in female subjects cease, a mucous expectoration occurs, profuse night sweats and diarrhœa set in, the body wastes away, the expectoration becomes gradually more purulent and abundant, the body is bent forward; as the tubercles soften, the guggling or rattle of the matter may be heard either with the naked ear or the stethoscope, the cough is cavernous, the respiration and rattle also become cavernous, and pectoriloquism is heard as soon as the softened tuberculous matter is thrown off, and the cavity becomes empty; the sound on percussion still continues dull, but now and then a peculiar metallic sound is evident. As the disease progresses towards the last stage, and the cavities acquire a large size, the respiration, voice and cough give forth the peculiar hollow, metallic sound or buzzing, termed amphoric resonance. The whole body now presents the appearance of extreme emaciation, the face is pale, cadaverous, and frequently tinged with a waxen or lemon hue, the lips and roots of the nails are bluish, the nose pointed, the voice becomes hoarse, the mouth and throat apthous, the feet œdematous, occasional delirium at night, and a continual failing of the physical powers, until death ensues.

Hæmoptysis, though not a necessary attendant upon phthisis, is of general occurrence during some part of its course: it may occur at any period of the disease, but most commonly it is one of the first symptoms.

Causes of Phthisis.—The causes of consumption

may be divided into, first, the *constitutional*; second, the *accidental*; and third, the *exciting*.

Under the first head may be included, first, hereditary scrofulous taint; second, hereditary impurities of the blood of a syphilitic, erysipelatous, or psoric character; third, imperfect organization of the thorax, feeble constitution; and fourth, a melancholy nervous temperament.

The most prominent *accidental causes*, are, confinement in close, crowded, and ill ventilated apartments, protracted mental depression, insufficient nourishment, unwholesome food, intemperance, damp and unprotected habitations, onanism, the habit of stooping, and thus contracting the capacity of the chest, tight clothing, late hours, over-excitement, abuse of drugs, especially mercury and opium, excesses in venery, want of exercise, and abuse of tobacco.

The *exciting causes*, are, atmospheric vicissitudes, suppression of the perspiration by cold, imperfectly subdued acute diseases of the pulmonary organs, repelled cutaneous eruptions, inhalation of irritating vapours, etc., external injuries. Of these proximate causes, Eberle, Laennec, and others, consider cold by far the most common and dangerous. It is probable, however, that cold of itself is by no means so injurious as these gentlemen have supposed, but that the sudden alternations from heat to cold which obtain in temperate latitudes, exert far more influence in engendering phthisis, than the severe but steady cold of more northern regions. Indeed, some recent writers have strongly recommended a change from temperate to cold latitudes, as more advantageous to consumptive subjects than a warm climate. In this opinion we do not coincide, since the highly condensed air of the former must act as a constant and powerful stimulus to the already irritable tubercles. We much prefer a warm, mild, and equable climate in these cases.

Therapeutics.—In all cases when it is well ascertained that tubercles exist in the lungs, either in a latent or partially developed state, the following course should be adopted, as far as circumstances will admit, viz.:

First, an immediate removal to an equable, mild,

dry, and healthy climate. In making this selection, we should choose the *interior* of the country, rather than the coast, in order, as far as possible, to be away from the influence of the breezes which blow from the ocean.

Second, constant exercise in the open air. By this we do not mean that snail-like moping around, with the body coiled up, and a countenance the picture of melancholy and despair; but that vigorous, free and cheerful exercise which invigorates and expands the physical powers, and cheers the mind. Exercise, to be beneficial, should be employed in such a manner as to bring all of the muscles into moderate and agreeable action, and as a pleasant recreation, rather than a necessary task. By this means the organism is strengthened, the circulation equalized, the "blue-devils" exorcised, and the pulmonary organs placed in the best possible condition to recover themselves.

In pursuing this course of physical exercise, regard should also be had to those gymnastic and other sports which tend to expand and strengthen the thorax. Too much cannot be said with reference to the importance of this subject, also the *erect position* of the body, and the habitual custom of taking deep and free inspirations; for the muscles of the chest, as well as of other parts of the body, waste away and become enervated, without constant exercise in a natural manner.

In connection with this course, we must strongly advise the frequent use of *breathing tubes*. Having experienced decided benefit in our own person from the employment of this kind of exercise of the lungs, and having often seen it adopted by others with prompt and marked advantage, we speak confidently of its efficacy in debility of the pulmonary organs.

Third, persons of a consumptive habit should make use of highly nutritious food. The articles which are particularly to be avoided, are *pork*, in all its diversified forms, as ham, sausages, lard, &c., all fish not having scales, like eels, catfish, clams, crabs, lobsters, &c., and oily and greasy food generally.

How far a free use of pork may exert an influence in generating tubercles, we know not, but the following fact is not without significance, viz.: The Jews and all other tribes and nations that are prohibited by their religion from using the swine as an article of food, *are almost uniformly exempt from scrofula and consumption.* The very common occurrence of tuberculous formations in this filthy animal, would seem to be presumptive evidence that it is peculiarly subject to scrofula. We commend therefore to the consumptive a strict adherence to the dietetic regulations which were advised by Moses of old to his brethren, the Hebrews, as being most conducive to health and longevity.

Fourth, as an important means for promoting a healthy action of the skin, and equalizing the circulation, too much cannot be written in praise of *external applications of cold water.* These applications should be employed daily, either in the form of baths, sponging, or the wet sheets ; in many instances the greatest service will be derived from using cold water applications to the chest in such a manner as to bring out an eruption.

The effect of this remedy is to impart tone and vigour to the cutaneous structures, and to allay in a decided manner nervous irritation.

Fifth, another valuable *preventive*, as well as *remedial* agent in lung affections, consists in the cultivation of a cheerful and happy disposition. The invalid must never brood over his ailments, for by gloomy ponderings upon his case, he is quite prone to exaggerate symptoms, imagine complaints which have no existence, and thus detract from his prospect of recovery.

Laennec ranks the depressing emotions as one of the most prominent accidental causes of phthisis, and we are quite satisfied that he has not over-estimated their importance.

Sixth, (and finally), we commend a strict avoidance of all excesses, whether in the pleasures of the table, wine, and liquors, or in the indulgence of any thing which over-stimulates and fatigues mind or body.

In conjunction with the above measures, some one of the following medicines may be occasionally exhibited with benefit ; making the selection, of course, according to the peculiar character of the indications which may be present, viz.: *ol. jecoris aselli, sulphur, hepar sulph., calcarea carb., mercurius, stannum, ferrum, silicea, sepia, phosphorus, acid phos., acid nit., lycopodium, lachesis, iodine, iod. potassæ, arnica, belladonna, sambucus* and *china.* Of these medicines the *oleum jecoris aselli* is probably the most valuable, and should receive more attention from the advocates of homœopathy than it has hitherto done. Holding its active principle, *iodine,* in a most excellent state of attenuation, the infinitesimal atoms of the drug with its oily vehicle are absorbed and conveyed to the lungs, where the most happy curative effects are often produced. We think the point clear, that *iodine* is the only real curative agent in these cases; although it is by no means improbable that its medium, the animal oil, which is composed principally of carbon and hydrogen, may serve the purpose of neutralizing a portion of the inspired oxygen, which would otherwise act upon the weakened lungs themselves. In administering this medicine, therefore, let it be borne in mind, that the *oil* is not the medicinal agent, but the mere vehicle by means of which the real remedy, *iodine,* is introduced into the system. Two drachms of the oil may be prescribed three or four times daily.

Sulphur and *hepar sulphur.* should always be selected when the pulmonary affection can be clearly traced to abruptly suppressed psora, whatever may be the general character of the symptoms. If, however, symptoms are present which point strongly to some other medicine, an alternation may be resorted to.

Consumption occasionally arises in those whose lungs are naturally weak and irritable, in consequence of violent and protracted syphilitic attacks. In these instances, the most suitable remedies are *mercurius, acid nit., potassæ iodide,* and *hepar sulphur.*

When phthisis is threatened during the progress of chlorosis, or in consequence of masturbation, or excessive venery, the appropriate medicines are, *phosphorus, acid phosph., calcarea carb., china, silicea,* and *ferrum.*

For uncomplicated scrofulous consumption, our most reliable remedies are, unquestionably, *oleum jecoris aselli, calcarea carb., iodine, sulphur, hepar sulphur., sepia, lachesis, phosphorus,* and *silicea.*

Administration.—The first, second, and third attenuations are most efficient in all stages of phthisis—the doses to be repeated from two to four times in twenty-four hours, until the required specific impression is produced.

It is to be regretted that as yet so few positive specifics have been discovered for the cure of tubercular phthisis, but we are sanguine in the belief that many such remedies will, sooner or later, be found. In the meantime let us be on the alert to attain these much coveted desiderata.

SECTION IX.

COUGH.

In most instances, *cough* is one of the symptoms of inflammatory action, either of the parenchyma of the lungs, or of some membrane connected with the respiratory organs; but coughs occasionally arise and reduce the patient to a very low state of hectic fever, without the presence of any inflammatory action, except that which is produced by the act of coughing, from an elongation and relaxation of the uvula, from the pressure of tumours and swellings in the throat, trachea, or thorax, from hypertrophy and other organic affections of the heart, and from accumulations of serum or pus within the thorax.

We have in several instances speedily succeeded in removing troublesome coughs, and of restoring patients to health, who were apparently in the last stages of pulmonary consumption, by clipping off a portion of an elongated uvula. It is not uncommon that protracted and troublesome coughs are promptly cured by the removal of tumours in the neck, by the puncturing of abscesses in the throat or chest, or by evacuating from the thorax an effused fluid. It behooves us, therefore, in all cases of cough, where the cause is not perfectly apparent, to make our investigations with reference to the above enumerated complications, in order that surgical measures may be resorted to on all suitable occasions.

It is to be feared that errors are sometimes committed by gentlemen of our school, in underrating the value and importance of surgery, as a means of curing disease. When the cause is of such a nature that our remedies are at best slow and uncertain, while a speedy and safe removal may be effected by a surgical operation, we should never hesitate in our choice. Even in cases like paracentesis abdominalis, or paracentesis thorasis, where only a troublesome symptom is removed, we often accomplish much good by placing the patient in the best possible condition for the favourable operation of remedial agents. But in the examples of obstinate tumours and abscesses, pressing unduly upon some part of the respiratory apparatus, the aid of the surgeon is often indispensable.

Many individuals are troubled with coughs in temperate latitudes from an inherent debility of the lungs, and a want of vigour to resist the stimulating influence of cold air. Such persons often succumb eventually from phthisis, without having experienced any actual inflammation of the pulmonary structure.

Others, from excesses of various kinds, acquire a predisposition to coughs, from the most trivial exciting causes.

Therapeutics.—Appropriate medicines for all ordinary kinds of cough, may be selected from those already referred to, when treating of the different affections of the respiratory organs.

CHAPTER XXIV.

DISEASES OF THE HEART AND ITS APPENDAGES.

The heart and its appendages are subject to several kinds of morbid action, which authors have described under the terms *angina pectoris*, *hypertrophy*, and *dilatation* of the heart, diseases of the *valves*, *carditis*, and *pericarditis*, and *palpitation*. Many of the symptoms of these affections are similar, but we shall endeavour, in the following brief description, to point out a sufficient number of signs to enable the physician to form a ready and accurate diagnosis in all cases.

SECTION I.

ANGINA PECTORIS.

Diagnosis.—At the commencement of the disease, the patient experiences occasional sharp pains in the region of the heart, especially after active exercise, or when putting the muscles of the chest upon the stretch. After a time, the pains recur more frequently, continue for a longer period, and are accompanied by palpitation, attacks of syncope, sense of suffocation, and tightness in the chest, and great difficulty of breathing. The attacks are usually excited by violent physical exertions, mental emotions, and deranged stomach, from abuse of stimulants and of indigestible food. In very severe cases, there are almost constant dyspnœa, pains extending down the arms and into the back, very frequent and alarming attacks of syncope and suffocation, pale and haggard, or livid and exceedingly anxious expression of countenance. If the disease is not arrested, the patient generally expires suddenly in one of these distressing paroxysms.

When *angina pectoris* proceeds from *hypertrophy* of the heart, we shall observe, in addition to the symptoms just named, powerful pulsations of the heart, which are visible at a distance, full and vibrating pulse, and dull sound on percussion.

If the disorder has arisen from *dilatation of the ven-*

tricles, there will be swelling and visible pulsation of the jugular veins, a loud and distinct sound on applying the ear over the fifth and sixth ribs, vertigo, frequent turns of syncope, palpitation and dyspnœa, pulse weak and tremulous.

When *angina pectoris* is connected with disease of the *valves* of the heart, the following signs will be present: great dyspnœa on the slightest exertion, frequent and violent palpitations, pulse feeble and irregular, livid and unnatural appearance of the countenance, œdematous swelling of the feet and ancles, and "a *permanent* sawing or rasping, or filing sound over the valves of the heart, especially after depletion and rest."—(*Swett.*)

Causes.—*Angina pectoris* may proceed from some organic disease connected with the heart, like ossification of the coronary arteries, or of the valves of the heart, dilatation or hypertrophy of the heart, obstructed circulation from an accumulation of fat about the organ, from the pressure of the tumours, or from asthma. Very often, however, it is a purely sympathetic affection, and entirely disconnected with any structural disorder of the heart or its appendages. In these instances, the nerves which supply the heart are affected in such a manner that slight exciting causes, as errors in diet, mental emotions, or ascending a flight of stairs, induce the paroxysms.

Therapeutics.—In the selection of remedies, strict regard should be had to the remote and exciting causes of each case. If the symptoms are the result of some organic affection of the heart, like those to which we have alluded, our prognosis must be, for the most part, unfavourable, and we can only reasonably expect to palliate the sufferings of the patient. But if the remote cause consists simply of a diseased condition of the *par vagum*, or of the cardiac nerves, which renders them liable to become morbidly excited from trivial causes, we may prescribe medicines with every prospect of ultimate success. The most reliable specifics in this malady, are *aconite, digitalis, hepar sulphuris, lachesis, nux vom., veratrum, sepia, sambucus, ipecacuanha, pulsatilla, arsenicum, aurum.*

The attenuations should be selected with reference

to the impressibility of the patient, and the medicine persisted in, at suitable intervals, during the continuance of the complaint.

SECTION II.

CARDITIS AND PERICARDITIS.

Diagnosis.—Inflammation of the fleshy substance of the heart, uncomplicated by disease of the pericardium, of the pleura, or of the aorta, is an occurrence so rarely met with, that some authors have described under one general head, the symptoms resulting from inflammations of the heart and its appendages. The signs usually present in carditis, often render our diagnosis very obscure, on account of their resemblance to affections of the lungs, and of the pleura, and of their frequent complication with the latter. Frank believes that much of the uncertainty which prevails respecting cardiac affections, is attributable to the general neglect of the profession in investigating the movements of the heart during disease, and in examining its morbid appearances in those who have died in consequence of diseases of the chest. "*Il n'est pas douteux que, si les hommes de l'art observaient avec la même attention les mouvements et les vibrations du cœur que les battements des artères, s'ils multipliaient leurs recherches sur les cadavres, ils viendraient à bout de dissiper les epaisses ténèbres qui environnent les maladies de l'organe central de la circulation.*"—(*Frank.*)

The ordinary symptoms of inflammation of the heart and its envelop, the pericardium, are acute pains in the region of the heart, increased by motion, or on assuming the horizontal posture, sense of fulness and oppression in the chest, palpitation, from the slightest exertion, or from mental excitement; rapid, difficult, and irregular respiration; short, dry, spasmodic cough; rapid, small, irregular, and intermittent pulsations of the heart and arteries; great anxiety, dread of suffocation, "absence of the respiratory murmur, and dull sound on percussion."—(*Hall.*) General febrile disturbance almost always accompanies the inflammation, although the heat is unequally distributed, some parts being intensely hot, while other parts are cold. The countenance is always expressive of anxiety and distress, the patient is desponding, irritable, and restless, and experiences alarming palpitations, faintness on rising up in bed, or on talking.

Causes.—Protracted grief, anxiety, or mortification, violent muscular efforts, external injuries, asthmatic, and other pulmonary affections, metastases of rheumatism, or gout.

Therapeutics.—Digitalis, aconite, bryonia, arnica, cannabis, pulsatilla, lachesis, spigelia, iodine, and *arsenicum,* are the medicines commonly employed in this malady.

Digitalis, on account of its specific power over the sympathetic nerve, and the cardiac plexus, is especially adapted to those cases of pericarditis which have been caused by violent emotions, and protracted grief, care, and anxiety. The special indications are, sharp stitches, or contractive pains in the region of the heart; uneasy sensations in the left side of the chest, often extending to the shoulder and arm; palpitations excited, by talking, movement, or on laying down, particularly on the left side; pulse rapid, weak, and irregular, or slow, soft, and intermittent; sense of oppression and anguish in the thorax; general weakness; frequent attacks of faintness; respiration slow, difficult, and unsatisfactory, or short, painful and sighing; frequent flushes of heat in the chest, face, and head, while the extremities remain cold; general feeling of anxiety and despondency. A drop of the second or third dilution should be prescribed, in water, every two hours.

Aconite is a suitable remedy, when the movements of the heart and arteries are more rapid and vigorous than in health, and when the congestion to the heart is accompanied by an unusual degree of erethism. The pains in the cardiac region are of a constrictive, oppressive or lancinating character; the breathing is short, anxious, and laboured; the pulse is rapid, strong, and intermittent; the action of the heart is exalted, and often irregular; febrile symptoms are strongly pronounced; the patient inclines to sit with his body bent forward, in order to relax the muscles of the thorax, and thus to obviate the liability of pain from this cause. The first or second dilution of *aconite* may be selected, and a single drop administered in water, every two, three, or four hours, as the nature of the case demands.

Bryonia will occasionally be required, in inflammations of the heart and its appendages, which are complicated by disorder of the pulmonary structures. It will likewise prove serviceable in cases which are connected with rheumatism or gout. The following are its indications: drawing and stitching pains in the chest, aggravated by breathing, or by movement; rapid, anxious, and painful respiration; dry, spasmodic, and painful cough; lancinating pains extending into the shoulders and back, between the shoulder-blades; oppression in the chest, which causes frequent sighing; determinations of blood to the chest, and head; rapid, weak, and intermittent pulse; anxious, depressed, and irritable. Its administration is the same as *aconite.*

Arnica is chiefly useful when the inflammation has been caused by external injuries, like contusions, wounds, &c. The special indications are, lancinating pains in the region of the heart; oppression at the chest; great difficulty of breathing; short, dry, and irritating cough; sharp pains through the heart, which cause faintness; irregular action of the heart; pains, and dyspnœa, increased by mental or physical exertion. It may be given the same as *aconite.*

Cannabis, pulsatilla, lachesis, iodine, and *arsenicum,* have been employed with success, in cardiac inflammations which have arisen from suppression of eruptions, or the drying up of old ulcers. They may be used at the second or third attenuations—the repetitions of doses to be governed by the urgency of the symptoms, and the medicinal or other effects produced.

Should the disease terminate in dropsy of the pericardium, our best remedies are, *arsenicum, apis mel.* and *iodine.* We prefer the first or second attenuations —a dose once in six hours until an impression is evident.

CHAPTER XXV.

DISEASES OF THE BRAIN AND NERVOUS SYSTEM.

SECTION I.

GENERAL OBSERVATIONS.

If the soul of man manifests itself through the healthy organism in a certain definite manner, and if these manifestations are modified precisely in accordance with the abnormal conditions which the organs and tissues may acquire, the importance of a correct understanding of the exact healthy functions of all the structures, and of their alterations during disease, will be duly appreciated. Unfortunately for science, the profusion of hypotheses, the arbitrary assumption of ancient ideas for facts, as well as the inherent difficulties attending the pathology of diseases of the cerebro-spinal system, have until recently retarded the onward progress relative to their nature and treatment. Until Sir Charles Bell demonstrated that the nerves which arise from the posterior column of the spinal marrow were devoted to *sensation;* those from its anterior column, to *muscular contraction;* while the middle column gives origin to the *respiratory nerves,* the most erroneous and contradictory notions were entertained respecting the functions and diseases of the nervous system.

Majendie, Flourens, Abercrombie, Hall, Solly, Serres, Bennett and Andral have also thrown much light upon the functions of particular portions of the brain; but much yet remains to be done in this important field of discovery, and it is only by banishing from our medical vocabulary all vague and obscure expressions, and contemplating the body as a complicated machine, actuated and kept in operation by an intelligence which pervades every part, and in conjunction with its material stimuli, giving rise to sight in the organ of sight,—hearing, taste, smell, digestion, assimilation, calorification, motion, &c., in their several organs;—and perceptions, memory, comparisons and ratiocination, by their operation upon a combination of organs, that we can arrive at accurate conclusions.

The cerebral organs may be affected throughout their whole extent, or in isolated parts alone; but whatever condition obtains, diseases of certain sections of the cranium usually give rise to peculiar and well defined symptoms. Thus, *compression* of the brain, whether from effused blood, serum or pus, depression of a portion of the cranium, or a congested and relaxed condition of the cerebral vessels, give rise to *coma*, with slow pulse and stertorous respiration: *organic lesions* of the brain, to *paralysis* of one or more parts of the body, depending upon the extent of the lesion and the part affected: *irritation* of the brain, to *convulsions:* disease of the *cortical substance* or *hemispherical ganglia*, to *delirium* and *mania:* of the *medullary* or *tubular structure*, to *convulsions:* effusion within the *ventricles*, to *dementia:* effusion upon the *surface* of the brain, to *lethargy:* inflammation of either *lateral lobe* of the *cerebellum*, to paralysis of the lower extremity of the *opposite side:* inflammation of the *middle lobe*, to erection of the penis, (*Hall:*) of the *arachnoid* and *pia-mater*, to *delirium: ramollissement*, to torpor of the *intellectual faculties* and loss of *muscular power*.

So strongly marked are these signs, that pathologists have made somewhat minute classifications of the diseases of the brain, as of the *arachnoid*, of the *pia-mater*, of the *cortical*, or the *medullary* part, the *base*, the *tuber-annulare*, the *hemispheres* and the *cerebellum*. But it is to be observed in most cerebral affections, that inflammations of particular structures rarely exist uncomplicated with more or less disease of the surrounding parts, and on this account we meet with a great diversity of symptoms during their progress. For this reason, if no other, it is more consistent to prescribe for the *totality of the symptoms* than for the mere *name* of the disease. By the former course we pursue a definite object, and apply our remedies with an assurance of success, even if we are in error respecting the pathology of the case; while by the latter method, we are liable to mistake the location and nature of the malady, and thus adopt a pernicious mode of practice.

For example, by mistaking the cerebral symptoms of a typhus fever for encephalitis, or the *anæmic* condition of the brain which obtains in true delirium tremens, in some cases of apoplexy, in epilepsy, and in ramollissement, for *acute inflammation*, and resorting to the usual remedies for the cure of the latter, viz.: copious venesections, the most disastrous results might be apprehended. It is now a well-ascertained fact, that delirium, coma, hydrocephalus, and one form of ramollissement, may result from an *anæmic*, as well as an *inflammatory* condition of the brain. Drs. Abercrombie and Marshall Hall recognise still another comatose condition independent of disease of the brain, and arising from exhaustion of the general system occurring during the last stages of certain diseases; but from the fact that this coma generally occurs after protracted bowel complaints where opium has been used as the principal remedy, we are of opinion that a real cerebral disease has been superinduced by the remedy.

For the cure of the symptoms above named, arising from an *anæmic* condition of the brain, tonics, stimulants and a nutritious regimen are deemed essential by the practitioners of the old school. Blood-letting and antiphlogistics in these cases, are fatal. But when the same symptoms arise from an *inflammatory* condition of the encephalon, a treatment directly the reverse, is supposed to be necessary to save life, like venesection, leeching, purging, blisters, &c. Now when we contemplate the great uncertainty attending the diagnosis in these two forms of disease, and the danger which must attend mistakes in treatment originating from errors respecting the peculiar condition of the brain, is it strange that people have no more confidence in allopathy?

We have before remarked, that morbific substances, in order to develop diseased action in the organism, must be taken into the blood and conveyed to those tissues upon which they exert a specific morbific influence, there producing those alterations (probably upon the sentient extremities of the nerves) which constitute disease. It is only necessary to refer to the examples to which we have alluded in another part of this work, to render this supposition entirely probable.

It is also equally evident, from the multitude of experiments by Müller, Majendie, Orfila, Pereira, Hahnemann, Trinks, Philips, Flourens, and Bichat, that poisonous drugs and all medicinal substances operate in the same manner in producing their specific poisonous or medicinal effects.

There are other causes constantly operating upon the system, of a character entirely different from those to which allusion has just been made, and which may with propriety be termed *spiritual* or *dynamic*. Thus, violent mental disturbance may cause epilepsy or apoplexy—chagrin and grief, biliary derangements, jaundice, and dyspepsia—sudden news, whether good or bad, diarrhœa—anger, fear, disappointment, and ill news, sometimes instantly destroy the appetite; fear and apprehension, predispose to contagious disorders; the sight of blood induces syncope; and of human suffering, pain and disorder in the stomach. In these cases, the unusual mental excitement determines an unnatural amount of blood to certain parts, the blood-vessels and nerves of such parts are oppressed, and disease results.

But it is of vast importance that these *spiritual* or *dynamic* causes be not confounded with those which are *material* and *imponderable*. Let us not deceive ourselves and the world, by classing them where they do not belong, simply because our limited knowledge of the sciences renders us as yet incapable of appreciating the nature and the precise mode of operation of the latter!

Although cerebral affections may arise under favourable circumstances, from the absorption of morbific and medicinal substances, and from spiritual or dynamic influences, yet the latter rank first in importance, especially in what are termed *chronic cerebral maladies*. In the treatment of brain diseases, therefore, too much importance cannot be attached to an accurate knowledge of these causes; for it is only by their prompt removal, together with a judicious application of remedial agents, that we can expect complete success.

The curious reader will find much to amuse, if not instruct, by tracing the medical history of cerebral maladies from Hippocrates to the present time. Throughout all of this period, notwithstanding the numerous changes of opinion respecting their nature, causes, &c., one striking fact will always be observed, viz.: that the *treatment* for all of these complaints has remained almost the same as first instituted by that very respectable heathen philosopher, Hippocrates, until the period of Hahnemann.

In proof of the singular tenacity with which the medical world has clung to the opinions of the ancients, we may cite the doctrines of eminent physicians as late as the time of Sydenham, who supposed the cause of many brain diseases, as lethargy, coma, paralysis, &c., to consist in a "*viscid condition of the blood and lymph, which obstructed the pores of the brain, and dulled the animal spirits. While the viscid blood forces its way into the brain, through the two carotids, it leaves in its passage a slimy matter, through which the animal spirits passing, stick by the way, and so the pores of the brain are obstructed.*"—(*Sydenham and Salmon, Prac. Phys.*, p. 203.)

Their indications of cure, were: first, "*to evacuate the redundancy of phlegm and choler, or to carry off that vicious acid which has created the viscosity of the blood.* Second, *to alter the present dyscrasia of the blood.* Third, *to open the pores of the brain now obstructed, and give a free passage to the spirits.* Fourth, *to strengthen the weakened parts, quicken the dull spirits, and increase their store or stock.*"—(*Ibid.*)

To fulfil these indications of cure, the fathers of allopathy adopted almost precisely the same treatment as that which prevails with their brethren of the present day, viz.: blood-letting, emetics, cathartics, "*to purge off the phlegm and choler,*" antimonials and alteratives, "*to cut up the gross phlegm, dissolve the coagulums of the blood and humours, and excite the animal spirits to a brisker and more lively air.*" Paracelsus and Van Helmont particularly commended *opiates* and *narcotics* in chronic affections of the brain. If we refer to the most recent writers on insanity and other cerebral affections, we shall find not only the same remedies retained, but the same diversity of opinions respecting the application of these remedies; some trusting to venesection and purges, some to tonics, while others depend upon *opiates* and *narcotics*.

In a book which is now before me, published in the year of our Lord, 1587, by "Andrew Boord, Doctor of Physic—an Englishman," our sapient author supposes that maniacs are possessed of devils, and advises for their cure, in addition to blood-letting, cathartics, &c., that they should be sent to Rome to be made whole. "For within the precincts of St. Peter's Church, without St. Peter's Chapel, standeth a pillar of white marble, grated round about with iron, to the which our Lord Jesus Christ did lie in himself at his delivery unto Pilate, as the Romans doth say, to the which pillar, all those that be possessed of the devil, out of divers countries and nations, be brought thither, and as they say at Rome, such persons be made there whole." It was a matter of doubt, however, whether the pillar or the priest (who accompanies the patient within the enclosure) effected the cure, though we believe the weight of argument was in favour of the priest.

The same writer supposes the cause of phrenitis to consist of "water or wind enclosed in the head," and the remedies were "to purge the head with sternutatories, and the bowels with physic."

Modern pathologists have discovered that maniacs are not possessed of devils,—that phrenitis is not owing to "wind being enclosed in the head,"—that coma, lethargy, and paralysis, are not caused by "viscid blood rushing into the brain through the two carotids, and leaving in its passage a slimy matter, through which the animal spirits passing, stick by the way," but they have demonstrated that inflammation, irritation, organic lesion, and compression, give rise to the phenomena which characterize the different diseases of the brain. But notwithstanding this change of opinion in a pathological point of view, the therapeutical doctrines remain the same as formerly, with the single exception of advising maniacs to be sent to the marble pillar at Rome.

Blood-letting, probably to let out the "*slimy*" part of the blood; emetics and purgatives, to "purge off the phlegm and choler," irritating and inflaming the intestinal canal in order to cure a disease located in the brain, and now and then an opiate to cover up symptoms when too troublesome, are still resorted to by gentlemen of the old school.

It is to be hoped that the time is not far distant when all such indirect and unreasonable practices for the cure of diseases, will be entirely superseded by the more *direct* and *philosophical* method of treatment which has been instituted by the father of homœopathia and his disciples.

Probably in no class of maladies has allopathy been so much at fault as in her classification of cerebral affections. Each author who has written upon the subject, has taken upon himself to promulgate pathological views different from those of his predecessors, and from these views to form new classifications and new modes of treatment. While some nosologists recognise inflammations of the arachnoid, of the pia mater, of the cineritious, or cortical substance, of the medullary, or tubular structure, of the different lobes of the cerebellum, of the tuber-annulare, &c., as distinct diseases, requiring different modes of treatment; others, as Frank,* describe inflammation of the hemispheres of the brain, the cerebellum, and their common envelopes, as a single disease, under the general term *encephalitis*, and demanding for its cure a definite course of treatment. Thus, "*L'inflammation du cerveau, du cervelet, de leur enveloppes communes, ne présente pas, selon la différence de son siége, des symptômes distinctifs sûrs et constants.*" So also Solly, in his work on the human brain, at page 322, remarks, "I have long felt convinced that there is no such thing as inflammation of the pia mater; independent of the brain, and that much mischief has accrued from our systematic writers treating of inflammation of the membranes of the brain as distinct from inflammation of the brain itself." The same writer lays down the following broad principles, viz., "that inflammation of the brain is a depressing disease, and that, as a general rule, general blood-letting is not often admissible.

* Traité de Médicine-practique, page 116.

That, although blood-letting may sometimes be attended with benefit at the time, the good derived from it is seldom permanent." Again, "*Il n'existe pas de signes certains qui annoncent le siége de l'encéphalite, qui caractérisent la phlogose superficielle et l'inflammation phlegmoneuse avec tendance à la suppuration. Ces variétés n'offrent pas des caractères differentiels assez constants pour distinguer la frènèsie de la céphalite. L'invasion subite de la douleur, la violence de la fièvre, la stupeur des organes des sens et de l'entendement, bientôt suivie de l'extinction de leurs facultés, ne prouvent pas l'inflammation de la pulpe cérébrale.—(Frank).*"

In view of these radical differences of opinion, and from the generally acknowledged fact, that no single structure within the cranium can become inflamed, without involving to a greater or less extent other portions of the cerebral region, we shall adopt the following classification: First, *encephalitis*, embracing acute inflammation of the hemispheres, the cerebellum, and their membranes; under which head we shall point out, as clearly as possible, the peculiar symptoms which are supposed to characterize affections of these different parts. Second, the diseases which occasionally result from encephalitis, as *ramollissement, hydrocephalus*, and *epilepsy*. Third, *apoplexy* and *paralysis*. Fourth, *delirium tremens*. Fifth, *insanity*.

SECTION II.

ENCEPHALITIS.

Diagnosis.—There are certain symptoms which are common to the first stages of all acute inflammations of the cerebral organs; and which, taken by themselves, afford no indication of the actual seat of the disorder. These symptoms are, a vague sensation of coldness in the first instance, perhaps succeeded by occasional flushes of heat, lassitude, anxiety, sadness, irritability, often alternating with great exaltation of the intellectual faculties; hilarity, sudden bursts of laughter, petulance, unwonted impudence and vulgarity; redness of the skin, heat, pain, pressure or tension in the head; strong pulsations of the carotid and temporal arteries; singing noises in the head, vertigo, weakness of memory, frightful dreams, fantastic visions when awake; trembling of the limbs, nausea, vomiting; eyes bloodshot, great sensibility to light; constant wakefulness; acuteness, or dulness of hearing; mouth and tongue dry; urine copious, yellow, and thin as water.

The symptoms which usually obtain in the second stages of these affections are, stupidity, coma, paralysis, eyes suffused and dull, besotted expression of countenance, strabismus, position upon the back, pupils dilated, suppression of urine, and general loss of muscular power.

The signs which are supposed to be peculiar to the first stage of inflammation of the *cortical* substance, or hemispherical ganglion, and the membranes of the brain, are, early derangement of the intellectual faculties, fixed pain in the upper part of the head; hot and dry skin, conjunctiva injected and red; eyes brilliant, ferocious, fixed, and intolerant to light; tone rough, violent, and defiant; face red and swollen; inclination to do himself or others injury; great exaltation of muscular strength; strong pulsations of the carotid and temporal arteries; constant wakefulness; continued and rapid motions of the head; impatience, irritability, and constant agitation.

The first stage of inflammation of the medullary substance of the brain, is recognised by the following symptoms: vague chills; deep-seated headache, or vertigo; vomiting, lassitude, trembling of the limbs; *convulsions* before any signs of mental disorder, anxiety, sadness, great agitation, arms continually raised towards the head, position mostly upon the back, noises in the head. This disease is so insidious in its approach, that *convulsions* may occur as the very first symptom. In instances like this, it is probable that inflammation exists in the medullary substance alone, without involving in the slightest degree the gray matter of the convolutions surrounding this part, or the envelopes of the brain. We are forced to this conclusion if we adopt the opinions of Bouilland, Solly, Duchatelet, Hall, and Bennett, who suppose the *cineritious*, or *cortical* substance of the brain, to be " immediately connected with the intellectual powers," while the medullary portion presides over the muscular powers of the organism. Therefore, after an injury to the head, if the intellect is only impaired, we may be certain that the hemispherical ganglion is the seat of the injury, while if, in addition, there are involuntary convulsive motions of the muscles soon after the accident, we may be equally sure that the medullary substance has also received detriment.

Inflammation of the medullary structure is more prone than either of the other cerebral inflammations, to terminate rapidly in softening, and for this reason it is incumbent upon physicians to exercise the greatest care in their investigations of this class of maladies, and to apply their remedial measures with due promptness.

The most prominent secondary symptoms of disease of this portion of the brain are, muscular paralysis, and loss of sensation in the parts affected.

According to Marshal Hall, " disease of a lateral lobe of the cerebellum induces paralysis of the opposite side, and chiefly of the lower extremity. Disease of the middle lobe of the cerebellum is denoted by erection of the penis. Disease of the medulla oblongata induces paralysis of the respiratory muscles, and consequently, when complete, instant death."

We have now enumerated those symptoms which are supposed to characterize the inflammations of the different cerebral structures, and in this connection, we call the attention of homœopathic practitioners especially to this subject, with reference to the therapeutical application of medicines. Flourens has demonstrated, by experiments upon birds, that *belladonna*, *opium*, and *alcohol*, uniformly exercise a specific action upon certain portions of the brain. Hahnemann and his disciples have also proved that large doses of these articles taken in health, uniformly give rise to those physical and mental manifestations which pathologists have shown to proceed from disease of these same. parts. When, therefore, in our provings of drugs, it is observed that the prominent symptoms are, derangement of the intellectual faculties, exaltation of the mental and muscular powers, eyes bloodshot, and expression furious and defiant, manner violent and overbearing, voice loud and rough, throbbing pain in the head, face red and swollen, we may be certain that a specific effect has been produced upon the *cortical* substance of the brain. If, instead of these symptoms, we are presented with convulsions, paralysis, and general depression of the powers of the system, we may infer that the drug has acted specifically upon the *medullary* portion of the brain. The same law obtains in relation to those symptoms which characterize diseases of the different lobes of the cerebellum of the medulla oblongata, of the different portions of the spinal marrow, of the nerves, and indeed of all other parts of the organism.

In our selection of remedies, therefore, we should always endeavour to choose those of which the action has been shown, by *pathological* facts, as well as by provings, to be positively specific upon the structure affected.

Causes.—Solly has very justly observed, in his treatise on the human brain, that "there is no single cause which so frequently produces inflammation of the hemispherical ganglion, or meningitis, as sudden emotion, whether of joy or fear. The latter is, however, much more common." Other causes are, fractures and contusions of the cranium; insufficient sleep; intense and protracted thought upon a particular subject, disappointed love or ambition; repelled eruptions, whether by natural causes or by the abuse of ointments; exposure to cold, or to a burning sun; abuse of opium, and spiritous liquors; metastases of rheumatism, gout, or erysipelas, and suppression of the lochial and other habitual discharges. It often arises during the progress of pneumonia, scarlatina, erysipelas, otitis, and bowel affections. The most common predisposing causes are, plethora, a passionate and excitable disposition, want of exercise, high living, and abuse of stimulants.

Therapeutics.—In the treatment of this class of diseases, it is of especial importance that due regard be paid to the causes which may have conduced to the attack. An encephalitis which has followed immediately upon the suppression of a lochial discharge, an habitual nasal hæmorrhage, or the retrocession of an eruption by improper external applications, not only requires a remedy which shall cover all of the *manifest* symptoms, but one which, at the same time, shall operate in such a manner as to bring back the original discharge, or eruption. If disappointment, pecuniary embarrassments, fright, or political or religious excitement, has been the exciting cause, the mind of the patient should be soothed and attracted into new and agreeable trains of thought. By these means we shall prepare the organism to receive our remedies in the most favourable manner.

The principal remedies employed in encephalitis, are, *belladonna, aconite, opium, hyoscyamus, stramonium, moschus, chamomela, laurocerasus,* and *ignatia,* for inflammation of the medullary substance alone: *moschus, plumbum, acid oxalic, nux vomica, opium,* and *oleander,* for paralysis: *rhus rad., rhus tox., bryonia,* and *belladonna,* for metastasis, or extension of rheumatism to the brain: *spigelia, cuprum acetat., tartar emetic, bryonia, sulphur, tabac.,* and *belladonna,* when the disease has arisen in consequence of repelled eruptions.

Belladonna will be required when the disease presents itself as follows: febrile symptoms, accompanied with dryness of the mouth, tongue, and throat; difficult deglutition, nausea, vomiting; confusion of the head; giddiness; dilatation of the pupils; injection of the conjunctiva; eyes suffused, brilliant, furious, and protruded; imperfect vision; gay delirium; increased secretion of urine, and frequent desire to evacuate the bladder; heaviness, pressure, or throbbing pain in the head; roaring in the ears; vertigo, with nausea.

When children are the subjects of attack, Dr. Bigel gives the following excellent indications for the use of *belladonna:* "The children constantly press their heads into their pillows, they are startled by the least noise or light, there are, snoring sleep, great heat of the head, face red and puffed, with visible beating of the arteries of the head and neck, swollen veins, and occasionally hydrophobic phenomena."

During the period of dentition, and directly after being weaned, children are particularly prone to attacks of inflammation of the brain. At this age, the child is exceedingly sensitive, and there is an unusual tendency of blood towards the brain; but if the signs of cerebral disturbance be closely watched, we shall find no difficulty in combating them successfully at the onset with *belladonna.* We have often employed this remedy with satisfactory results when the following phenomena were present:

External indications.—Face hot, red, and swollen; eyes red, sparkling, and fixed, or half open and distorted; pupils contracted; visible throbbing of the carotid and temporal arteries; veins of the head distended; constant boring with the head into the pillows; paralysis of one or more parts; convulsive movements; rapid, small, or intermittent pulse; subsultus tendinum; distortion of the features; grinding of the teeth; tongue bright red, and cracked; urine scanty or suppressed.

Physical sensations.—Sharp, throbbing, or confused pain in the head; great restlessness and agitation; intolerance to sound and light; thirst; head and face very hot; limbs cold, with internal burning heat; roaring or humming in the ears; deafness; inability to speak or to swallow; nausea and vomiting during the course of the disease; sparks, flashes, or visions before the eyes.

Mental and moral symptoms.—Great sensitiveness of the nervous system; violent delirium at night; profound sleep; mania; hydrophobic symptoms.

Belladonna is likewise especially necessary in inflammations of the brain, proceeding from metastases of scarlatina, measles, erysipelas, and smallpox.

Its specific action is upon the cortical substance, the tubercula quadrigemina, and the membranes of the brain. When febrile symptoms are strongly pronounced, it should be preceded by *aconite*, or given in alternation with it.

Administration.—We advise from the first to the third attenuation for adults, and from the third to the sixth for children. As a general rule, the dose may be repeated every two hours until the required impression is produced upon the inflamed structure.

There is no proof that *aconite* affects specifically

either the brain or its envelopes. In autopsical examinations of those who have died from having accidentally taken poisonous doses, no traces of inflammation have been found in the cortical substance, or the membranes of the brain, and but slight marks of action in the medullary structure. The prominent symptoms to which large doses give rise, are, "numbness and tingling of the parts about the mouth and throat, and of the extremities, vomiting, contracted pupil, and failure of the circulation."—*Pereira, Materia Medica*, vol. ii., p. 153. The intellectual powers remain unaffected, and neither convulsions nor stupor usually occur.

Dr. Lombard, of Geneva, in his clinical practice, and in his experiments on animals, found that the internal exhibition of *aconite*, generally had the effect of "rendering the pulsations less frequent, without irregularity, and, consequently, that it exerted a decidedly sedative effect upon the heart; whence he infers that it is a proper remedy in inflammatory affections in general."

Others have observed, that its *primary* effect was to stimulate the action of the heart and arteries, and cause a universal glow over the surface; while the *secondary* effect was decidedly sedative upon the circulatory vessels.

Its effects are so manifest upon the action of the heart and arteries, that its use will be of eminent service in all those cases of encephalitis, or congestion, dependent upon a plethoric state of the system, or organic disease of the heart. It should also be given during the existence of active febrile symptoms, in all cerebral affections, and generally in alternation with some positive specific, in order that the malady may be met at all points. Attenuation and repetition of doses the same as *belladonna*.

Opium. It is conceded by both schools, that *opium*, when exhibited in moderate doses, exercises upon the human constitution two different effects—a *primary*, and a *secondary*—which are of directly opposite characters. The first of these effects is invariably stimulant, as is evinced by such phenomena as increased force and frequency of the pulse, dryness of the mouth and throat, a pleasant glow upon the skin, exaltation of the mental faculties and of the muscular system, a sense of intoxication, and temporary retention of the stools.

The *secondary* manifestations are, general diminution of sensibility throughout the body, a feeling of relaxation and calmness, tremulousness in the limbs, disinclination to exercise, pulse full and slow, drowsiness, dryness of the mouth and throat, thirst, nausea, and, finally, if a large dose has been taken, slow and laborious respiration, spasmodic contractions of the muscles, eyes half closed, pupils dilated or contracted, and insensible to the light, bloated, suffused, and besotted expression of countenance, cold and clammy extremities, respiration gasping, rattling, stertorous, face pale, sunken, and deathlike, rigidity of the jaws, entire insensibility to external impressions, pulse thready, and almost entirely imperceptible.

Wood and Bache suppose " that the active principle of *opium* is conveyed into the circulation, and operates upon the brain, and probably upon the nervous system at large, by *immediate contact with their interior structure.*"—*Wood & Bache's U. S. Dis., p.* 476.

Opium is generally supposed to cause death by suspending the " cerebral influence necessary to sustain the respiratory function ; and it is supposed, also, that the heart ceases to act in consequence of the cessation of respiration."—*Brodie.*

From these facts, we infer that the specific action of *opium* is principally upon the *medulla oblongata,* although the other symptoms indicate that there has been some action upon other parts of the brain, and also upon the skin, and lungs.

In autopsical examinations of those who have died from the effects of this substance, extravasated blood has been found in the brain, distention of the sinuses, and of all the cerebral vessels, but it is probable that many of these appearances are results of the impeded respiration, the imperfect decarbonization of the blood, and the impaired circulation which have arisen from a paralysis of that portion of the cerebral mass which presides over the respiratory functions, rather than from any specific operation of the *opium* upon these different structures.

Opium, in small doses, has always been observed to excite the venereal propensities, and has been used for this purpose for a long period by the Turks, Chinese, and Egyptians. This fact, viewed phrenologically, affords another proof of its specific action upon the cerebellum.

In proof that the active principle of *opium* is *absorbed*, and operates by *actual contact* in producing its specific effects, we quote the following from Pereira and Barbier: "The odour of *opium* is frequently recognisable in the secretions, exhalations, and breaths of persons poisoned by it, and the secretions, in some cases, appear to possess narcotic properties."

My own opinion, derived from post-mortem examinations of those who have been poisoned by opium, and from the effects to which it usually gives rise, is, that it exercises, first, a specific action upon the cerebellum and medulla oblongata. If the drug be taken in moderate doses, this action is in the first instance, *excitant*, producing venereal desires, erections, accelerated respirations, circulation, and augmented muscular force; and secondarily, *sedative*, as is shown by the languid, relaxed and calm state of the whole system, the diminution in the number of respirations, and in the action of the circulatory vessels. If taken in very large doses, the parts appear to be paralyzed at once, and all of those organs the functions of which are dependent upon the integrity of this part of the brain, cease to act.

Another specific effect of opium is upon the skin, as is evinced by the perspiration and its odour, and the eruption to which it occasionally gives rise.

Nor is it at all improbable that it may operate somewhat upon the par vagum, or the lungs themselves.

The most prominent indications, therefore, for the use of opium, are, exaltation of the physical and mental powers, succeeded by depression and calmness, dry throat and mouth, agreeable reveries, dreams, pulse at first rapid and full, afterwards slow and feeble, drowsiness, disinclination to muscular exertion, slow, irregular and stertorous respiration, profound coma, pallid, sunken and ghastly face, immoveable, contracted, or dilated pupils, rigidity of the jaws, cold and clammy extremities, complete insensibility to external impressions, and sometimes convulsive twitchings, extinction of the pulse, interrupted and gasping respiration, and finally death. It may be administered in the same manner as *belladonna*.

Hyoscyamus, *stramonium*, and *musk*, are applicable in cases attended with complete loss of sense, convulsive or spasmodic movements; closed eyes, low muttering delirium, constant movements with the hands, dilatation of the pupils, rapid and anxious respiration, frequent sighing.

If inflammation of the brain has arisen in consequence of a suppressed otorrhœa, *sulphur* should be employed. In those cases which occur in children from teething, *chamomela*, *belladonna*, and *aconite*, are our most reliable remedies.

In cases of metastases or extensions of rheumatic inflammations to the brain, *rhus rad.* and *rhus tox.* are our best remedies.

Cuprum acetat, should be given, in cases which have arisen from repelled eruptions.

When encephalitis threatens to run into dropsy of the brain, *mercurius sol.* is the best remedy to counteract the tendency to effusion.

If the disease has arisen from exposure to the sun, repeated doses of *camphor* are highly recommended.

Administration.—Our attenuations may range from the first to the sixth, and the doses repeated every two, three, or four hours, according to the severity of the symptoms.

SECTION III.

RAMOLLISSEMENT DU CERVEAU.—SOFTENING OF THE BRAIN.

It is not yet decided whether *ramollissement*, or *softening of the brain*, proceeds from inflammation, or is a disease, *sui generis*. Many of the French pathologists suppose it to be the result of inflammation; while others, as Rostan, believe it to be a disease, *sui generis*. Abercrombie believes it may arise from either inflammation, or from a condition of the cerebral structure analogous to those parts which have become gangrenous in other parts of the body, while Solly supposes that it may arise from inflammation, from a total failure of the circulation, and from "local and general anæmia." Dr. Burnett recognises two kinds of cerebral and spinal softening, an inflammatory and a non-inflammatory, and "which may always be distinguished from each other by means of the microscope."

Inflammation of the tubular structure is more prone to terminate in softening than any other portion of the brain, and it is usually very insidious in its approach.

Diagnosis.—Softening of the brain may supervene suddenly upon an attack of acute inflammation, like hydrocephalus, or it may make its appearance in a gradual and imperceptible manner. Some of the characteristic symptoms of ramollissement are, insensibility, dilated pupils, slight muttering delirium, paralysis, contraction of the flexor muscles, constipation, and a urinous smell.

Those cases which have arisen from an anæmic condition of the brain, or from an obliteration of the arteries which supply this organ, are usually slow in their progress, and manifest themselves by a gradual failure of the memory, drowsiness, an œdematous state of the body, occasional wandering of the mind, especially during the night, general languor, slow, dragging, and imperfect articulation, constipation, loss of energy and ambition, and an almost entire absence of pain or febrile symptoms.

Ramollissement, from whatever cause it may proceed, is seldom cured. As remedies, however, we suggest *opium, hyoscyamus, china, secale cornutum, carbo vegetabilis, belladonna, nux vomica.*

SECTION IV.

ACUTE HYDROCEPHALUS.

Diagnosis.—This is a malady almost peculiar to infancy and childhood. The symptoms which indicate its approach, are neither very uniform nor regular. Indeed, so various and uncertain are these symptoms, that some writers suppose the effusion to be dependent upon a debilitated condition of the membranes, analogous to dropsy, while others attribute it to inflammation in all cases.

It may appear suddenly, with most of the phenomena which we have designated as characteristic of encephalitis, viz., febrile symptoms, quick pulse, fits of screaming, expression bold and furious, eyes bloodshot and brilliant, great heat of the head, nausea, vomiting, noise and light painful, convulsions, ending in coma and death, in a few days. In cases of this description, there exists unquestionably acute inflammation of the meninges of the brain, and the effusion commences almost simultaneously with the inflammation.

In other instances, the disease approaches insidiously, presenting no marked symptoms for some days. The child will perhaps be observed to be petulant, to complain of some pain in the head, to become easily fatigued, to have occasional flushes of heat, to be restless at night, occasionally to grind the teeth, to have lost the appetite, and to prefer the recumbent position. After these symptoms have continued for an indefinite period, the more serious signs of effusion present themselves, as general diminution of sensibility, less frequent and more irregular pulse, greater debility, constant inclination to keep the bed, or to be held in the arms, dilatation or contraction of the pupils, frequent sighs, strabismus, or an unnatural expression of the eyes, turning inwards of the feet and hands, slight convulsive twitchings of the face, upper lip, and arms, automatic movements of the hands towards the head, rolling of the head from side to side, constant motion of the lips, convulsions, paralysis, and coma.

Chronic hydrocephalus, is usually the result of a very slight inflammatory action, which has progressed very slowly and insidiously. The indications which mark this affection are, gradual emaciation, feebleness, unnatural enlargement of the head, occasional giddiness, and now and then strabismus.

Therapeutics.—The medicines which we would suggest in this affection are, *belladonna, digitalis, nux vomica, phosphorus, stramonium, tartar emetic, veratrum* and *aconite.*

During the first stage of the acute variety, our most

reliable remedies are, *aconite* and *belladonna.* They should be given as often as once in two hours, until a manifest effect has been produced, after which we may repeat as circumstances require.

If the inflammation has not been promptly subdued by the use of *aconite* and *belladonna,* but signs of effusion manifest themselves in the form of "deep red, or almost brown face ; eyes rolling in their orbits, sometimes closed, and at others wide open ; lips dry ; tongue covered with a brownish yellow fur ; tension and swelling of the belly ; constipation ; generally, retention of urine, or difficulty in passing it ; respiration quick, anxious, and sighing ; deglutition difficult ; skin of the whole body dry and burning, *bryonia* acts surprisingly."—(*Bigel.*)

Helleborus nig., has been successfully employed in many apparently hopeless cases, which were attended with coldness, and insensibility of the surface ; rapid and feeble pulse ; convulsions and spasmodic rigidity of the limbs ; face pale and swollen ; constant rolling of the head from side to side ; moaning ; general prostration.

After decided marks of effusion obtain, *digitalis, mercurius sol., belladonna, veratrum* and *arnica* deserve our consideration.

Nux vomica and *stramonium* will be required when great agitation, flushed face, convulsions, strabismus, haggard and staring look, involuntary twitchings of the muscles, dilated or contracted pupils, groaning and crying, and opisthotonos, are present.

Phosphorus and *tartar emetic* will be found useful in hydrocephalus, depending upon metastasis of some disease to the brain, and in cases occurring in worn out constitutions.

Administration.—The first, second, and third attenuations should be used, and the doses repeated once in from four to six hours.

SECTION V.

EPILEPSY.

Diagnosis.—The symptoms of epilepsy are exceedingly variable. Sometimes premonitory symptoms are present, like headache, giddiness, ringing in the ears, *aura epileptica*, or prickling sensation extending from the extremities to the head, drawing inwards of the thumbs towards the palms of the hands, and sensation of fulness of the head; but more frequently the subject is struck down without any warning. When the attack comes on, the patient falls suddenly; there are violent convulsive movements, with loss of consciousness; the face and eyes become distorted; the tongue is often bitten, and in consequence we see blood and froth issue from the mouth; stertorous and difficult respiration; the muscles of one side are often more agitated than those of the other, and pulse weak, frequent and irregular; after the paroxysms have subsided, the patient usually sleeps profoundly for eight or ten hours, and sometimes remains for a considerable period in a feeble and languid state, with headache and occasional delirium, but more commonly he very speedily recovers his usual state of health and vigour.

The seat of epilepsy is supposed by some to be in the tubular structure of the brain, while others suppose that it may arise from irritation of the spinal marrow, but nothing is known with certainty upon the subject. The pathology of epilepsy is still involved in obscurity.

Causes of Epilepsy.—Organic affections of the brain, abnormal osseous deposites within the cranium, ill formed cranium, diseases of the heart, fractures of the skull, violent mental disturbances, secondary syphilis, mercurial affections, derangement of the stomach and bowels, onanism, suppressed eruptions, habitual discharges, and excesses in the use of liquors; prolonged abstinence from sexual intercourse, as well as its immoderate indulgence; and the sight of other epileptics.

Prognosis.—Epilepsy which occurs in infancy and childhood, from fright or suppressed eruptions, is curable. When the cause is abstinence from sexual intercourse, a cure may often be effected, by marrying: on the other hand, those cases which proceed from organic affections within the cranium, from long continued masturbation, and from disease of the heart, more especially if they occur after the age of twenty-five years, or if they have continued for several years, are generally incurable. As a general rule, *idiopathic* epilepsy is more difficult of cure than the *symptomatic*.

Therapeutics.—When called to a person labouring under an epileptic attack, we should at once loose all of the clothing, in order that the blood may have free circulation to and from the head, as well as in other parts of the body. We should also place a cork or some soft substance between the teeth, to save the tongue and lips from being wounded by the convulsive movements of the jaws. The patient should be placed in bed and restrained just sufficiently to prevent him doing himself personal injury during the convulsions. When the paroxysm is preceded by an *aura*, the attack may sometimes be warded off by tying a ligature firmly just above the part where the *aura* commences.

It is a general impression amongst homœopathic practitioners, that anti-psorics alone are capable of effecting a permanent cure of epilepsy. This is true with regard to those cases which are connected with syphilis, mercurial affections, and impurities of the blood, but when the disease has been caused by injury to the cranium, by mental excitements, by onanism, or by excesses in liquors or venery, it is apparent that a different course of treatment is requisite.

The most important remedies in the treatment of epilepsy are, *belladonna, sulphur, mercurius, stramonium, aconite, china, ignatia, coffea, phosphorus, arnica, opium, nux vomica, hyoscyamus, agaricus, ipecacuanha, cicuta, silicea, argentum, cocculus, cuprum, camphor.*

Belladonna.—Hartmann has found this remedy specific for the following symptoms, viz.: "great irritability of the whole nervous system, so that the patient is startled at the merest trifle; he becomes peevish and sensitive, and is affected by tremors and twitchings in the muscles; restless sleep, which is disturbed by frightful dreams; hyper-sensibility of the eyes, sparks and flashes before the eyes; also dyplopia and myopia, stammering speech, with congestion of blood to the head, and nervous distention; vertigo, with roaring in the ears; convulsions of particular muscular parts, subsultus, distortion of the face," &c. *Belladonna* will be generally applicable in those cases which have been induced by fright, or other mental emotions.

Sulphur and mercurius are proper when there is reason to suspect a psoric or syphilitic taint as the cause of the malady. These remedies should be persevered in until all trace of the impure taint has been eradicated.

Stramonium, ignatia, hyoscyamus, or *coffea* may be administered during an attack. These remedies are appropriate in cases caused by chagrin, fright, or mortification.

Camphor is indicated in epileptic attacks caused by taking cold, or by vexation,—particularly if congestion of the brain is threatened ; when caused by fright, *artemisia*, at the first or second dilution, has been found curative ; when occurring in sensitive children, during the period of dentition, *chamomela, coffea*, and *hyoscyamus* are the specifics ; in the epilepsies of nervous and impressible subjects, with distortion of the limbs and face, bloodshot eyes, foaming at the mouth, livid face, and protracted loss of consciousness, *cicuta* and *stramonium* are our best remedies ; epilepsy induced by unusual excitements, worms, exposure to a high degree of heat, and attended with sudden loss of consciousness, and of muscular power, screams, violent convulsive movements of the limbs, gnashing of the teeth, frothing at the mouth, livid face and forehead, bloodshot eyes, and irregular spasmodic twitches in various parts of the body, may generally be cured by *hyoscyamus, ignatia* and *cocculus ; nux vomica* is an invaluable remedy when the complaint proceeds from abuse of stimulants, venereal pleasures, sedentary habits, undue mental exertion, disordered stomach, or worms ; in the epilepsies of drunkards, *opium* may often succeed *nux* with advantage ; frequently recurring epileptic fits have often been permanently cured by Dr. Dunsford, with *argentum nit., belladonna, agaricus, moschus*, and *silicea ;* when the fit arises during the course of an eruptive fever, in consequence of a retrocession of the eruption, caused by cold, we may employ *ipecacuanha, cuprum*, and *belladonna*.

China and *phosphorus* should be given in epilepsy which has followed protracted masturbation, or excesses in venery. The latter may also be used in cases proceeding from osseous deposites within the cranium.

Opium and *nux vomica.*—For the epilepsies of inebriates these medicines are important, and will often effect permanent cures, after the previous habits of intemperance are corrected.

When the cause consists of an injury to the head, *arnica* is our chief remedy—this medicine should be used externally as well as internally.

If the paroxysms have been caused by fright, grief, chagrin, or from some sympathetic emotion, we may often prevent an attack (homœopathically) by exercising the patient with some more potent mental influence, which shall supersede the original cause. It was upon this principle that Boerhaave cured a number of epileptics, at the hospital for orphans of Harlem, who had been attacked in consequence of fright from seeing an epileptic brought into the hospital during a paroxysm. In these instances Boerhaave had a red-hot poker kept ready, in order, as he assured these girls, that he might apply it to their heads, as soon as there was any indication of an attack. The fright caused by this *idea* entirely overwhelmed the other cause, and an immediate cure was generally the result.

Administration.—We commonly advise the lower attenuations, and administer the remedy once or twice daily, until a cure is effected.

SECTION VI.

APOPLEXY.

Apoplexy may occur as an idiopathic, or as a symptomatic affection, and in an inflammatory or an adynamic form. We may also, with propriety, divide it into three varieties, the *sanguineous*, or extravasation of blood upon the brain, the *serous*, or effusion of serum, and finally the *simple* apoplexy, produced by abnormal distention of the vessels of the brain. The symptoms will vary according to the extent of the effusion, and the part of the brain in which the extravasation is located. If the fluid is so situated as to make pressure upon the hemispheres, there will be a sudden loss of consciousness, coma, and stertorous respiration. If the effusion occurs upon the surface of the vertex of the brain, the symptoms, according to Abercrombie, will be moderate in the first instance, but as the effusion increases, comatose symptoms come on, and the patient succumbs; when the effusion occurs near the base of the brain, there is no coma or loss of consciousness, but we find loss of speech and paralysis. It is most common at the age of fifty or sixty years, but it sometimes occurs in subjects of twenty five or thirty years.

Although this formidable malady is, in general, sudden and overwhelming in its attack, yet, fortunately, in the great majority of cases, especially of the inflammatory form, there are well pronounced premonitory symptoms for days, and sometimes for weeks preceding its onset, such as vertigo, drowsiness, throbbing pain, or sensation of numbness in the head, frequent flushing of the cheeks, unusual heat in the head, and disinclination to bodily or mental exertion. These symptoms, therefore, should always receive prompt attention, when occurring in those who are predisposed to apoplexy, in order that the threatened danger may be averted in due time.

Causes.—Apoplexy occurs most frequently in large towns, amongst the opulent and luxurious. The impure air of cities, acts as a powerful predisposing cause, and, in connection with the numerous vices prevalent in a patrician society, as want of exercise, high living, excesses in the use of stimulants, and the pleasures of love, affords a solution of the fact of its more frequent occurrence in towns than in the country.

The most common proximate causes of *sanguineous*, and of *simple* apoplexy, are, want of exercise, excesses in eating, drinking, love, suppression of an habitual nasal hæmorrhage, unnatural fulness of the blood-vessels of the brain from any cause, violent mental emotions, excessive study, and great physical exertion.

The most favourable condition for the occurrence of serous apoplexy, is, general debility and innervation, whether from insufficient nutriment, excessive mental or bodily labour, sickness, old age, long continued intemperance, abuse of drugs, or the depressing emotions.

Frank asserts that it is not rare to find *serous* and *sanguinous* effusion in the same brain, and he has detailed several instances of this kind which have fallen under his own observation.

Diagnosis.—Inflammatory apoplexy is for the most part confined to individuals of a sanguine temperament, plethoric, with short thick necks, vigorous circulation, and a great amount of animal heat. The attack is often preceded by vertigo, unusual heat about the head, face red and full, eyes injected and troubled with muscæ volitantes. The invasion of the malady is so sudden, that the patient is struck down instantly, deprived of all consciousness and power of voluntary motion. The respiration becomes stertorous, the cheeks and lips puffed out at each expiration, the pulse slow and full, pupils dilated, face red or livid, or purplish, throbbing of the carotid and temporal arteries, eyelids convulsed, either closed or half open, paralysis of the muscles of one side, or of the face only, and distention of the veins of the head and neck. After a time the breathing becomes less stertorous, the pulse more soft, and some signs of returning consciousness indicate convalescence; or, as more often happens, these symptoms become more grave, and the vital forces continue to fail, until the patient sinks under the disease.

Some of the marks which characterize *serous* apoplexy, are, general appearance of debility, face pale and haggard, pulse below the natural standard in frequency and fulness, surface cool and clammy, pupils contracted or dilated, loss of consciousness, and paralysis of one or more parts.

If the patient recovers from the more serious symptoms of this malady, there usually remains for a long time, a paralytic condition of one or more parts of the body.

Therapeutics.—We commend the following medicines in apoplexy: *belladonna, opium, rhus toxicodendron, coffea, phosphorus, laurocerasus, acid hydrocyanic,* and *protoxide of nitrogen.*

Belladonna.—External indications.—Profound coma;

stertorous respiration; face swollen, bluish or dark-red; spasmodic movements of the lips; distention of the veins of the head and neck; visible throbbing of the carotid and temporal arteries; dilatation of the pupils; injection of the conjunctiva; grinding of the teeth; suppression or involuntary discharge of urine; paralysis and immobility of one limb, or of one side of the body.

Physical sensations.—If the patient is sufficiently conscious to note his sensations, *belladonna* will cover confusion of the senses; vertigo; throbbing pains in the head; loss of memory; heaviness and pressure in the head; cramp-like pains in the face and limbs; dimness of sight; double vision: deep-seated pain in the orbits; roaring in the ears; hardness of hearing; loss of taste, or putrid taste; constipation; lameness and weakness of the extremities; painful sensitiveness of the whole surface to the touch; drowsiness, disturbed sleep; great sensitiveness to cold; aggravation of the pains by movement or by contact.

Mental and moral symptoms.—Despondency; dejection of spirits; apathy; irritability.

Administration.—In grave cases, a drop of the second potency may be given every half hour, or every hour, until the effect is manifest. When there is only a predisposition to the malady, a drop once in six or eight hours will suffice.

Opium.—External indications.—Face red, bloated, and swollen, or pale and sunken; expression of countenance stupid and besotted; distortion of the mouth; dropping of the under lip; eyes half closed, pupils dilated, and insensible to light; irregular and snoring respiration; profound coma, with stertorous and rattling respiration; convulsive and spasmodic motions; bluish colour of the lips and nails; general relaxation of the muscles; coldness of the extremities, with heat in the head.

Physical sensations.—Stupidity, imbecility and dulness of the mental faculties and senses; drowsiness; vertigo; giddiness; buzzing in the ears; heaviness, pressure, and tightness in the head; congestion of blood to the head; visions; dryness of the mouth; paralysis of the muscles of the throat and tongue;

constipation, or involuntary stools; suppression of urine; numbness and insensibility; weakness; languor; general diminution of power throughout the organism.

Mental and moral symptoms.—High spirits, succeeded by depression; calmness; agreeable reflections; pleasant fancies; taciturnity; courage; confidence; contempt of danger, and finally by coma, with stertorous breathing.

Administration. — A drop of the third dilution in water, or on sugar, and repeated according to the urgency of the case.

Rhus toxicodendron and laurocerasus are applicable in some cases of adynamic apoplexy, after *belladonna* or *opium.* It is specific for the secondary effects, which have not been removed by the last named medicines; like great prostration; paroxysms of fainting; bruised pains in the affected parts; numbness; stiffness; paralysis; cramps; great sensitiveness to cold air; tingling and twitchings in the limbs; irresistible drowsiness.

Administration.—A drop of the third dilution once in six or eight hours.

In the adynamic apoplexy of old people, *phosphorus* is a valuable remedy. The symptoms which point to its use are, general appearance of debility and prostration; face pale and sickly; eyes sunken; torpor of the mental and physical powers; coldness; paralytic weakness; tremor of the hands, and feeble pulse.

Administration.—Same as *rhus.*

Coffea, ignatia, and *nux vomica,* may be exhibited to remove the premonitory symptoms of adynamic apoplexy. The vapour of the nitrous oxyde gas may be inhaled with advantage in cases which are characterized at the commencement by great exhilaration, increase of muscular force, constant desire for locomotion, and succeeded by profound sleep, or sleep disturbed by visions. This remedy should be administered in such a manner as to produce a decided impression.

SECTION VII.

PARALYSIS.—PALSY.

Paralysis is characterized by a partial or total loss of voluntary motion or of sensation. In some cases both sensation and voluntary motion are destroyed. These symptoms occur without coma, loss of consciousness, or much derangement of the intellectual powers, if we except an occasional weakness of memory. It may follow apoplexy, or arise from disease of the spinal marrow. When it succeeds to an apoplectic attack, there is usually a paralysis of one side of the body, which is termed hemiplegia. Palsy of the lower part of the body, or paraplegia, may arise from disease of the brain, or spinal marrow, though most commonly the former organ is the seat of the affection. Partial or local palsy affects some particular part of the body, as an arm, wrist, or the face. The muscles of the face are most often affected. This variety may arise from the pressure of a tumour, from mechanical injury, or from disease of the *portia dura*. We sometimes see a palsied state of the *wrists*, which has been termed *lead palsy*, from the supposition that it owes its origin to the absorption of lead into the system. We have no doubt but that the absorption of lead may induce this palsy of the wrists; but in most of the cases which have fallen under our observation, we have been unable to trace the cause of the malady to this drug. On the contrary, we have in several instances known it follow long exposure to cold and wet, in the act of driving. In three instances this result has occurred in individuals in perfect health. In one instance, the exposure took place after a course of blue pills.

Diagnosis.—When there is only a loss of voluntary motion, the part affected wastes away, and becomes soft from want of use, while sensation may remain natural, or, as sometimes happens, there will be a morbid sensibility, or a bruised and painful feeling in the part affected. I have known this morbid sensibility in two or three cases to be exceedingly troublesome, rendering it impossible for the patient to move, or be moved, without great pain. In some cases, there is an entire loss of sensation, as well as voluntary motion. Often, when the sensibility of the part is only partially destroyed, formication is experienced in the parts affected.

The loss of muscular power and of sensation will in all instances bear a direct ratio to the extent and severity of the original affection and the part affected.

Therapeutics.—Rhus toxicodendron, arnica, nux vomica, ruta, sulphur, electro-magnetism. All of these medicines, with the exception of *ruta* and *sulphur*, are made use of as chief remedies by allopathic, as well as homœopathic practitioners.

Rhus may be used in cases of paralysis, when there is great sensitiveness to cold air; general debility; tingling or itching in the paralyzed parts; languor; constant desire to lie in bed; fainting fits.

Arnica may be given to paralytics with feeble or impaired constitutions, whose pains are aggravated by motion or talking; with painful sensitiveness of the whole body; tremors of the limbs; relaxation and general debility; *hemiplegia.*

Nux vomica is suitable for paralysis occurring in sanguine or choleric individuals. The indications for its use are, paralysis, especially of the lower extremities; trembling of the limbs; painful contractive sensations; cramps and spasmodic twitchings in the parts; languor; heaviness and stiffness of the limbs; great sensitiveness to cold air; paralysis which has been induced from abuse of stimulants, coffee, or narcotics; or where the predisposing cause has been want of exercise, with severe and protracted mental labour.

Ruta has been highly extolled as a remedy for rheumatic paralysis of the tarsal and carpal joints. It is also indicated in local paralysis, which has followed surgical operations, or which is owing to injury or pressure upon some particular nerve.

We have found *sulphur* of eminent service in cases of paralysis, accompanied by great irritability and sensitiveness of the rectum, and causing excruciating pains during every attempt at an alvine evacuation.

In all of those cases of palsy which have resisted

our treatment by internal remedies, we should have recourse to *electro-magnetism*. This agent, when properly and perseveringly applied, will often effect cures after all other means have failed. This potent remedy should always be applied, however, under the direction of a judicious physician; for it is an agent capable of doing serious injury when improperly employed.

We also suggest *baryta carb.*, *cocculus*, *lachesis*, *plumbum*, *pulsatilla*, *bryonia*, *conium maculatum*.

Administration.—The remedies may be exhibited at from the first to the third attenuations,—a dose once or twice daily.

SECTION VIII.

DELIRIUM TREMENS.—MANIA À POTU.

Dr. Solly, in his treatise on the human brain, classifies delirium as an anæmic affection of the brain. Amongst other reasons for this conclusion, he asserts that in all cases which he has examined after death, he "has invariably found the hemispherical ganglion pale and bloodless; the venous canals were generally full; and occasionally the arachnoid thickened, as if it had been the subject of chronic inflammation." A judicious distinction is made by this author, and some others of recent date, between the delirium which is produced by the sudden withdrawal of stimulants after a long and free indulgence, and that which may be excited in any person by an excessive temporary use of stimulants. The former he terms *true* delirium tremens, which depends upon an anæmic condition of the hemispherical ganglion; and the latter, *delirium ebriosorum*, depending upon a congested state of the same structure.

Dr. Solly enumerates the following as a few of the marks of distinction between the two maladies. "The head and skin generally are cool and moist in delirium tremens, dry and hot in delirium ebriosorum. The pupil varies in both according to the stage; in the early stage of both it is generally contracted, in the latter stage dilated. The conjunctiva red and injected in delirium ebriosorum; the reverse in delirium tremens.

The mental derangement in the former is more allied to an exalted, excited state of intellect; in the latter it approaches fatuity and depression. The tongue is generally pale and furred in delirium tremens, sometimes unnaturally clean and red; in delirium ebriosorum it is usually dry, and sometimes brown, but this is no certain guide. The pulse is most uncertain; but, upon the whole, there is less power in the beat of the artery, and that more varied, in delirium tremens than in delirium ebriosorum."

Diagnosis.—True delirium tremens is characterized by a wild expression of countenance; eyes fixed intently and earnestly upon some imaginary object in the room; constant endeavours to grasp or to avoid these visionary images; motions sudden and rapid; tremour of the hands and limbs, also of the tongue when protruded; tongue flabby and moist; pulse nearly natural; skin cool and often covered with perspiration; constant desire to move about; inability to concentrate the thoughts for any length of time; entire inability to sleep; mind wandering and delirious; bowels regular; face bloated; absence of thirst, heat, and other febrile symptoms; general appearance of debility.

Delirium ebriosorum may be recognised by the unnatural heat and dryness of the skin; face flushed; conjunctiva red and injected; expression fierce and excited; pulse frequent and full; tongue dry and red, or brown; boisterous delirium; increase of muscular strength; strong pulsations in the carotid and temporal arteries; pupils first contracted, afterwards dilated; inability to sleep night or day.

Causes.—Excessive and protracted use of poor liquors, abuse of opium, and other narcotics. The proximate cause of the malady is the sudden withdrawal of the accustomed stimulant. Delirium ebriosorum arises from an excessive temporary use of liquors. Alcohol, being decidedly specific in its action upon the brain, is manifestly capable, when abused, of producing an inflammation of this organ, and, consequently, the symptoms which characterize delirium ebriosorum. A *long continued* abuse of this stimulant induces an anæmic condition of the brain and nervous system, thus developing the legitimate *secondary* effect of the article, while its *temporary* abuse induces the legitimate *primary* effects which we observe in delirium ebriosorum.

Therapeutics.—Opium, nux vom., belladonna, hyoscyamus, stramonium, ether vapour, chloroform, protoxide of nitrogen.

Opium.—External indications.—Skin cold and covered with sweat; tongue moist and red; wild and staring expression; motions rapid and constant; grasping at imaginary visions; pulse rather below the natural standard; tremour of the hands and limbs; unsteadiness in moving about; face pale and bloated.

Physical sensations.—Tormented with frightful or fantastic visions; giddiness; confusion of ideas; inability to compose or to concentrate the mind, or to sleep; sensation of numbness or prickling in different parts of the body.

Mental and moral symptoms.—Delirium; frightful or fantastic visions; confusion of ideas; stupefaction; gloomy feeling; inclination to commit suicide.

Nux vom.—External indications.—Trembling of the limbs; spasmodic twitchings in different parts of the body; countenance pale and bloated; tongue white and moist; vomiting; surface covered with sweat.

Physical sensations.—Constant uneasiness, anguish, and desire to run away; troublesome visions; pressure and burning at the stomach; constipation; vertigo; headache; cold extremities; head cold or hot; sensation of debility or faintness.

Mental and moral symptoms.—Silent; apprehensive of death; confusion of ideas; depression of spirits; desire to be in the open air.

Belladonna is well adapted for the cure of delirium ebriosorum, occurring in individuals of a full, plethoric habit, and presenting the following symptoms: congestion of blood to the head; heat and pain in the head; flushed face; injected eyes; boisterous delirium; insomnia; strong pulsations of the carotid and temporal arteries; great nervous erethism; tongue and mouth red, hot, and dry; thirst; trembling of the limbs; cramplike pains; starting suddenly from sleep; failure of memory; pain in the neck and limbs; sparks before the eyes; visions.

Stramonium and hyoscyamus may be exhibited in cases complicated with epileptic paroxysms, when there are, convulsive movements; subsultus tendinum; fainting fits; muttering delirium; picking at imaginary objects; suppression of the secretions; extreme irritability; constant and rapid motions; contraction and stretching of the limbs; irascible; noisy, and difficult to manage.

Administration.—In urgent cases, the remedies may be given at the second or third attenuations every hour until the symptoms begin to yield.

The vapour of *sulph. ether,* of *chloroform,* and the *nitrous oxyde gas,* may be *inhaled* with advantage in cases which are characterized in the commencement by great mental exhilaration; increased muscular force; constant desire to move about rapidly, to dance, to sing, to leap, to fight, or do something extravagant; flushed cheeks; accelerated respiration; frequent pulse, succeeded in a short time by profound sleep, or sleep disturbed by visions; general insensibility to external impressions, with pallid and deathlike expression of countenance.

These remedies are admirable specifics in this affection, and we have known their exhibition in several instances of serious mania à potu, effect the most speedy and happy cures. They should never be administered except through the advice, and under the personal superintendence of a medical man.

SECTION IX.

INSANITY.

If it be true, that the cortical substance of the brain is the exclusive seat of the intellectual faculties, it follows, that diseases of this structure must be succeeded by more or less mental disturbance.

Insanity is supposed to be hereditary, and, so far as a general similarity between parent and child, relating to physical conformation and temperament, is concerned, there may be an hereditary influence; but the inheritance by children of the mental and moral imperfections of parents, appears to us to admit of much doubt. When the infant enters the world, his physical organization is complete, and all of the organs exercise their functions in a healthy and uniform manner, while for a long period there are but few, if any, of those manifestations denominated intellectual. On the contrary, the intellect, as it gradually manifests itself in the child, even until its full development in the adult, constantly exhibits the influence and the impressions which have been produced by circumstances, as early associations, parental example, education, habits of action and thought, poverty, riches, hardships, indulgence, &c. The proximate cause of insanity is not a derangement of the mind, but an actual disease of the *cortical substance of the brain,* and, in order to avoid the consequences of this diseased condition, it is only necessary to avoid all of those causes capable of producing inflammation or irritation of this structure. So, in effecting a cure, it is necessary to act with our medicines upon the *organ diseased,* rather than upon the mental aberration.

My respected preceptor, Dr. Brigham, in his sixth Annual Report to the Managers of the New York State Lunatic Asylum, inculcates the importance of early physical and moral education, in order that insanity may be averted in those who are physically predisposed to it. Doctor Brigham observes: "Great pains should be taken to form a character not subject to strong emotions, to passions, and caprice. The utmost attention should be given to securing a good bodily constitution. Such children should be confined but little at school; they should be encouraged to run about the fields, and take much exercise in the open air, and thus secure the equal and proper development of all the organs of the body. They should not have the intellect unduly tasked. Very early cultivation of the mind, and the excitement of the feelings by the strife for the praise and the honour awarded to great efforts of mind and memory, are injurious to all children, and to those who inherit a tendency to nervous diseases, or insanity, most pernicious. In after life, persons thus predisposed to insanity, should be careful to avoid engaging in any exciting or perplexing business or study, and should strive, under all circumstances, to preserve great equanimity of temper."

The impression has always obtained, until within the last century, that insane persons were possessed of evil spirits, and that all remedial measures must be directed towards expelling from the body the tormenting demon. It is only of very recent date that correct doctrines have been inculcated in regard to the true nature and seat of this grievous malady; but the researches of Pinel, Esquirol, and Connolly have conduced much to enlighten the profession upon this previously mysterious subject, and to point out successful modes of treatment.

The different varieties of mental alienation have been classified as follows:

1.—MANIA,

Consisting of an entire perversion and derangement of the intellectual and moral qualities. The patient seizes at the same time upon topics the most dissimilar, passing from one to the other without order or arrangement, and reasons, draws inferences and forms opinions, without any regard to logic or common sense. The intellect is deranged on all subjects, and the moral qualities indicate their perversion, by ferocity, unnatural hatreds, rage, quarrelsomeness, continual desire to do mischief, and an urgent propensity to carry into immediate effect any fancy which may strike the imagination. At the same time the patient is perfectly conscious of his identity,—has a kind of an idea of right and wrong, and is fully aware of what he is doing: but the mind operates through a diseased organ, the healthy equilibrium is lost, vague and absurd fancies take the place of reason, and the individual is impelled to obey the dictates of his diseased imaginings. Mania is usually unaccompanied by fever, except, perhaps, at its very commencement, although there is a great exaltation of the mental and muscular powers. It has also been observed that maniacs are capable of enduring the most severe bodily inflictions, and the most intense cold, without evincing much consciousness of pain,—also extreme and protracted hunger and thirst, without serious inconvenience.

Dr. Brigham remarks, that "insanity often commences in a very insidious manner. Some appear to be deranged only as regards their feelings or moral qualities. They are noticed to be different from what they formerly were; to be more restless and sleepless, or unnaturally morose and irritable. Some manifest an unfounded dread of evil, say but little, shun society, and are suspicious of their dearest friends and relatives, while others are unusually vivacious and pleasant, or quarrelsome and abusive. Such changes of character and habits, will usually be found to be subsequent to some reverse of fortune, loss of friends, or sickness, and should excite alarm. Persons thus affected, will converse rationally, and in company, or before strangers, will conceal their peculiarities, and thus are known to be insane but to very few, until some violent act leads to an investigation, and then it is found they have long been partially deranged. This is the case with most of those who commit suicide. Often insanity exists, in a slight degree, for months, and is only noticed by the most intimate friends or relatives, and then *suddenly* assume an alarming form, leading, in some instances, to homicide, and in others, to self-destruction."*

Frank asserts, "that mania may alternate with hypochondria, melancholia, or dementia. That it may be continued, remittent, or intermittent. Intermittent mania returns every eight days, every month, every three months, every year, every two years, &c." According to the same author, "mania may terminate by various crises: mucous or bloody stools, vomitings, ptyalism, leucorrhœa, epistaxis, re-establishment of the menses or of suppressed hemorrhoids, varices, eruptions, erysipelas, and boils. It may terminate by continued or intermittent fevers. It may degenerate into melancholia, or dementia. The diseases with which maniacs finally succumb, are cerebral fever, apoplexy, inflammation of the meninges, phthisis pulmonalis, and ulceration of the intestines;" complete exhaustion, also, of the physical and mental forces, is a common termination of insanity.

*Dr. B.'s Eighth Annual Report.

2.—MONOMANIA,

Is characterized by derangement upon some particular subject which constantly occupies the thoughts to the almost entire exclusion of everything else. When the patient's attention is diverted from the subject of his insanity, he reasons correctly and converses rationally upon all other topics presented to him; and even upon the subject of his derangement, he reasons consistently upon his false data. Monomania may be of a gay or of a sad character, but in a majority of instances, the monomaniac dwells upon a painful train of ideas. Sometimes a prey to the most absurd fears and dreads, as of poverty, being violently killed, suicide, homicide, of having committed the unpardonable sin, or of some serious impending calamity; sometimes he imagines himself a clock and stands in a corner of the room through the day, swinging his arms like a pendulum; or an animal, and imitates, as far as he is able, its peculiarities; or that he has no legs or arms, and therefore refuses to walk or help himself; or that he is full, and therefore cannot eat or drink any more; or, like J. J. Rousseau, that all men are his enemies, and are seeking to ruin him. At other times he imagines himself to be the Saviour, or a great prophet, or the emperor of the world, or some renowned statesman, philosopher, or general, and swells about issuing orders suitable to his fancied dignity.

Monomania may exist in a light form for a long period, without attracting particular attention. We have at the present time, under our care, two patients who have tormented themselves a good part of the time, for years, and have reduced themselves to a wretched state of health, with the dread of committing suicide or homicide, and yet they have had the firmness to conceal their morbid condition from their friends. We have known other individuals who have been thrown into phthisis pulmonalis, by silently brooding for a long time over some apprehended misfortune, like loss of property. The mind, like the body, requires rest and diversion; one set of muscles cannot be constantly exercised without becoming impaired in their functions, nor can the mind dwell upon a single train of ideas exclusively and for a long time, without becoming deranged.

This malady, like mania, may be continued, remittent, or intermittent. The cure is generally preceded by some crisis, either physical or moral. The physical crises are, eruptions, sweats, vomitings, and diarrhœas, tumours, fevers, acute inflammations of the brain. The moral crises consist of all those emotions or passions which, by violently impressing the brain, are capable of exciting a new action which shall supersede the morbid affection. Under this head may be ranked, sudden and startling news, fright, rage, violent grief, &c.

3.—DEMENTIA.

In this variety of insanity, the intellectual faculties are all impaired—the power to concentrate the thoughts, to arrange and compare ideas, or to draw inferences, is lost. The past is a blank to the unfortunate victim, and thus, family, friends, home, the associations of early years, as well as the cares and pleasures of maturity, are all forgotten. Yet the irritation of the cerebral structure often incessantly impels the patient to move about, and to give utterance to the random and incoherent images which are constantly passing through his brain. Some are silent and almost insensible to everything around them. If articles are presented or topics of interest broached for their attention, apparently no impression is produced, but the mind still pursues its incoherent wanderings.

This form of insanity is more difficult of cure than either of the others, for the causes are usually so gradual and insidious that the cerebral mass becomes hopelessly disorganized, or the meninges permanently thickened and adherent to the cranium, before serious alarm is taken. If, however, the malady is attacked within the first few months or the first year, hopes of cure may be entertained. Dr. Brigham asserts that "insanity is rarely cured after it has uninterruptedly continued two years, though there is always hope if the patient is vigorous and the form of insanity varies."

Causes.—In examining the tables of the supposed causes of insanity, as published in the reports issuing from the different insane hospitals of Europe and America, we find a very great variety; but we agree with Dr. Brigham that the general causes of insanity may, with propriety, be divided into moral and physical. Under the head of physical causes should be included, injuries to the brain, from falls, blows upon the head, &c.; all morbid or medicinal substances which, when absorbed, exert a specific action and are capable of powerfully impressing the cerebral organs, like irritating gases, as carbonic acid, and nitrous oxyde gas; vapours, like ether vapour and chloroform; also alcoholic liquors, opiates, and other narcotics; mercury, electric shocks, sun strokes, excessive labour, violent exertions, straining, masturbation, protracted sea sickness, exposure to violent heat, sudden exposure to cold water, other diseases, repelled eruptions, excesses in sexual pleasures, drying up of old ulcers, or of accustomed issues, turn of life, suppression of the menstrual or lochial discharge, metastases of rheumatism, gout, or other disease, syphilis.

The *moral* causes comprise, over-exertion of the intellectual powers, violent emotions, excessive and protracted grief, mortification, disappointed love and ambition; jealousy, remorse, anxiety, exclusive and protracted thought upon a single subject, or a single train of ideas, religious enthusiasm, vivid and unrestrained imagination, improper mental education.

Amongst the physical causes enumerated, it is well known that many of them exercise a decidedly specific action upon the brain, as for example, opium, belladonna, alcoholic liquors, the nitrous oxyde, and carbonic acid gases, the vapours of ether and chloroform, &c. Opium eating is set down in works upon insanity as one of the causes of the malady, and yet this remedy has often effected cures, both in the hands of the allopathist and the homœopathist. The vapours of ether and chloroform have caused insanity, and they have also effected cures. Alcohol causes one kind of derangement, (delirium tremens,) and yet it is an efficient remedy in effecting cures, in the hands of all practitioners. Taking these facts into consideration, we can easily explain the modus medendi of these cures, viz., the application of remedies in accordance with the only true principle of cure, *similia similibus curantur.*

Want of sleep is ranked by Dr. Brigham as the "most frequent and immediate cause of insanity, and one of the most important to guard against."

Dr. B. dwells upon this cause with much earnestness, and endeavours to *impress* upon all, the vast importance of "securing sound and abundant sleep." "Long continued wakefulness," says Dr. B., "disorders the whole system. The appetite becomes impaired, the secretions diminished or changed, the mind dejected, and soon waking dreams occur, and strange phantoms appear, which at first may be transient, but ultimately take possession of the mind, and madness or death ensues."—(*Sixth Annual Report of the New-York Lunatic Asylum, by Dr. Brigham.*)

Pathology of insanity.—Induration of the brain from long continued sub-acute inflammation, is a frequent cause of insanity. In recent and slight cases of this malady, the intellectual faculties exhibit no very prominent derangement, but as the induration progresses and extends, the hallucination becomes more strongly pronounced, until eventually complete fatuity is the consequence. Solly believes that chronic inflammation of the dura mater is a very frequent cause of insanity. In post-mortem examinations of those who have died demented, Esquirol has observed softening or increase of the density of the brain, adherences of the arachnoid, thickenings, atrophy and defective organization of the brain or cranium.

In monomania, Pinel, Frank, and Esquirol assure us "that organic lesions of the lungs and abdominal viscera, are more frequent than alterations of the brain."

The latter writer supposes displacements of the transverse colon, to be amongst the most common of these derangements, and this is supposed to account for the constipation and the pains in the epigastric region, which are usually present in this variety of insanity.

Many cases have been reported, in which no organic lesions have been found after death, either in the brain or the abdominal cavity, and on this account some authors recognise a *nervous* or *vital* monomania. It is probable, however, in all cases of mental derangement, that either the brain or its membranes are in a diseased condition, although our ordinary modes of examination may not enable us in all cases to detect it.

Therapeutics.—Our means of cure are, *moral* and *medicinal.* We have seen that a majority of the proximate causes of mental alienation consists in undue exercise of the emotions and passions. It is then reasonable to suppose that suitable moral influences may conduce much towards removing the morbid impressions.

Our general course of moral treatment should consist in calming and soothing the mind, and by presenting an entirely new train of associations and ideas, gradually divert the mind from its morbid channel, until the diseased encephalon shall recover its tone, and the impressions made upon it, produce their legitimate results. So important is it to abstract the mind from all accustomed associations and thoughts, that it is a matter of extreme difficulty to cure deranged persons so long as they are permitted to remain with their friends or in their usual residences. For this reason alone, an early removal to an insane hospital should be insisted upon, in order that proper restraints may be imposed, and the ideas directed in such a manner as to fill the mind with new impressions to the exclusion of the old ones.

In order to accomplish this object effectually, it is essential to investigate the peculiarities of each particular case, so that new and different trains of thought may be perseveringly kept before the patient.

We take occasion in this place to translate the admirable remarks of Frank upon this point: "The physician should endeavour to substitute a new passion in the place of the dominant one: for example, hope for despair, mildness for rage, etc. He should carefully prohibit monomaniacs from listening to mystical lectures or conversations, and all religious discussions. In the mean time, when the delirium consists in the fear of the judgments of God, or want of confidence in his mercy, we can sometimes cure the patient by instructing him in the true principles of religion. But it is not necessary to insist, if the melancholic, instead of relishing the solid reasons which we give him, finds in these conversations a new aliment to his delirium. The consolations of religion are always useful to persons whom reverses of fortune, domestic chagrins, unfortunate love, etc., have plunged into a melancholic state. We have seen a case of melancholia with propensity to suicide, fixed by excess of study and of onanism; the patient suffered moreover much from hypochondria. Voyages, distractions, and rigid diet produced only momentary relief. The consolations of religion, a rigorous observance of continence and of other christian virtues, gradually operated a cure. We have re-examined this patient at the end of six years: he enjoys perfect health, and when a sad idea comes to darken his imagination, the most simple practice of religion suffices to restore to his mind calmness and serenity. Religion is capable of operating similar cures daily; it acts upon the heart of man with much more force than all the arguments of philosophy. But its happy influence is unknown to the incredulous, and as we do not think that the proofs of religion can be submitted to the discussion of a lunatic, we reserve the succours contained in the evangelical moral, to pious minds, or at least to believers, whom different causes have plunged into melancholy. As for unbelievers, we can only offer them beautiful maxims, and the cold consolations of philosophy."—(*Medecine Practique; par J. P. Frank.*)

Monomaniacs may sometimes be cured, however, by indulging them in their delusions, and encouraging them in the hope of being able to remove the cause. The late Dr. George McLellan once had a case in point: a highly intelligent merchant was firmly possessed with the idea that there was a living eel in his stomach, and he so tormented himself with the delusion, that he became seriously ill, and was obliged to abandon his business. He had employed many eminent physicians, who all ridiculed his delusion, and endeavoured to convince him of its absurdity, but all to no effect; the idea continued firmly fixed, and his general health continued to suffer, when as a last resort, and in disgust at the ignorance and obstinacy of all physicians, he called in Dr. McLellan, who, on investigating his case, decided to indulge the patient in his delusion, and accordingly assured him that he had a monstrous living eel in his stomach, but that he could give him a medicine which would destroy the animal, and carry it off by way of the bowels. Accordingly a long prescription was written, amounting to a powerful drastic purgative, and the patient directed to take it. At its operation, the attendant was advised to slip a mutilated eel into the vessel, and convince the invalid that it had passed from him. The stratagem succeeded admirably, and the man was directly restored to health, mental and bodily.

Frank mentions the case of an individual "who did not wish to urinate for fear of producing a new deluge : he was told that if he persisted in his sad resolution, a fire would occur and burn up the universe. He hastened to urinate, and his delirium vanished." Another monomaniac believed himself damned : one of his friends, habited as an angel, entered his chamber during his sleep, holding in one hand a flambeau, and in the other a glistening sword. He announced to him, in behalf of God, the pardon of his crimes, and the patient was restored to health. Another monomaniac imagined that there were rabbit-burrows in his head. To cure this illusion, they made a crucial incision in his scalp, and showed him bloody rabbits, which they told him had retired by the wound."

Much, however, must depend upon the peculiar circumstances attending each particular case, in applying our moral treatment; but as a general rule, uniform kindness, respectful treatment, proper discipline, and a perseverance in all of those means which tend to direct the mind into new channels, like games, music, gymnastic exercises, mechanical or agricultural labour, exhibitions, etc., will enhance very materially our success in the treatment of this class of maladies.

The employment of baths are highly recommended by some authors. As the daily habit of general bathing is considered at the present day not only essential to health, but to personal cleanliness and decency, we deem it as unnecessary to allude to the habitual attention to this important duty, as it would be to allude to the importance and propriety of other personal habits, like washing the hands and face, or changing the linen. Tepid or cold baths may be employed, as the condition of the patient demands; but as the healthy function of the skin is so often deranged in insanity, and as nothing conduces so much to restore and preserve this function as frequent bathing, its importance will be readily appreciated. During the first stages of mania, or at other periods when there exists great excitement, with hot skin and frequent pulse, the cold shower-bath, or the cold dash, may be employed with decided advantage. Some discrimination, however, is requisite in using these more powerful applications.

The most certain specifics which we possess for the cure of insanity, are, *opium, belladonna, nux vomica, aconite, ignatia, hyoscyamus, stramonium, pulsatilla, veratrum, platina, conium, helleborus, aurum mur.*

Opium is suitable in cases of *dementia,* attended with stupefaction of the senses; general loss of mind and sensation; indifference to pain or pleasure; strange visions; laborious respiration; constipation; face pale, or red, or brownish; diminished temperature of the skin; full and slow pulse; spasmodic motions and trembling of the limbs.

Belladonna.—External indications.—Furious and violent derangement, or merry and silly craziness; face red and hot; expression gay, or ferocious with fixed look; eyes brilliant, pupils dilated; head hot; spasms; startings; sanguine choleric temperament; impressible nervous system.

Physical sensations.—Vertigo; headache from congestion of blood to the head; sleeplessness, with great uneasiness and anguish; frightful dreams, starting one suddenly from sleep; spasms or stiffness of the limbs; constant inclination to change the position of the limbs; visions; thirst; general sensation of uneasiness and discontent.

Mental and moral symptoms.—Furious mania; rage; or sadness, despair, and fear of death.

Pathological anatomy.—Congestion of the vessels of the brain; injection of the vessels of the dura mater, pia mater, and substance of the brain with black blood.

Nux vomica is suitable for ***suicidal monomania***, attended with great anguish, and desire to go from place to place ; also in nervous *hypochondria*, arising from derangement of the stomach and liver ; also mental derangement, arising from abuse of liquors; from mortification ; from excessive study ; from suppressed hæmorrhoids. It is sometimes useful to remove the constipation which is so frequently present in insanity.

When there are frequent and full pulse, hot and dry skin, thirst, and other febrile symptoms, with congestion of blood to the head, and a general exaltation of the muscular and mental powers, *aconite* may be employed to remove this condition.

Ignatia is recommended in *melancholy* and *fixed mania*, occurring in individuals of a mild disposition, sad or cheerful, and occasioned by fright, despair, anguish, grief, chagrin. A relaxed, exhausted, and feeble condition of the body also requires it.

Pulsatilla is indicated in puerperal melancholy, and when it occurs during pregnancy, with anxiety, pain in the head, sleeplessness, pressure at the heart, general uneasiness, vague desire to escape, incoherent talk, sadness and distrust.

Stramonium is applicable in derangement with spasmodic symptoms ; in puerperal mania ; in timid mania, with staring look, desire to escape, screeching, frightful visions, heat, redness and moisture of the skin ; in loquacious mania, with great mirthfulness, laughter, high-flown speeches, and ridiculous motions ; also in *religious monomania*, with great depression of spirits, despair of salvation, and desire to converse upon the subject. It is also sometimes useful in "rage, with furious delirium."

Veratrum is proper in hypochondriac, suicidal, and religious melancholy ; in puerperal mania ; in mania with lewdness and lascivious speeches, and in some cases of furious mania. This remedy is especially indicated when the derangement partakes of an intermittent character.

For the treatment of suicidal monomania, accompanied with extreme depression of spirits, unrefreshing sleep from frightful dreams, dread of some impending calamity, loss of ambition and energy, diminution of virile strength, and a constant disposition to dwell upon imaginary ailments, *muriate of gold* is a remedy worthy of the very highest consideration. Indeed, in cases of this description, no other medicine can bear any comparison with it.

Platina is excellent for females of excitable temperament, and with strong sexual desire. It has cured melancholy, with great timidity and depression of spirits, all persons seeming to be demons; or with vanity; trembling of the hands and feet; anguish at the heart; absence of mind; dread of death; furor uterinus; constipation; small and feeble pulse.

There are other remedies which may be consulted in the different varieties of insanity, like the vapours of ether and chloroform, the nitrous oxyde gas, &c. But as we have not had sufficient experience in the use of these, we shall not now attempt to point out the symptoms which demand their use.

Administration.—As a general rule, the above medicines may be given at the first or second attenuations, every twelve or twenty-four hours until there is a medicinal aggravation, or an amelioration of the symptoms.

SECTION X.

INFLAMMATION OF THE SPINAL MARROW, AND ITS MEMBRANES.

Under this head we include *tetanus* and *hydrophobia.*

1.—TETANUS.

We understand by the term tetanus, sudden morbid contractions or cramps of many muscles of the body, with rigidity and loss of voluntary motion in the affected parts. This morbid contraction and rigidity may affect the muscles of almost every portion of the body, or it may be confined to the muscles of a single part, like the lower jaw, when the affection receives the name of *trismus;* or to the extensors of the back, giving rise to *recurvation* of the body, when it is termed *opisthotonos;* or to those of the front part of the body, causing *incurvation*, termed *emprosthotonos;* or to the muscles of the side, causing a *lateral* curvature, and called *pleurothotonos.*

Tetanus is much more common in hot than in temperate latitudes, and generally selects for its victims individuals of a nervous and irritable temperament, or those whose constitutions have been impaired by the abuse of stimulants, or exposure to a vitiated atmosphere.

There are two varieties of tetanus, the *traumatic*, and the *idiopathic*. The usual exciting causes of the former are, punctured and lacerated wounds, causing injury or partial division of the nerves; and of the latter, general debility of the nervous system from long continued illness, or protracted derangement of the different functions of the organism.

Diagnosis.—This malady generally commences with uneasiness at the præcordia; stiffness and tension in the muscles of the back of the neck, back, and loins, and some difficulty in deglutition and in articulation. This contraction and stiffness gradually increases; the sensation of uneasiness in the chest becomes changed to violent and painful contractions about the ensiform cartilage; the pains and cramps extend to the back, jaws, and limbs; the appetite fails; the countenance assumes a flushed and anxious appearance; the bowels are constipated; the mind remains sound until the last stage of the disease, and the body will be rigidly drawn into such a position as will enable us to decide what particular class of muscles are affected, and which of the varieties of tetanus is present.

Traumatic tetanus is always a dangerous affection, but hopes of cure may be entertained when unusual pains in the wound or cicatrix, with pains extending along the limbs in the direction of the contracted parts, occur simultaneously with the first symptoms of the complaint. But if the symptoms continue to make steady progress, while the original wound is cicatrized, and no pain or disturbance is experienced either at this point, or extending from it, the case may be looked upon as highly dangerous.

Idiopathic tetanus proceeds from constitutional causes, and is far less dangerous than the *traumatic* variety. Its approach is also more gradual, and attended with less pain, but when the contraction and rigidity of the parts take place, they remain in this condition a longer time than in the other form of the disease. The violent contractive pains about the ensiform cartilage, and in the nape of the neck, which are so characteristic of traumatic tetanus, are also absent in this variety. Indeed, we have seen cases where no pains or uneasy sensations were experienced in any part of the body, except from the constrained positions of the parts affected with the morbid contraction.

Causes.—Punctured and lacerated wounds, which partially divide one or more nerves, is one of the most common causes. The admission of cold air into wounds, sudden check to the perspiration after long and fatiguing exercise under a hot sun, the irritations of splintered bones, or other foreign substances in contact with nerves and tendons, amputations, and blows upon the spine, are all occasional causes of traumatic tetanus.

The exciting causes of idiopathic tetanus are, suppressed menstruation, or other habitual discharge, low fevers, over-exertion of mind or body, too close confinement in small and ill ventilated apartments, sitting in unnatural and constrained positions, tight lacing.

Therapeutics.—A preliminary step in the treatment of tetanus, should always be to remove, as far as possible, whatever causes may have operated towards inducing the disease, or which may continue to exert an irritating effect after its full formation. The causes of this character are, the presence of irritating spicula of bone, of needles, of dirt, of rust, or any other foreign substance, in contact with the nerves and tendons; abuse of stimulants, the wearing of too tight clothing, foul air, exposure to sudden changes of temperature, especially from intense heat to coldness and humidity. When there is reason to suspect the presence of a foreign body in a cicatrized wound, after the appearance of tetanic symptoms, we should at once cut down and endeavour to extract the obnoxious substance; and in case nothing can be found, to apply spirits of turpentine, or some escharotic, in order to ensure suppuration in the wound. This important surgical resource should always be resorted to in cases of this description, for it is not an uncommon occurrence to perceive the immediate disappearance of incipient tetanic symptoms, on the removal of a foreign substance from the wounded part.

The remedies most appropriate in the treatment of tetanus, are, *nux vomica, belladonna, arnica, stramonium, cicuta, hyoscyamus, opium, pulsatilla, sulphur.*

Nux vomica, from its decidedly specific action upon the spinal marrow, and its membranes, as well as from its pathogenesis, and the appearance of individuals who have been poisoned with it, is evidently a remedy of importance in this dangerous malady. It is especially called for when the spasms are frequent and short, consciousness is perfect, and there are cramp-like pains in the region of the stomach, constipation, and loss of appetite, and when the patient has been addicted to the abuse of stimulants.

Belladonna, succeeded by *pulsatilla,* may be given in idiopathic tetanus which has arisen from deranged menstruation, or other causes connected with the utero-genital system, and where the extremities are for the most part affected with the morbid contractions. It may also be sometimes given in the last stages of traumatic tetanus, when there is delirium, dilated pupils, and great mental anguish.

Arnica should be used both internally and externally, in all injuries which threaten to lead to tetanus. This remedy possesses the power of warding it off, when it might otherwise have occurred without its use, and should always be resorted to when danger is anticipated from a wound.

When we find great rigidity of the extremities, contraction of the thumbs or fingers, wild and fixed look, painful and difficult respiration and deglutition, we may give *stramonium* in alternation with *hyoscyamus* or *cicuta.*

Many writers speak in favourable terms of warm baths in the treatment of this affection. We have seen the most unequivocal advantage follow general bathing, and a thorough application of fomentations to the affected parts, and to the spine. We can call to mind two cases where life was apparently saved by the persevering application of these hot fomentations, together with frictions along the course of the spine.

We take occasion in this place to suggest to the profession the use of the saliva of rabid animals as a remedy in this affection. It has been found by Majendie and Brechet, that if this saliva be introduced under the skin, or into the blood of animals, that the animal so impregnated contracts the hydrophobia. Why should it not then be employed in those maladies which are characterized by symptoms similar to those of rabies?

Other medicines which may demand attention are, *veratrum, moschus, phosphorus, china, ignatia, lachesis, acid hydrocyanic, camphor, plumbum.*

Administration.—We advise from the third to the sixth attenuations in this affection—a dose every hour until the system responds in a satisfactory manner, after which we must be governed by circumstances.

2.—HYDROPHOBIA.

The term hydrophobia, or dread of water, is given to that dreadful malady which follows the bite of a rabid animal, and the introduction of its saliva into the blood. A dread of water is commonly a prominent and characteristic symptom of the disease, but it is by no means one which is invariably present. Cases are reported by Hunter, Frank, and Eberle, in which no unpleasant consequences followed the use of drinks, from the commencement to the fatal termination of the disorder. We, ourselves, have seen a rabid dog that would, without hesitation, plunge into water and drink during the whole course of the disease, without exciting spasmodic contractions, or any other disagreeable symptom.

Rabies originates spontaneously in animals of the canine species, like the dog, the fox, the wolf, &c., and appears to consist of a morbid deterioration of the saliva. The precise nature of this deterioration, or of the specific poison which this fluid contains, is at present entirely unknown; but in regard to its specific action upon some portion of the nervous centres, there remains no doubt, although morbid anatomists have hitherto failed to detect the peculiar diseased appearances to which it gives rise. Perhaps this may be accounted for when we call to mind the proneness of pathologists to regard congestion of the blood-vessels, redness, effusion, softening, or induration, as the only morbid appearances indicative of previous disease, while in point of fact, if we may trust the pathological investigations of Dr. Hugh Bennett, by means of the microscope, "important changes may take place in the cerebral substance, spinal marrow, &c., inappreciable to the naked eye, but clearly discernible with the microscope."—(*Ed. Med. and Surg. Jour.*, vol. 58, p. 58 and 60."

The redness of the fauces and œsophagus which is often observed in men and animals dead of hydrophobia, is attributable rather to the irritation consequent upon the intense and unindulged thirst which was present during the attack, than to any specific action of the virus upon these parts.

The virus of rabies is formed and is active, for the most part, in the saliva, but a sufficient quantity is absorbed into the general circulation to produce the morbid impression upon the spinal marrow which constitutes the chief fact of the disease. Could we confine the virus to the saliva of the mouth, and prevent its admission into the circulation, no evil effects would result; but place the smallest quantity in a position where absorption can take place, and it will be conveyed with unerring certainty to the part which possesses a specific affinity for it, and there produce its legitimate morbid impression.

Some writers suppose that the poison does not enter the general circulation, because the N. American Indians, the inhabitants of the country of Mantone, &c., often eat the flesh of hydrophobic animals with impunity; but this proves nothing, for the lacteals and absorbents of the digestive apparatus, reject this substance as an irritant, and it is carried off with the fæces, without producing any impression.

McIntosh believes that tetanus is often mistaken for hydrophobia, when dread of liquids is one of the symptoms of the former; and when we reflect that the teeth of dogs usually inflict such punctured or lacerated wounds, as often give rise to tetanus, the opinion seems plausible.

Hydrophobia usually makes its appearance in from twenty to sixty days after the bite, although well authenticated cases are recorded in which the virus has remained dormant in the system for years, when it has finally developed itself from some constitutional disturbance, and the patient has succumbed with all the symptoms of hydrophobia.

Diagnosis.—At an uncertain period, varying from three to nine weeks from the reception of the wound, the first symptoms of hydrophobia make their appearance, usually in the bitten part, which presents a livid and slightly swollen appearance, and attended with burning heat or shooting pains which dart from the seat of the injury to the neighbouring parts. These symptoms are speedily succeeded by rigours, lassitude, great depression of spirits, anxiety, watchfulness, irritability, giddiness; eyes red, brilliant and sensitive to light, uneasy sensations at the stomach, tension at the chest, difficulty of deglutition, and slightly oppressed respiration. As the disease advances, the cramps about the throat, neck, and chest, become more and more violent, until the mere sight of a liquid, or of a shining substance, will produce the most painful paroxysms: there is a viscid saliva constantly secreted which compels the victim to be continually spitting, while at the same time he is tormented with a dryness in the mouth and throat, and an intense thirst, which he is unable to allay, on account of the spasmodic contractions which occur whenever drinks are presented to him. The skin is hot and dry, the cicatrix opens and presents an unhealthy appearance, the respiration becomes more and more difficult, the voice becomes changed, the pulse nearly natural, the body affected with tremours or slight spasmodic twitchings, vague pains extend up from the lower part of the spine to the head, and finally the countenance becomes pale and haggard, the eyes sunken yet still brilliant, there are palpitation of the heart, wandering delirium, constant inclination to bite, extreme anxiety and uneasiness, sinking of the pulse, loss of voice, clammy sweat, and finally, the sufferer sinks into a lethargy, or into convulsions, and dies.

The disease commonly terminates in from two to eight days from its first approach.

Therapeutics.—The most certain *preventive* means after the bite of a rabid animal, is to excise immediately and thoroughly, the wounded part. This severe measure can only prove available unless resorted to within a very short period—say fifteen or twenty minutes after the infliction of the bite. If a longer time than this has elapsed, we should advise free incisions upon the wounded points, and after they have bled freely, and been suitably washed and cleansed, the application of the caustic alkali. Some surgeons speak in high terms of the application of the red-hot iron, of the butter of antimony, of corrosive sublimate, of chloride of zinc, &c.; but in my opinion, the prompt use of the knife, and of caustic potash, will prove more efficient and less painful than the other applications. Nor do I give this advice from theory alone, for I had occasion, some five years since, to test the *practical* operation of these severe measures upon my own person. In July, 1844, I was bitten in the leg, without provocation, by a dog which came tearing past me at a furious rate, with fierce and brilliant expression of the eyes, tail pendant between the legs, foam at the mouth, and hair standing erect upon the back. Without any delay, I excised the bitten part, and applied the caustic potash to the wound, in the most thorough manner; after which, I dressed and bound up the limb, congratulating myself on my promptness, and probable escape from this most dreadful malady. Inquiries were now instituted to ascertain something respecting the course and the whereabouts of the "mad dog," when to my surprise, and indeed I may say indignation, I was informed that the animal was not rabid, but "dreadful ugly." The course adopted, however, was a prudent and safe one, and I should most certainly do the same again under similar circumstances, on the principle "that an ounce of prevention is worth a pound of cure." As the matter actually turned out, I was tormented with a painful limb for two or three months unnecessarily; but had the animal proved to have been rabid, then the result would have been the saving of my life.

No specific has yet been discovered for the cure of hydrophobia, although many articles have been at different periods brought into notice by the old school, as for example, *mercury*, *burnt lichen*, and *black pepper*, the *purple-flowered anagallis*, *oil of valerian*, *opium*, *musk*, *ignatia*, *camphor*, *cantharides*, *stramonium*, *nux vomica*, and *belladonna*.

Professor Munch has given the last named medicine to several who had been bitten by rabid dogs, and not one was attacked with rabies. Hahnemann also administered it with success, both as a prophylactic and as a curative remedy.

In consulting the pathogenesis of *belladonna*, we find amongst the most prominent symptoms to which it gives rise, are dryness and constriction of the mouth and fauces, accumulation of a tough mucus about the mouth, deglutition difficult or even impossible, injected and glassy eyes, articulation difficult, voice changed, giddiness, trembling and weakness of the whole body; mouth and jaws spasmodically affected, intense thirst, nausea, and finally, previous to death, "a feeble pulse, cold extremities, subsultus tendinum, tremours, deep coma or delirium, and sometimes convulsions."

From the above description, it is apparent that this medicine induces a close correspondence to the most marked symptoms of hydrophobia, and therefore it is entitled to our earnest consideration, when called to cases of this description.

When the disease is fully formed, and there are, severe convulsions, with sense of impending suffocation, dryness of the mouth and fauces, extreme difficulty of deglutition, dread or horror even at the sight of liquids, delirium, rage, and fury, we may likewise consult *stramonium*, *nux vomica*, *hyoscyamus*, *lachesis*, *cantharides*, and *veratrum*.

The medicines may be administered in the same manner as advised in *tetanus*.

SECTION XI.

CHOREA.

Chorea occurs, for the most part, in girls of feeble constitutions and of irritable nervous temperaments, and between the ages of five and fourteen. The disease is recognised by almost constant involuntary movements of the muscles affected, while in the waking state, either with or without derangement of the intellect. From its resemblance to raphania, it has been sometimes confounded with it. It also presents many marks of similarity to epilepsy and hysteria, and is probably somewhat analogous to these maladies in its location and nature. The affection is not usually attended with danger, and terminates at the period of puberty; but when it has existed for a number of years, accompanied by perversion of the intellectual faculties, permanent idiocy, or at least an impaired understanding, may result. Finally, the disease may occasionally occur at any period of life, and in individuals of both sexes.

Diagnosis.—Generally, for months previous to the occurrence of the involuntary motions which characterize this disease, it will be found that the child has suffered from constipation, oppression in the region of the stomach and chest, vertigo, and other bad feelings in the head, appetite morbidly increased or depressed, occasional flushes of fever during the night, palpitation of the heart, nervousness, irritability, and coldness of the feet. The involuntary motions commence by slight twitchings in the muscles of the face, which soon become strongly pronounced and extend to a greater or less extent to other parts of the body, as one entire side, or one arm or leg. When the limbs are affected, the walk becomes awkward and unsteady, and the arms fail to obey the commands of the will, while involuntary gestures and motions are continually made without reason or point, thus causing the individual to present a most ludicrous appearance. The patient may remain in this condition for years, without the occurrence of any other serious consequences, unless the intellect becomes impaired, when a total loss of mind may result. Some cases are attended with difficult respiration, dysuria, vague pains in the limbs, confusion of ideas, and failure of memory.

Causes.—A naturally delicate constitution or one which has been impaired by abuse of medicines, and a nervous temperament, are conditions most favourable to the production of chorea. Probably, the most frequent exciting cause is the repercussion of some chronic cutaneous eruption. Many facts are on record which go to prove this; as, for example, the cases cited by Hahnemann, Stapf, Pouchet, Frank, &c., where the malady has arisen in consequence of sudden drying up of tetter, plica polonica, herpes, scald-head, psora, or some habitual discharge. Other exciting causes are, the depressing passions, fear and terror, masturbation, irritation of the bowels from worms and fæcal accumulations, cold, insufficient nutriment, and excessive loss of blood.

Therapeutics.—In all cases of chorea the patient should be removed to the country, where she may enjoy pure and salubrious air, abundant exercise, and a plain, but highly nutritious regimen.

The remedies for chorea are, *stramonium, belladonna, cuprum acetat, sulphur, calcarea carb., hyoscyamus, rhus, nux vomica, ignatia, lycopodium, phosphorus, china, ferrum.*

If the disease has been caused by fright or terror, and we find great contortions of the face, eyes, and limbs, head thrown back, or drawn frequently to the left side, oppressed respiration, wild and staring expression, convulsive laughter or weeping, restlessness, convulsive twitchings of the muscles, anxiety, pale face, features sunken, small pulse, and delirium, we may select one of the following medicines: *stramonium, belladonna, hyoscyamus,* and *ignatia.*

When the symptoms have followed the drying up of chronic cutaneous eruptions, *cuprum acetate, sulphur* and *lycopodium,* will be called for; if they have set in after measles, *calcarea carb.* is proper; if the cause can be traced to onanism, *phosphorus* and *china* are applicable; if they have arisen from constipation, and collections of fæcal matter in the intestines, *nux vomica* and *sulphur* are the best remedies; if the malady has been induced by excessive loss of blood, or by general debility, we advise, *ferrum*, *china*, *acid phosph.*, *acid nitr.*, and *rhus toxicodendron*.

Administration.—In chorea, the whole nervous system is in a morbidly impressible condition, and will generally respond readily to the higher attenuations. We usually commence with the twelfth dilutions, and administer a dose once or twice daily, until a suitable impression is made upon the symptoms.

SECTION XII.

HYSTERIA.

Sydenham, Stahl, Van Swieten, Sprengel, and Frank, regard *hysteria* and *hypochondria* as substantially the same affection. The two maladies unquestionably bear a very close resemblance to each other in many respects; as, for example, the almost infinite variety and similarity of the symptoms which they present, and the proneness of the subjects of both diseases to exaggerate trivial or even imaginary ailments into disorders of magnitude.

But there are marks of distinction between them equally important, which refute conclusively the opinion respecting their identity.

Pure hypochondria almost invariably occurs in individuals of a lymphatic and bilious temperament. Their dispositions are generally gloomy and morose, and ever inclining to "look on the dark side." Hope, confidence, cheerfulness, enter but sparingly into their dispositions; they are not addicted to "building castles in the air;" never behold anything bright, agreeable, or desirable in the future; but, looking with distrust and aversion upon mankind, and obstinately fixing their thoughts upon some dreadful impending calamity, which they are sure will overtake them sooner or later, they either drag out a miserable existence, suffering mentally almost every evil, or terminate their woes by suicide.

Hysteria, on the contrary, usually occurs in females of a nervous, or nervous-sanguine temperament, with cheerful, lively, and ardent dispositions, vivid imaginations, and highly impressible organizations.

Hypochondria is uniform and continuous in its course, and presents but slight variations from day to day. Hysteria occurs in paroxysms, with intervals of greater or less duration, of passable bodily health and excellent spirits.

Hypochondria is always connected with disorder of the stomach and liver. Hysteria is owing to an irritation or erethism of the whole nervous system.

Writers have always regarded the seat of hysteria as in the uterine and sexual organs, because it has usually been associated with derangement of the functions of these organs. It occurs after the period of puberty, in females of a nervous, or nervous-sanguine temperament, with strong sexual propensities, and is accompanied with deranged menstruation, dysuria, sexual excitement, or pains in the pelvic region. Yet the malady is, in my opinion, one of a purely nervous character, consisting of an erethism of the whole nervous system, and capable of being brought into active operation by any exciting cause which may operate upon the economy, like deranged menstruation, the depressing emotions, fright, terror, mortification, dread, chagrin, disappointed love, undue excitement of the sexual organs, &c.

This peculiar irritable condition of the nervous system may exist for an indefinite length of time, without any actual development of proper hysteric symptoms, provided the above named *exciting* causes do not operate.

Diagnosis.—Sometimes the first symptoms of hysteria are flatulency, pains, or distressing sensations in the stomach, bowels, chest, head, and back ; faintness, vertigo, bitter taste, eructations, dysury, anxiety, depression of spirits, difficulty of breathing, sense of suffocation from something like a ball rising in the throat, (or globus hystericus), ringing in the ears, delirium, or loss of consciousness. Symptoms of this kind take place in individuals of a feeble and purely nervous temperament, and the *delirium* and *loss of consciousness* appear to take the place of *convulsions.*

In others, of a nervous-sanguine temperament, with robust constitutions, the convulsive paroxysms come on by slight twitchings of the muscles of the mouth and eyes, with wild expression, eyes rolled up, convulsive laughing, crying, or sobbing, constant attempts to pull out the hair, to strike the breast or some other part, and to bite ; difficult and laborious respiration, succeeded in a short time by the most violent convulsions.

In other instances the paroxysms are preceded by a croupy-cough, or colic pains, or pains in the head, chest, back, or pelvis.

In some cases the paroxysm takes place suddenly, without any warning symptoms, and the patient may suffer a series of dreadful convulsions, with only brief intervals of consciousness, for many hours, and then be restored speedily to all her mental and bodily faculties.

It would be useless to attempt a detail of all the phenomena which may occur in hysteria, and we shall in conclusion only observe, that the peculiar condition of the nervous system upon which the disease is dependent, and the convulsive paroxysms to which this morbid state gives rise, should command our principal attention in the treatment of the malady.

Causes.—The predisposing causes are, a delicate, nervous temperament, too much confinement in close and heated apartments, the frequent perusal of exciting works of fiction, attendance on theatrical exhibitions, tight lacing, want of exercise, premature tasking of the mind to the neglect of the body, habitual indulgence in lascivious thoughts, nervousness, luxurious living.

Amongst the exciting causes may be mentioned, violent mental impressions of any kind, whether produced by the sight of disagreeable objects, or the smell of disagreeable odours, or the hearing of sudden noises, discordant sounds, or by terror, fright, anger, rage, grief, chagrin, mortification, and disappointed love or ambition.

Hamilton supposes the presence of irritating and indigestible substances in the intestines is a common exciting cause of hysteria.

Other exciting causes are, sudden suppression of the menstrual discharge, too profuse evacuations and leucorrhœa.

Therapeutics.—For the cure of hysteria arising from a torpid state of the bowels, and an accumulation of undigested fæcal matter, and attended with putrid or sour taste, bitter or acid eructations, flatulency, fulness, distention and pain in the epigastrium, constipation, nausea, weakness, languor, faintness, headache, giddiness, confusion of ideas, strong tendency to convulsions, *nux vomica* and *sulphur* are the proper remedies.

When the attacks appear to have been excited by derangement of the uterine functions, the most suitable remedies will be *pulsatilla, sabina*, and *silicea.*

If the exciting cause has been terror, fright, anger, disappointment, mortification, or any violent mental excitement, *ignatia, hyoscyamus, aurum, belladonna, coffea,* will each cover most of the symptoms.

Administration.—The remedies should be administered at the third dilution, during the paroxysm, by placing a drop upon the tongue at short intervals, or by smelling; but during the intervals, a drop once in twelve hours, until the desired impression is produced.

SECTION XIII.

NEURALGIA.

By the term neuralgia, we designate all of those painful affections, in different parts of the body, of a purely nervous character. This disease may attack every system of nerves, and every structure of the organism, whether external or internal. Different names have been given to it, derived from the particular structures affected, but as the real nature of the disease is always the same, in whatever part it may be located, and as the points of its attack are almost innumerable, there is a manifest difficulty and impropriety in endeavouring to effect a minute classification. The most common seat of neuralgia is in the first, second and third branches of the fifth pair of nerves, and in the portio-dura. When the disease is confined to the facial portions of these nerves, it is recognised under the name of *tic douloureux ;* when its location is in the nerves of the stomach, *gastrodinia ;*

when in the first branch of the fifth pair of nerves, *nervous headache;* when in the nerves of the feet and legs, *neuralgia pedis;* when in those of the mammæ, *neuralgia mammæ;* when to those of the heart, *angina pectoris,* &c. But as these various names only tend to complicate our classification, and render complex what is in reality simple, we shall treat of all these nervous attacks under the general appellation of *neuralgia.*

Diagnosis.—The following are the general characteristics of neuralgia : sudden paroxysms of exceedingly acute pain in some particular nerve, with violent lancinating pains extending along the ramifications of the nerve in different directions, attended with turgescence of the blood vessels in the vicinity of the part chiefly affected, but without fever. The pains are so sudden and severe as to resemble electric shocks, and they often give rise to spasmodic contortions or twitchings of the muscles of the face when the branches of the fifth and the facial branch of the seventh pair of nerves are the seat of the pains. The pains are sometimes aggravated by the slightest movement, or by the gentlest touch, although *firm pressure causes no pain.* The particular nerve or nerves involved, can always be pointed out with exactness, because the principal seat of the attack is always in some portion of a nerve, and radiates thence along its different ramifications ; and from this circumstance surgeons have occasionally excised with success portions of nervous trunks to effect cures ; but this severe measure should never be resorted to, when suitable homœopathic specifics can be so readily procured.

In facial neuralgia, there are often lachrymation ; increased flow of saliva ; spasmodic twitchings of the mouth, cheeks, and eyelids ; spasmodic closing of the eyelids ; unusual heat and tension in the side affected ; stiffness in the jaw and neck ; increase of pain by light, noise, motion, touch, talking, or eating ; heat or coldness of the body ; vertigo ; and confusion of ideas.

When the head is the seat of the attack, we may have violent periodical pains in some part of the head, darting along the nervous ramifications ; nausea ;

vomiting ; extreme sensitiveness to the touch, cold air, sounds and light ; humming in the ears ; sense of heat and fulness in the affected part ; floats before the eyes on the slightest attempt to use them ; aversion to food ; confusion of ideas ; disinclination to converse, or to listen to others.

When neuralgia affects the superior or inferior extremities, back or mammæ, the symptoms will be fewer on account of the less number of sympathetic connections existing between these parts. In these instances, the violent lancinating pains, occurring in paroxysms, and increased by the slightest contact, and by motion, and unaccompanied with actual inflammation, are the symptoms which especially mark the complaint.

For the symptoms of neuralgia affecting *internal* organs, we refer our readers to the articles upon gastrodinia and angina pectoris.

Causes. — Pathological researches have as yet thrown but little light upon the nature of neuralgia. Many excellent observers have instituted rigid autopsical examinations, in order to ascertain its precise nature and location, but their labours for the most part have proved fruitless ; since no lesions or other marks of diseased action have been discovered, either in the nerves or their envelopes, at all sufficient to account for the symptoms.

Dr. Macculloch believes neuralgia to be a *malarious* disease ; this opinion is founded upon the fact of its frequent occurrence in marshy districts, and in locations where intermittent fever abounds. It is probable, however, in these cases, that the miasmatic influence operates merely to *excite* or to call into active operation a diseased condition of the nerves, latent it is true, but already existing. The malaria operates in these instances, as the *immediate exciting cause*, and in a manner similar to impure air, errors in diet, excessive mental or physical labour, abuse of narcotics or stimulants, over-excitement, fatigue, exhaustion, great loss of fluids, and the depressing emotions. The remote cause and the real nature of the disorder remain unexplained. A conclusive fact in refutation of the views of McCulloch respecting the malarious origin of the disease, is its common occurrence in New England, where intermittent fevers do not prevail.

Neuralgic pains sometimes arise from the pressure of tumours and exostoses, the irritation of decayed and ulcerated teeth, and also from mechanical injuries. In these instances we may generally remove the cause by surgical means, and thus cure the disorder.

Therapeutics.—The specific medicines for the cure of neuralgia, are, *arsenicum, belladonna, colocynth, nux vomica, aconite, china, arnica, bryonia, calcarea carb., hepar sulph., phosphorus, acid hydrocianic, pulsatilla, sepia, sulphur, spigelia, stramonium, mercurius.*

Arsenicum.—External indications. — Temperament, leuco-phlegmatic, lymphatic, or bilious and choleric, or nervous, with disposition to melancholy; general appearance of debility and exhaustion; countenance pale and sunken, or bloated and red; features distorted; lips bluish; twitchings of the muscles of the face, lips, and eyelids; tongue white; coldness of the extremities; anasarca; emaciation; trembling of the limbs; cramps in the extremities; pulse small.

Physical sensations.—Paroxysms of excruciating pain in the head, particularly in the forehead over the root of the nose,—over the left eye,—in one side of the head,—in one eye: pains aggravated from the slightest movement or touch; scalp sensitive to touch or to motion of the hair; roaring in the ears during the pain; mouth dry; thirst or adypsia; bad taste in the mouth; aversion to food; nausea, eructations, hiccough; pressure, heat or burning, or cramplike sensations in the stomach; drawings and cramps in the arms and legs; cramps in the fingers; rigidity of the hands; violent lancinating pains in different parts of the body, aggravated by movement or touch, attended with paralytic weakness, contractive sensations, faintness, coldness, shuddering and trembling.

Mental and moral symptoms.—Fits of violent anguish; fear; dread, with tremours; impaired memory; inability to think or collect the thoughts; dizziness; vertigo; general uneasiness.

Administration.—A dose of the second or third trituration, every half hour until an aggravation or amelioration of the symptoms occurs.

Belladonna.—This medicine is well adapted to the "diseases of women and children, whose nervous systems are in a state of erethism." The *external indications* are, sanguine and choleric temperament; general appearance indicative of a full and plethoric habit; cheeks red and swollen; eyelids spasmodically closed; spasms and startings in different parts of the body; distortion of the face; trembling and rigidity of the limbs.

Physical sensations.—Great sensitiveness to cold air and light; headache, compelling to close the eyes; acute throbbing pains in the forehead; semi-lateral headache; pains aggravated by movement, noise, light or cold air; lancinating pains in the orbit; spasms of the eyes; violent stitches in the parotid gland, extending to the external and internal ear; roaring in the ears; paroxysms of tearing, digging toothache; toothache of pregnant females; neuralgic pains darting from the side of the face to the teeth and ears, of a tearing, or lancinating, or digging character, with heat and redness of the part affected; toothache occurring after eating, from contact with cold air, from study, from pressure upon a decayed tooth, from eating, and from swelling and ulceration of the gums; darting pains in the lower jaw, and in the glands of the affected parts, from a decayed and hollow tooth; toothache with drawing in the ear; neuralgia affecting the crural nerve; cutting, darting, and tearing in the left thigh when sitting; lancinating pains in the right thigh when sitting; tearing and lancinating pains in the region of the tibia, extending to the calf of the leg and sole of the foot; neuralgic pains in the back and shoulders.

Mental and moral symptoms.—Anguish; despondency; great irritability; vertigo; confusion of ideas; delirium; inclination for firm pressure upon the head, which affords relief, while slight touches increase the pains.

Administration.—A drop of the second or third dilution on sugar or in water every half hour, until a decided impression is produced.

Colocynth.—Dr. Watzke remarks as follows respecting the therapeutic action of *colocynth* in neuralgic affections :—" The curative sphere of action of colocynth in the new system, is almost confined to a few *neuralgia* and *hyperæstheniæ*, and of these, almost exclusively those which affect the *trigeminus*, the *cæliac plexus*, and the *lumbar and femoral* nerves. First: the hemicrania and prosopalgiæ which colocynth cures, proceed from an exaltation of sensibility dependent on rheumatic, gouty, or gastric irritation, or on congestion of the fifth pair of nerves, in all cases on a purely functional affection of the sensitive filaments. Colocynth is of no use in organic prosopalgiæ, from growing out of the teeth, hypertrophy of the bones of the skull or face, tumours, &c.

"Second: the neuralgia of the cœliac plexus and its branches, are particularly likely to be quickly and permanently removed by *colocynth* when they occur as substantive affections, not caused by derangements of the stomach, but by cold, vexation, or anger, occurring during the period of evolution ; complicated with spinal irritation and neuralgia of the great nerves of the thigh, with hæmorrhoids, chronic diarrhœa, or vermicular symptoms."

Colocynth is adapted to dry, bilious and choleric-melancholy temperaments. It is especially suitable in cases of neuralgia, confined to certain parts of the *left* side of the body. The paroxysms are usually attended with spasms, twitchings, and contractive sensations ; and the lancinations are sudden, violent, and extend to a distance from the starting point.

Administration.—A drop of the third dilution in water, every hour, until its effects are apparent.

Nux Vomica.—External indications.—Temperament sanguine or choleric; disposition lively, artful and malicious ; face pale or highly coloured ; contractions of the hands and feet; coldness of the body, especially after drinking; trembling of the limbs; fainting fits, spasmodic twitchings in different parts of the body ; better adapted to *males* than *females.*

Physical sensations.—Periodical and intermittent pains ; excessive sensibility of the affected parts to external impressions of all kinds; periodical headache every morning after rising, increasing until noon, then gradually diminishing until night, when the pain ceases; the pains are drawing, tearing, compressive, affecting the whole head, or the forehead, or the part just above the root of the nose; headache accompanied with confusion of ideas, nausea, bitter eructations, vomitings, constipation; scalp painful and sensitive to touch or cold air; tearing pains in the facial and infra orbital nerves; ringing in the ears; toothache in sound and decayed teeth; pains of a sticking, drawing, tearing, jerking, or digging character, aggravated by cold air and drinks, by study and meditation, and relieved by rest and warmth; toothache from cold, and from extraction of a tooth; drawing toothache in several teeth; looseness of the teeth; swelling of the gums; drawing toothache in a hollow tooth, with pains extending to the face and temples; gastrodynia attended with violent, cramp-like, contractive and tearing pains in the stomach; pleurodinia; contractions and cramps in the hands, feet and limbs; coldness of the hands and feet; painful contractive sensations throughout the body; faintness; languor, and indisposition to mental or physical exertion.

Mental and moral symptoms.—Great sensitiveness to external impressions; melancholy; sadness; apprehension; anxiety; petulancy; indisposition to mental exertion.

Administration.—This medicine may be employed in the same manner as *Belladonna.*

We have occasionally employed *Aconite* with advantage in neuralgia, accompanied with great erethism of the vascular system, flushes of heat, congestion of the head, chest, and heart. Whenever the function of the heart appears to be affected in neuralgia, this remedy will generally prove useful.

When neuralgia has arisen from excessive loss of the fluids of the body, we may refer to *china, phosphorus, calcarea carb.,* and *sepia.*

When the disease appears to be connected with scrofula, exostoses of the bones, chronic cutaneous affections, abuse of mercury, constitutional syphilis, glandular and other tumours, reference should be made to *sulphur, mercurius, hepar sulph., sepia and aurum muriaticum.*

In neuralgic attacks of the heart, or stomach, or

uterus, our best remedies are *nux vomica, acid hydrocyanic, pulsatilla and colocynth.*

Neuralgia from mechanical injuries, will commonly yield to *arnica, aconite* and *calendula.*

For a more particular description of the neuralgic symptoms pertaining to special organs, and the mode of treatment, we refer to the diseases of the different organs and tissues in other parts of this work.

Administration.—A wide range of attenuations should be employed in neuralgia, in order that we may adapt our remedies precisely to the degree of erethism present in each particular case. When the pains are very acute, the dose may be repeated every hour until relief is obtained, or until a medicinal aggravation admonishes us to discontinue the medicine.

CHAPTER XXVI.

DISEASES OF THE URINARY AND GENITAL ORGANS.

SECTION I.

NEPHRITIS.—INFLAMMATION OF THE KIDNEYS.

Diagnosis.—Inflammation of the kidneys commences with the ordinary febrile symptoms, like slight chills, hot and dry skin, thirst, frequent and hard pulse, either accompanied from the first, or speedily succeeded by deep-seated, aching pain in the region of the kidneys, which soon becomes acute and pulsative; urine scanty and high-colored; entire inability to lie upon the healthy side or upon the stomach; position mostly upon the back when reclining, or on the affected side, with the dorsal and lumbar muscles flexed; inability to lie upon the diseased side with the muscles extended; severe pains upon rising up to the erect posture, or from the concussions arising from riding, walking, or running; when the disease is strongly pronounced, there are, absolute inability to walk, or even to stand upon the feet; pressure over the inflamed kidney does not cause pain, but any motions which call into exercise the deep-seated dorsal or lumbar muscles, excite acute pain; the inflammation generally attacks the left kidney; both kidneys are rarely affected at the same time in the first instance; the pain at first is aching, compressive and dull, but often becoming, in severe cases, violent and lancinating; the pains extend along the ureters to the bladder, or follow the spermatic cord to the testicles; the urine is very scanty, bloody, purulent or red, or watery; constant desire to urinate; there are nausea, eructations, vomitings, flatulence, constipation; pains in the rectum, from contiguous sympathy; tenesmus; swelling and heat over the affected side; when complicated with calculi, there will be retraction of the testicle; numbness of the thigh; anxiety, and more severe constitutional disturbance.

Nephritis may readily be distinguished from lumbago, inflammation of the psoas muscle, and neuralgia, by the character and direction of the pains which follow the ureters to the *vesiculæ seminales*, or the spermatic cords to the testicles; also by the nausea, vomiting, constant desire to urinate ; the partial, and in some cases almost entire suppression of the urinary secretion ; the sympathetic pains in the rectum ; and the increase of pain whenever any of the muscles which bear upon the kidneys are extended.

The terminations of nephritis are, resolution, suppuration, induration, schirrus, or gangrene. The duration of the acute stage is usually from six to nine days, when one of the above terminations usually obtains.

Its termination in resolution is indicated by a gradual return of all the functions to a more healthy state ; increased secretion of urine, which deposits an abundant sediment ; moderate and general perspiration ; subsidence of the pains ; ability to lay on either side, or to walk without difficulty.

When suppuration has taken place, the pains become less severe ; there are chills, or shiverings ; dull throbbing in the region of the kidneys ; sometimes appearance of pus in the urine ; a sensation of numbness and weight in the affected side ; a partial subsidence of the febrile symptoms ; and occasionally an abscess, which may be recognised by swelling and fluctuation in the part.

The purulent matter may be discharged by the ureters into the bladder, or find its way between the lumbar, or the internal crural muscles, to the thigh, or it may find its way by ulceration into the cavity of the spleen, the liver, or the colon, or it may burst externally.

In these cases fistulous passages are apt to remain for a long period, giving issue to the pus and urine.

In a very few instances, after the acute symptoms have subsided, there remains a *chronic induration* of the kidneys, which in the end degenerates into a true *schirrus*. In other rare instances, when the inflammation has been exceedingly violent, and suitable remedial measures have not been employed, the vitality of the part becomes destroyed, and *gangrene* is the result. The occurrence of gangrene is recognised by the pale, sunken, and deathlike expression of countenance, cold, clammy sweats, universal prostration, constant vomiting, delirium, small and frequent pulse, absence of pain, hiccough, and dark and fœtid urine. Whenever either of the last described occurrences take place, no hopes of cure should be entertained.

Causes.—External injuries, strains from violent exercise or lifting heavy weights, the irritation of calculi, sudden check to the perspiration from cold, abuse of medicinal or morbid snbstances which operate specifically upon the kidneys.

Therapeutics.—Frequent external applications of cold water over the inflamed kidney will be of great service in abstracting the superfluous animal heat, and thus allaying the inflammation. The water should be applied quite cold, and repeated until the temperature of the part is permanently diminished, and the pain has in a measure subsided.

The specific medicines are, *cantharides*, *cannabis*, *tussilago petus.*, *aconite*, *copaibæ*, *terebinthina*, *belladonna*, *arnica*, *nux vomica*, and *pulsatilla.*

As soon as we are called to a case of nephritis, we should have immediate recourse to *aconite*, either alone or in alternation with one of the other specifics, and continue it until the febrile symptoms have subsided. In slight cases, *aconite* alone as an internal remedy, together with thorough external applications of cold water, will suffice.

If the inflammation be of a severe grade, and there are tearing, drawing, and pulsative pains in the region of the kidneys, extending to the bladder and testicle, constant desire to urinate, scanty secretion of high-coloured urine, inability to lay on the affected side, tenesmus, colic-pains, urine tinged with blood, painful micturition, *aconite* in alternation with the third dilution of *cantharides*, or *cannabis*, or *terebinth*, or *tussilago petus.*, or *bals. copaib.*, may be exhibited.

Arnica is suitable for inflammation of the kidneys, caused by external injuries, concussions, sprains from lifting, &c.

When there is reason to suspect that suppuration is about commencing, *sulphur*, *sepia*, and *lycopodium*, may be used with advantage.

SECTION II.

CYSTITIS.—INFLAMMATION OF THE BLADDER.

Diagnosis.—Inflammation of the bladder commences like nephritis, with shiverings or chills, frequent pulse, hot and dry skin, anxiety, thirst, urine scanty and high-coloured, nausea, vomiting, eructations, and constipation. In a short time, the patient experiences deep-seated lancinating pains in the hypogastric region, frequent desire to urinate, each effort giving rise to increased pain, great anxiety, and uneasiness. As the inflammation extends, the pains become more severe, and there are a continual burning sensation in the bladder, with painful pulsations; acute pain on making pressure in the vicinity of the inflammation, and when attempting to urinate; sense of weight in the hypogastric region; acute or dragging pains in the loins, the ureters, the perineum, and the anus; swelling and distention of the abdomen; great difficulty in voiding the fæces, on account of the sympathetic inflammation of the rectum; all movements of the muscles which bear upon the bladder excite increased pains; and finally rigours, cadaverous expression, cold extremities, delirium and convulsions. If the inflammation be confined to the neck of the bladder, there will be an almost entire suppression of the urinary discharge; constant ineffectual and exceedingly painful efforts to urinate; and violent pain in the perineum. If the ureters become involved, pains are frequently felt as high as the kidneys; the secretion of urine becomes more deranged, the suppression is more decided, and the attempts to void the urine still more painful. When the whole interior surface of the bladder is affected, the urine is red and tinged with blood, and a severe burning and throbbing pain is experienced. Occasionally the external surface of the organ becomes inflamed, either on one side, on its anterior or posterior, or its superior or inferior part; in which cases the symptoms will be in correspondence with the location of the malady.

Cystitis may terminate in *chronic inflammation of the bladder*, in *resolution*, *suppuration*, or *gangrene*.

The signs which indicate these different terminations, are similar to those described under *nephritis*.

Causes.—Injuries resulting from child-birth, from the use of instruments during accouchement, from blows, concussions and falls, from gravel, stone, abuse of diuretics, metastases of erysipelas, rheumatism, or gonorrhœa, the use of stimulating injections into the urethra, prolonged retention of urine, introduction of catheters and sounds into the bladder, suppression of the menses, and extension of inflammation from neighbouring parts.

Therapeutics.—*Aconite*, *cantharides*, *cannabis*, *thuya occiden*, *terebinthina*, *copaibæ*, *tussilago petus.*, and *asparagus*, are our best specifics. They may be employed at the first, second and third attenuations, either alone or in alternation with *aconite*, and the doses repeated as the urgency of the symptoms shall require.

SECTION III.

DIABETES.

Numerous hypotheses have been offered respecting the seat and nature of this singular malady, but neither of them appears to afford a satisfactory explanation of all its phenomena. The affection has been referred to a morbid condition of the kidneys alone, also to derangement of the stomach, of the liver, to a defect in the fluids, to suppressed perspiration, to an imperfect animalization of the blood, to the retrograde action of the lymphatics, and to an unnatural waste of the body, thus calling into increased activity the digestive and assimilative functions to supply the waste. Galen, who saw but two cases of diabetes during his life, supposed that it was caused by an inflammation of the kidneys, " which made them draw much serum from the emulgents." Aretæus attributed it to a feeble and relaxed condition of the kidneys, " which weakens the retentive faculty." Actius believed that the cause consisted in "an afflux of sharp or salt humours, which continually stimulated the veins to expulsion." Van Helmont attributed it to a paralysis of the muscles of the bladder. Willis, who first pointed out the saccharine character of the urine, thought it was caused by "the dissolution and over-lax frame of the blood, whereby it loses its serum before it has done its office." Sylvius says: "the disease arises from a sharp volatile salt, either received from without, or inbred in the parts." Cullen, Sydenham, Rollo, and Home, regarded the affection as "dependent primarily on a disordered state of the digestive organs, in conjunction with a defect in the assimilating functions."

This last opinion is probably the correct one, and much credit is due to Bouchardat for having first pointed out the changes which certain aliments undergo in consequence of this disordered state of the digestive apparatus. Dr. B. broached the opinion, that "in diabetes, starch was converted in the intestines into sugar, which passed into the blood and urine." Hence, a diet composed chiefly of neutral azotised substances, to the exclusion of starch, has been recommended for the cure of this disease, and, in some instances, with success.

It may, then, be safely assumed, that the primary cause of diabetes consists, first, in a morbid state of the digestive and assimilative organs, which favours the formation of *dextrine*, or *sugar*, from the starchy or farinaceous substances introduced into the alimentary canal, and its absorption into the blood and urine. The following are a few of the reasons for this opinion: Diabetes is usually attended from the first, with a disordered state of the digestive organs, as is indicated by uneasy sensations in the stomach after eating, impaired or morbidly increased appetite, eructations, nausea, vomiting, bad taste, and dryness of the mouth and tongue.

The function of the stomach is exceedingly complicated, and is inflamed, perhaps, more than any other organ of the body, by the numerous natural or artificial circumstances which constantly operate upon living beings. When the organism is in a sound condition, and no disturbing causes exercise an influence, the digestive apparatus elaborates thoroughly a certain amount of chyle, and the assimilative organs take it up and appropriate it in a certain manner. But these functions may be impaired, suspended, or even unduly increased, by moral and physical causes. Ill news, grief, chagrin, mortification, disappointment, anger, fear, dread, apprehension, and disagreeable sights, often suspend both digestion and assimilation. These functions may also be impaired or suspended from the abuse of drugs, stimulants, tobacco, coffee, tea, sedentary habits, excessive bodily fatigue, want of sleep, the irritation of vitiated bile, or of the gastric fluid, or of acids, excesses in eating, or the use of indigestible food, inflammation, &c. They may also be morbidly increased by tonics and stimulants, like bark, the preparations of iron, the bitter infusions, wine, alcoholic liquors, cordials, and condiments.

In the malady under consideration, the digestive organs are in a peculiar condition. The thirst is intense, and the appetite voracious, yet the digestive function is perverted, the aliments are imperfectly converted into chyle, a superabundance of saccharine matter is elaborated, while the activity of the absorbents is astonishingly increased.

That farinaceous aliments are really converted into sugar in the stomachs of diabetic patients, is evident from the fact that traces of it have been detected in the matters ejected by them after the use of farinaceous food. It is also proved from the circumstance, that when this kind of food is withheld, both the secretion of urine and its saccharine character is materially diminished.

Matteucci has demonstrated, that "starchy substances, when introduced into the stomach and intestines of diabetic patients, are converted into dextrine, or sugar, by the saliva, or pancreatic juice, and are then absorbed directly into the blood, either in this form, or after having been converted into lactic acid."

The experiments of Dutrochet, Cuna, and Matteucci have proved that different liquids may pass through the stomach, membranes, skin, and other animal tissues, by *absorption*, *imbibition*, *endosmose*, or *exosmose*, the activity and direction of these phenomena depending upon the character and position of the fluid used, and the physiological condition of the structure acted on. Thus, "azotised neutral substances dissolved in the stomach by the acid liquid, or by the catalytic action of pepsine, pass into the blood merely by the imbibition of the coats of the capillary bloodvessels of the stomach." Water, and alcoholic drinks, introduced into the stomach, are also absorbed; they do not pass beyond this viscus, nor are they to be found in the chyle, yet they reach the blood."

In diabetes, the digestive organs appear to have lost the power to elaborate healthy chyle, and also the absorbents of resisting the entrance of the saccharine fluids formed by this perverted action. Whether the nature of this morbid condition is of an inflammatory or non-inflammatory character, whether dependent upon exalted action or laxity, loss of tone or paralysis of the affected parts, is somewhat problematical, although we incline to the opinion, that the disease is essentially dependent upon a relaxed and enfeebled condition of the digestive and assimilative functions.

But an objection will be urged to the above views, because the quantity of sugar found in the urine of diabetic persons is not at all proportionate to that of the fecula taken as aliment; but this argument falls to the ground when we reflect that the *uric acid* and the *urea* derived from the rapid metamorphosis of the tissues, is likewise converted into sugar, and passes, with the fluids arising from these changes, through the blood and kidneys, thus contributing to make up the enormous quantity of saccharine fluid which is observed in this affection. Prout has shown that the constituent elements of *urea* and *sugar* are the same, and exist in similar proportions; from which fact, we can readily comprehend the change from one substance to the other, and the affinity exercised by the saccharine fluid circulating in the blood, upon the urea arising from the transformation of the tissues.

Second. As a consequence of this primary derangement of the digestive and assimilative functions, the saccharine fluids formed, are transmitted rapidly through the blood, absorbing, during their course, the changed urea, and, finally, eliminated by the kidneys. It is the office of the kidneys to separate from the organism all substances incapable of further use, whether such useless substances are the product of the natural secretions, or of the transformations of the tissues. Now, as sugar is a substance foreign and injurious to the blood, it is taken up as fast as formed, and conveyed speedily to the kidneys, which separate it, after which it passes off through the bladder. This is evident from the fact, that when a solution of sugar is injected into the veins of an animal, it does not remain in the blood, but makes its appearance very speedily in the urine. It is on this account that it is so difficult to detect sugar in the blood of diabetic patients, although traces of it have been found by Dr. Capezzuoli, not only in the blood, but in the contents of an abscess of a diabetic patient.

When more saccharine matter is absorbed than can be speedily eliminated by the kidneys, it is highly probable that it passes off through the liver, the salivary glands, the pancreas, and even into abscesses, rather than remain in the mass of the blood.

Third. The kidneys themselves being constantly acted upon by a fluid unlike their natural stimuli, become irritated, their vessels enlarged, and thus excited into unnatural activity. This fluid also often gives rise to an inflammation about the orifice of the urethra.

Diagnosis.—In tracing the progress of diabetes, and noting carefully the symptoms which are especially characteristic, it will be found that a very intimate connection necessarily exists between these symptoms and the pathological conditions above described.

In the first instance, there are indications of derangement of the digestive apparatus, as morbid appetite, distress in the stomach after eating, flatulent distention, acidity, eructations, nausea, heartburn, lassitude, and debility.

When the disease is fully formed, the prominent symptoms are, urgent and insatiable thirst, voracious appetite, hot and harsh skin, and the elimination of an unusually large quantity of urine abounding in saccharine matter.

As the disease advances, the tongue is clammy and white, or clean and red; there is distress after eating; a peculiar hay-like odour issues from the body and lungs; there are pain and weakness, and sometimes swelling, in the loins; anxiety; peevishness; despondency; impaired memory; vertigo; constipation; inflammation about the glans penis and the orifice of the urethra; rapid and great emaciation; loss of strength; impotence; coldness of the extremities; difficulty of breathing; dropsical effusions; weak and frequent pulse; great prostration of all the powers.

Diabetic urine is of a straw colour, of a disagreeable odour, and a sweetish taste. The quantity voided in different cases varies very much, some patients voiding as much as fifty or even one hundred pounds in twenty-four hours, while others pass only eight or ten pounds during the same period. The average quantity voided in twenty-four hours may safely be placed at about fifteen pounds.

Diabetes usually continues for months, and sometimes for years, before it terminates fatally. Hitherto it has been almost invariably fatal; but may we not hope that the discoveries which have been recently made, and which are still being made, in organic chemistry, as well as in the practice of medicine, will enable us yet to understand and conquer this singular and intractable malady?

Therapeutics.—If the theory which we have advanced respecting the nature of diabetes is correct, it follows as a consequence, that one of our most important therapeutical indications consists in pointing out a proper system of dietetics. We have seen that through a perverted action of the digestive apparatus, all the farinaceous or starchy substances consumed become converted into sugar, and thus afford *material* for the perpetuation of the malady. A rigid abstinence from everything of a feculent nature should therefore be insisted on, while, at the same time, a diet as nutritious as possible should be enjoined, consisting of beef, mutton, venison, fowls, game, fish, animal soups, jellies, and articles of this nature. We commend most strongly as valuable auxiliary means in this affection, sea voyages, and frequent applications to the whole surface of the body, of salt water. The free use of ice, gradually dissolved in the mouth, will also prove serviceable in allaying the intense thirst which consumes the patient.

The internal remedies which have been found most successful in this disease are, *acid phosphoric, carbo vegetabilis, nux vomica, acid muriatic, baryta muriate, belladonna, uva ursa, rhus rad., conium mac., digitalis,* and *opium.*

Our experience has been so limited in the homœopathic treatment of diabetes, that we shall refrain from extending our observations respecting the especial indications and the practical employment of each particular remedy, but refer our readers to the provings, and mode of employment, by different medical men, for further information and suggestion upon the subject.

SECTION IV.

ENURESIS.—INCONTINENCE OF URINE.

Diagnosis.—This affection may be recognised by a partial or total loss of power to retain in the bladder the secreted urine. When the loss of voluntary power over the muscles concerned is total, the urine continues to dribble away as fast as secreted, becoming thus an incessant source of trouble and annoyance.

If the loss of power be only partial, the urine can be retained until a given amount is accumulated, when the patient is suddenly compelled to yield to the pressing demand, *sans ceremonie.* In other instances, the incontinence is troublesome only during sleep, and appears to be excited by dreams, constrained positions, &c.

The malady is unaccompanied by febrile symptoms or pains, and usually occurs as a symptom of some other disease.

Causes.—Complete enuresis may be caused by paralysis of the sphincter of the bladder from constitutional causes, from external injuries, from tedious and protracted labours, from the pressure of tumours, from calculous deposits, and from abuse of diuretics.

Partial enuresis is a common complaint amongst

children, and is particularly troublesome in the night during sleep. It has too often been attributed to habit, and negligence of proper efforts to restrain the discharge on the part of children, and for this reason, external applications, in the form of "spanking," and "essence of birch," have been employed, but so far as our knowledge extends, without advantage. The disease in these cases is undoubtedly associated with irritation at the neck of the bladder, originated by acrid urine, gravel, the irritation of worms in the rectum, etc.

Therapeutics.—*Cantharides, cannabis, uva ursa, nux vomica, cicuta vir., sulphur, calcarea carb., pulsatilla,* and *rhus*, are the chief remedies.

For the cure of paralytic enuresis, recourse should be had to *cantharides, nux vom., rhus* and *uva ursa.*

When the disease occurs in children, our best remedies are, *cantharides, calcarea carb.,* and *sulphur.* When from external injuries, difficult accouchements, or the irritation of calculi, we may prescribe *arnica, pulsatilla, rhus,* and *cicuta virosa.*

Administration.—The remedies should be used at the first or second attenuations, and a dose given once or twice daily as long as necessary.

SECTION V.

SUPPRESSION AND RETENTION OF URINE.

The causes capable of giving rise to suppression or retention of urine are so various and diversified, and the circumstances attending the course and progress of different cases so numerous, that our description must necessarily be confined to the more prominent symptoms and occurrences connected with the malady.

By the term *retention of urine*, we mean to include all of those cases in which the urine is secreted by the kidneys as usual, but where the power to evacuate the bladder is lost; while *suppression of urine* corresponds with the affection known as *ischuria renalis,* in which the secreting function of the kidneys is either partially or totally destroyed.

Ischuria renalis is always attended with danger, from the peculiar tendency which exists in the brain to take on diseased action. When there is an entire suppression of the urinary secretion, from paralysis of the kidneys, coma and effusion upon the brain occur very speedily. In cases of this description, the saliva, the sweat, the pulmonary exhalations, the bile, the pancreatic and gastric fluids, become impregnated with a fluid possessing the appearance, taste and odour of urine. It has also been observed, that the liquid effused upon the brain, possesses a decidedly urinous smell. In cases of the disease dependent on inflammation of the kidneys, we shall have febrile symptoms, hot and dry skin, thirst, nausea, vomiting, rapid pulse, tenderness of the abdomen on pressure, swelling and pain in the region of the kidneys, frequent desire to urinate, and the passage of the small quantity secreted, causing great pain, urinous taste in the mouth, urinous odour of the sweat, anxiety and general uneasiness. If the suppression be total, the symptoms will be still more grave, and there will be early indications of serious cerebral disorder, in the form of delirium, rapidly succeeded by coma and effusion.

On the other hand, in suppression, depending upon paralysis of the kidneys, the febrile symptoms may be very slight, and there may be an entire absence of pain and uneasiness in the region of the kidneys or in the abdomen, and no desire to urinate. In these instances, the danger is no less imminent than in the other variety, for fatal oppression of the brain almost invariably ensues, if the malady persists more than two days. Cases, however, are recorded, of almost total suppression for two or three months, in which the patients have been restored to health, but such instances are of rare occurrence, and should only be considered in the light of exceptions to the general law of the disease.

Suppression now and then occurs from the presence of calculi or gravel in the structures of the kidneys, thus causing a mechanical obstruction to the healthy performance of their functions. In these cases the foreign bodies may operate by causing inflammation, spasms, induration, or ulceration. They give rise to swelling, pains, sensation of weight and uneasiness in the vicinity of the kidneys, to numbness of the thighs, retraction of the testicles, abdominal tenderness, constipation, frequent inclination to urinate, pain and tenesmus in passing water, anxiety, irritability, febrile symptoms, nausea, vomitings, hiccoughs, pain in the lumbar region, pain and tension in the perineum, scalding in the urethra, pulse full and frequent, difficulty of breathing, sighing, delirium, convulsions.

Ischuria may be distinguished from retention of urine from the circumstance, that in the latter disease, the bladder is distended and rises up above the pubis, offering to the pressure of the hand a firm and resisting body, while in the former complaint this viscus is empty, falls down below the pubis, and affords no resistance or fluctuation.

Retention of urine may arise from inflammation, from stricture of the urethra, from paralysis of the bladder, from enlargement and inflammation of the prostate gland, from mechanical injuries to the bladder, from abuse of stimulating diuretics, from inflammation of the rectum, from the pressure of tumours, from displacements of the uterus, from calculi, from the lodgement of gravel or a stone in the ureters or in the urethra, from thickening and obstruction of the ureters, from too long continued retention of the urine, and from spasms.

The general symptoms of *retention* are, distention of the bladder, and its elevation above the pubis, pains in the region of the bladder, with pressing desire and frequent ineffectual attempts to urinate, anxiety, general uneasiness, and more or less constitutional disturbance.

As retention is generally but a symptom of some other malady, we are often presented with constitutional disturbances during an attack, in no way dependent upon this affection. We may cite as examples of this kind, diseases of the brain and spinal marrow, which may have preceded the retention for months, protracted calculous affections, chronic inflammations of the bladder and of the prostate gland, constitutional effects of onanism, retroversion of the uterus, and the effects of previous mechanical injuries. From these facts it is apparent that there may exist an almost endless variety of symptoms during the progress of the different cases of retention which are constantly occurring.

When the malady arises from simple *inflammation* of the neck of the bladder or of the bladder itself, not complicated by any previous disease, the symptoms are, hot skin; frequent and hard pulse; thirst; pain in the region of the bladder and in the perineum, increased by pressure; restlessness; anxiety; constipation; frequent inclination to pass water, with violent, painful and ineffectual straining; shooting pains extending up the ureters towards the kidneys, or along the spermatic chords towards the testicles; headache; nausea; oppression at the præcordia; and general feeling of fulness and distention of abdomen.

Retention caused by *paralysis*, on the other hand, is accompanied by but few of these symptoms. Indeed, many cases are recorded, where the accumulations of urine have reached an enormous amount, before the patients were aware of it. Other instances are mentioned where the distention has been so gradual and painless as to cause it to be mistaken for ascites, and in more than one instance of this description, *paracentecis abdominalis* has been resorted to as a curative means. In cases like these, fifteen or twenty pints have occasionally been drawn off by the catheter at a single operation. It is not an uncommon result in these over-distentions, for the bladder to become united by adhesive inflammation to the umbilicus, and afterwards to discharge itself through this part by ulceration. The same occurrence sometimes takes place into the rectum, vagina, and even into the abdominal cavity. In these cases, the danger from peritoneal inflammation, and from gangrene, is imminent.

Retention may arise from *spasmodic contractions* about the neck of the bladder, giving rise to most violent and painful attempts to urinate, bearing-down pains, frequent painful erections, great sensitiveness of the urethra and perineum. In this variety of retention, it is always very difficult and sometimes absolutely impossible to pass a catheter, without previously allaying the irritation by fomentations or by the employment of suitable medicines.

Spasmodic retention, although sudden and violent in its onset, is not usually a dangerous affection. The essence of the disease consists in an irritation about the neck of the bladder, and is dependent upon inflammation of the prostate, of the rectum, of the urethra, or some other neighbouring structure, from which it has been propagated by contiguous sympathy.

But the most difficult cases of retention with which the physician meets, are those caused by strictures of the urethra, and enlargements of the prostate gland. The practitioner, during his professional career, will sometimes be called to cases of each of these maladies, where nothing but an incision into the membraneous portion of the urethra, through the stricture, or the puncture of the bladder, will save life. In these cases, great judgment, decision, and surgical skill, are indispensable to the safety of the patient. This will be conceded when we think of the rapidity with which retention may terminate in fatal cerebral disease, ulceration, and gangrene. By these observations, we by no means desire to deter the physician from the employment of every medicinal means in his power, so long as they can be applied without endangering the life of the patient; but there is a point beyond which we cannot safely pass without resorting to one of the operations just alluded to, and in making up a correct decision upon this point, the best judgment and the highest professional knowledge are requisite. I cannot better illustrate this subject than by detailing the history of a case which came under my observation during an early part of my professional career:

Mr. B., aged forty years, of robust constitution, had been operated upon fourteen years previously, for stricture in the membraneous part of the urethra. An incision had then been made through the strictured part, a catheter introduced and allowed to remain a good portion of the time for several weeks, but for some unknown reason, the opening made by the knife did not heal, and a fistulous passage was formed, through which the urine has passed for the most part of the time since that period. For two or three years previous to his coming under my care, this fistulous passage had been gradually contracting, and he experienced, at times, retention, which could only be obviated by baths, fomentations, injections, relaxing medicines, and the skilful use of the probe. Several times, however, I succeeded in relieving him of the attacks, by these means; but on one occasion, being in the country, and having contracted a cold from wetting his feet, the retention recurred, accompanied with unusual inflammation and tumefaction in the fistulous tract. Persevering efforts were made by his medical attendant, to allay the inflammation, relax the parts, and to draw off the water by means of catheters and probes, for nearly two days, but without success. The symptoms now becoming very urgent, he returned home and placed himself under the care of Dr. Brigham and myself. We found great distention of the bladder, constant desire to urinate, bearing-down pains in the region of the bladder, expression exceedingly anxious and care-worn, eyes sunken, mouth and throat dry, thirst, pulse rapid and feeble, great prostration, nausea, hiccough, delirium, frequent sighing, exhalation from the surface of the body of a urinous smell, coldness of the extremities, and a sluggish and unhealthy appearance at the orifice of the fistula.

After resorting to the usual remedies in such cases, and making repeated attempts with the catheter and probe, we decided, although it was then midnight, that an incision must be made through the perineum without further delay. This was speedily effected, and the patient's life thus saved, while had we delayed a few hours more, gangrene or congestion of the brain would probably have resulted.

We also have in mind, a case of retention, from enlargement of the prostate, which proved fatal in consequence of an absolute refusal, on the part of the patient, to submit to the operation of puncturing the bladder. In this instance, the swelling and inflammation of the gland were so great, together with a constant tendency to spasmodic contraction of the neck of the bladder, whenever the catheter came in contact with the part, that all efforts at introduction, aided by baths, fomentations, and relaxants, were of no avail.

Here, a timely puncture of the bladder, would have saved the patient's life.

We are well aware of the practical skill and tact necessary to effect an introduction of a catheter in these cases, and of the importance of securing the services of a skilful and experienced surgeon; but cases sometimes occur which baffle the most eminent surgeons in their attempts to pass a catheter by an enlarged prostate.

Retention sometimes occurs from *obstruction of the ureters*, by gravel, calculi, by thickening and induration of their walls, by hydatids and other unnatural formations, by the pressure of tumours in their vicinity, and by occlusion from adhesive inflammation. The following signs indicate the existence of this variety of disease: unusual fulness, pain and sensation of weight in the vicinity of the kidneys, tension along the track of the ureters, nausea, vomiting, retraction of the testicles, pain along the spermatic cord, collapsed state of the bladder, no resistance to the introduction of the catheter, absence of urine in the bladder, and more or less constitutional disturbance. When the obstruction is complete, the ureters and the kidneys become so much dilated that urine to the amount of two or three pints, sometimes accumulates in them, before congestion, ulceration, or gangrene supervene.

Retention not unfrequently arises in females, from a retroversion of the uterus, from the presence within the vagina of polypi, hydatids, of schirrous enlargements, from injuries arising during difficult accouchements, from the irritation caused by acrid secretions, from the presence of hardened fæces in the rectum, and from adhesion occurring between the walls of the vagina, in consequence of inflammation and sloughing of the mucous membrane.

Causes.—The most frequent proximate cause of retention, is *inflammation* of some portion of the bladder. Amongst the more prominent causes of this inflammation, are, metastases of gout and rheumatism, abuse of diuretics, mechanical injuries, injections, venereal diseases, calculi, acrid urine, strains, and extension of inflammation from neighbouring parts.

The causes which rank next in importance, are

strictures of the urethra. They occur at all periods of life, and always require the interference of the surgeon for their removal.

Enlargement of the prostate gland, is a frequent cause of retention in old men. The remote cause can generally be traced to excesses in sexual indulgence during early life. This gland may become enlarged from mere inflammation and engorgement of its structure, or from schirrus degeneration. Affections of the prostate are usually called into activity by undue exposure to cold and wet, by abuse of stimulants, and by neglect of timely urinary evacuations.

Other causes, some of which have already been alluded to, are, retroversion of the uterus, obstruction of the ureters from foreign bodies, occlusion of the ureters from adhesive inflammation, paralysis of the bladder, from injury or disease of the brain or spinal marrow, from undue retention of urine, from mechanical injuries, from abuse of drugs, from metastases of gout, thickening of the mucous membrane of the bladder, tumours and excrescences near the neck of the bladder, repercussed eruptions, pressure upon the bladder by tumours in its vicinity, schirrus of the bladder or rectum, accumulations of hardened fæces in the rectum, suppression of the menses, phymosis, ulcers, external injuries, blows, contusions, and falls, leucorrhœa and gonorrhœa.

Therapeutics.—In all cases of suppression or retention, where there can exist a possible doubt in regard to the true nature of the case, we should avail ourselves, without delay, of the use of the catheter. If this instrument passes without difficulty into the cavity of the bladder, and no discharge of urine follows its introduction, we may be certain that the cause and seat of the difficulty is not in this viscus; while if a free discharge takes place through the catheter, affording immediate relief to the distention, pain, and other unpleasant symptoms which had previously existed, we may be assured that the bladder, the prostate gland, or some part of the urethra, is the seat of the complaint.

To ensure an accurate diagnosis, then, we in the first instance ascertain whether or not a catheter can be passed into the bladder.

Second. If it can be, whether easily or otherwise.

Third. How large an instrument can be passed.

Fourth. If a discharge of urine follows the introduction.

Fifth. If the operation is attended with pain.

Another important step in forming our diagnosis, consists in procuring from the patient or his friends, a minute history of his case, and every circumstance connected with the individual, which might have a bearing upon it. Thus, if we are called to an old man, whose malady has approached gradually, who has had no febrile symptoms and little pain, where no resistance is offered to the introduction of a full-sized catheter, and where a large quantity of urine flows off, affording immediate relief to the uneasy feelings, we may with confidence pronounce the cause, *paralysis of the bladder*. The same law obtains in cases of retention succeeding injuries, or diseases of the spinal marrow.

If we have a case where the catheter passes into the bladder with great difficulty, on account of some obstruction near its neck, we then inquire whether there exists a stricture, a spasmodic contraction of the neck of the bladder, or an enlarged prostate gland. The following circumstances will enable us to decide the question satisfactorily:

Stricture approaches gradually, as is indicated by the gradual contraction of the stream of urine, the frequent and sometimes constant presence of a gleety discharge, and a sensation, after passing water, as if a few drops still remained behind.

Enlarged prostate occurs, for the most part, in old men, is attended with pulsative pain over the bladder, weight in the perineum, constant inclination to urinate, with much straining, fever, and general uneasiness. By introducing the finger into the rectum, we may often detect the enlargement by actual touch.

Spasmodic contraction of the neck of the bladder usually proceeds from inflammation of some neighbouring structure, as the prostate gland, the rectum, and the urethra. Spasms of this part may arise also from the irritation of gravel and calculi. The previous history of the case will enable us to decide as to the real cause of the spasmodic affection.

Retention, from stricture of the urethra, can only be permanently cured by the gradual dilatation of the contracted part by bougies. Temporary relief may sometimes be afforded by the use of medicines, but the only permanent cure is by artificial dilatation. But much may be done towards effecting cures in cases of diseased prostate, by a judicious employment of specific medicines. Many cases of this description owe their origin to scrofula, or to a venereal taint, or to abuse of mercury, or to schirrous degeneration, for which reason our prescriptions should be made with reference to these peculiar states of the system, as well as to the more immediate symptoms of the complaint.

With regard to the other causes of retention, the importance of a minute investigation into all the circumstances of each case, cannot be too strongly insisted on; for much of our success will depend upon an early removal of those causes which have operated to induce the retention, and which perhaps continue to exist to perpetuate the malady.

If a retention has been caused by a metastasis of gout or rheumatism, our selection of remedies should be made with reference to these general diseases, as well as to the more urgent local symptoms. If the cause can be traced to a displacement of the uterus, to impacted fæces in the rectum, to inflammation of any of the surrounding tissues, to the presence of ascarides in the rectum, to excrescences about the neck of the bladder, to imperforate hymen, to unnatural adhesions within the vagina, to the impaction of a stone in the urethra, our attention should be immediately directed towards the removal of these remote causes.

The following medicines will cover all of the symptoms which occur in suppression or retention of urine: *cantharides, cannabis, uva ursi, solidago virga aurea, acid phosphoric, rhus rad., aconite, pulsatilla, nux vomica, arnica, belladonna, oleum terebinthina, tussilago pertuss., camphora, agnus castus, arsenicum, sulphur, iodine, electro-magnetism.*

Cantharides and *cannabis* are indicated in *suppres-*

sion from chronic inflammation of the kidneys, and in *retention* from long continued irritation of the neck of the bladder. They may also be employed in suppression and retention from acute inflammation of the kidneys and bladder, after the febrile symptoms have been subdued by *aconite*. Hahnemann advises them in retention from paralysis of the neck of the bladder, and in cases of *chronic retention* arising from thickening and induration of the mucous membrane.

Arnica is our best remedy when the functions of the kidney and bladder have been impaired or suspended by mechanical injuries, falls, contusions, sprains, blows, and concussions, or by the irritation of calculi.

Rhus rad., *belladonna*, and *solidago virga aurea*, are applicable when the disorder has proceeded from metastases of gout or rheumatism. These medicines may be alternated with *aconite* when the inflammatory symptoms run high.

Agnus castus is an excellent specific in retention in consequence of *paralysis* of the bladder. *Nux vomica*, *tussilago*, *arsenicum* and *oleum terebinth.* are remedies which should command attention in paralytic retention.

Spasmodic retentions are readily cured by *camphor*, *belladonna*, and *aconite*.

When gravel or calculi are the exciting causes of the affection, we advise the employment of *uva ursi*, *solidago virga aurea*, and *belladonna*.

Affections of the prostate gland may be met by *pulsatilla*, *sulphur*, *aconite*, *rhus rad.*, *arsenicum* and *iodine*.

Retention from onanism, or excesses in venery, are treated best with *acid phosphoric*, *agnus castus*, *cantharides*, *cannabis*, *rhus rad.*, and *arnica*.

Administration.—The lower attenuations should be employed in these affections, and the doses repeated every two, three, or four hours, until the medicinal effect is perceptible. Auxiliary to the above medicinal treatment, we make a thorough use of warm baths, fomentations, bland, diluent drinks, injections by the rectum, and lastly, though by no means the least important means, *electro-magnetism*. This powerful remedy should only be employed after the inflammatory symptoms have been reduced, and then with extreme care and moderation.

SECTION VI.

DYSURIA.

Diagnosis.—In this complaint the urine can be voided at will, but it usually passes away in a small spiral, or divided stream, or drop by drop, each act being attended with burning and cutting pains at the neck of the bladder. There is a frequent inclination to urinate, and sensations of pressure and tenesmus, which constantly urge the patient to void his urine. The inflammation is confined to the neck of the bladder, and does not often give rise to constitutional disturbance.

Causes.—Perhaps the most frequent cause of dysuria is the absorption of *cantharides.* This substance exercises a specific influence so decidedly upon the neck of the bladder, that even a sufficient quantity may be absorbed from the external application of blisters to cause the malady. Other causes are, stimulating injections, abuse of stimulants and condiments, onanism, extension of gonorrhœal inflammation, cold, turpentine, worms in the rectum, gravel, and calculi.

Therapeutics.—*Camphor* is the specific against dysury caused by the absorption of *cantharides.* When arising from other causes, *cannabis, uva ursi, digitalis, solidago virga aurea, cantharides,* and *terebinth,* are worthy of confidence.

Administration.—*Same as in retention,* &c.

SECTION VII.

URINARY CALCULI.

There is not space in a manual of this description for the careful consideration which is demanded for this disease by its importance; but we shall endeavour to glance hastily at the most prominent doctrines at present in vogue, with a view of attracting attention more particularly to the subject, rather than from any expectation of affording a satisfactory explanation of the phenomena attending the formation and development of calculous concretions. Chemistry has indeed afforded us much accurate knowledge respecting the composition of the different varieties of calculi, but we still remain in ignorance of the real causes and nature of the abnormal action, the peculiar condition of the organism requisite to originate this action, and of the specific medicines capable of effecting cures. The data upon which modern physicians have founded their prescriptions, may be more scientific and accurate than those of the ancients, but we are not aware that the practical results which they have obtained are in any degree more decided or favourable. The ancient allopathists attributed the formation of stone to the union of the "*terrestrial and tartarous parts of the blood with the clamminess of the viscous lympha, that continually flows by with the urine, and further compacted together by the salts with which the urine is loaden.*"* And for the cure, they prescribed *venesection, opiates, mercurials, diuretic infusions* and *decoctions, and* "*lithontriptics,*" or "stone-dissolving remedies." Modern allopathy attributes calculous depositions to a superabundance of uric acid, of the phosphates of lime, magnesia, and ammonia, oxalate of lime, &c., in the blood and urine, and they also prescribe blood-letting, opiates, mercurials, diuretics, and "*stone-dissolving remedies,*" but with no more success than their heathen predecessors. To what extent homœopathy may be able to combat this formidable disease, time alone can determine; but so far as the limited observations and experience of our practitioners extend, in this class of affections, our method of practice has been highly satisfactory. Our system is especially adapted to correct those peculiar diatheses upon which the formation of calculi depend.

Calculous affections have been observed to prevail in some countries more than others: even in some portions of the same country they may be common, while in other sections they will be unknown. The disease is rarely seen in very cold or very hot latitudes. English surgeons assert that it never originates in the East Indies, and it is supposed to be of very rare occurrence in the northern kingdoms of Europe.

* Salmon.

Children and old people are most subject to the disease, and it seizes especially upon those in whom gout is hereditary. Indeed this gouty diathesis is so common in individuals afflicted with calculi, that many suppose that the urine exercises but little if any influence in their formation, but that metastases of gout to the mucous membrane of the urinary passages, determine the formations of these calculous concretions.—Thus, Frank, in his "Traité de Prac. de Med.," p. 367, vol. ii," says: "The attacks of calculous affections, like those of gout, are preceded and accompanied by languor of the stomach, nausea, oppression, eructations, borborigmi. In inveterate gout, this phlegmasia gives rise to calcareous concretions, formed of a material combined with uric acid, and which do not differ from urinary calculi except in consistency and form. Suppose now that fixed gout, which produces calcareous concretions in the articulations of the great toe, attacks the mucous membrane of the bladder, *may it not become the source of calculi in this viscus?*"

Calculi have been found in the brain, lungs, liver, spleen, gall, bladder, uterus, the articulations and the soft parts of nearly every portion of the organism, but the urinary organs are by far the most common seat of these formations. Several years since I saw taken from the upper part of the left lobe of the lung of a miller, two concretions of a chalky appearance, but hard and tough, and of the size of a goose-egg. Concretions of lithate of ammonia are also common in all parts of the body, in gouty patients.

Prout has divided the mechanical deposits from the urine into three classes: First, *Pulverulent, or amorphous sediments.* Second, *Chrystaline sediments, usually denominated gravel.* Third, *Solid concretions or calculi, formed by the aggregation of these sediments.*

The sediments of the first class are held in solution by the urine until it is discharged from the bladder, when they are gradually deposited in a state of fine brown or yellow powder. These sediments are generally composed of "two species of neutral saline compounds; viz., the lithates of ammonia, soda, and lime, tinged more or less with the colouring principle of the urine, and with the purpurates of the same bases, and constituting what are usually denominated *pink* and *lateritious* sediments; and secondly, the earthy phosphates, namely, the phosphate of lime, and the triple phosphate of magnesia and ammonia, constituting, for the most part, sediments nearly white. The two species of sediments are frequently mixed together."—(*Prout.*)

The sediments of the second class, or *gravel*, are found in the urine in regularly crystallized grains, varying in form and colour in accordance with the constituents of which they are composed. The lithic acid crystals are much the most common, and may be distinguished by their red colour. The crystals of the triple phosphate of ammonia and of magnesia are of a white colour, while those of the oxalate of lime are black or dark green.

Prout supposes that two-thirds of the whole number of calculi originate from lithic acid; and when we bear in mind the constant presence of this acid in the urinary organs, and its proneness to form hard, inodorous concretions of a yellowish or brown colour, the supposition will not appear unreasonable.

Chemists have described many different varieties of calculi, amongst which the following are the most common:—

First, The *lithic* or *uric acid calculus*, formed by concentric lamellæ, presenting a light brown or reddish colour, and a general appearance something like wood. These calculi are infusible by the blow-pipe, but may be slowly evaporated, until a slight residue of white ash remains. They are soluble in alkaline solutions, which, on this account, are supposed to be valuable as remedial agents, but they are not dissolved by muriatic or sulphuric acids. The lithic acid diathesis prevails in childhood and at about the age of forty or fifty, and the urine voided in these cases is generally *acid*, and the sabulous sediment of a *red colour*.

Second. The calculi of most common occurrence after the variety last described, are those composed of a triple combination of *phosphoric acid*, *magnesia*, *and ammonia*. They are of a lightish gray colour, indistinctly laminated, with an "uneven surface and covered with small shining crystals." This variety is not soluble in alkaline solutions, but may be partially dissolved by muriatic, nitric, and sulphuric acids, and imperfectly fused by the blow-pipe. The urine in these cases is very fetid, and the sediment deposited of a white colour, "resembling mortar." Sir Astley Cooper asserts that this kind of calculus is very apt to be reproduced after lithotomy, and on this account advises the postponement of operations in these cases until the morbid diathesis is corrected.

Third. Not a very uncommon variety is the *mulberry calculus*, of a dark brown colour, uneven surface, and very compact, heavy and hard. It consists of *oxalate of lime*, and is partially soluble in muriatic and sulphuric acids, but the alkaline solutions have no effect upon it.

Fourth. The *phosphate of lime calculus* is in a few instances found pure, but usually it exists in combination with uric acid and phosphate of magnesia and ammonia. It is laminated, polished, of a pale brown colour, soluble in muriatic or nitric acid, and may be fused by the blow-pipe. They are of small size, and are generally found in the *prostate gland.*

Fifth. The *cystic oxyde calculus* is another variety of rare occurrence, of a yellowish hue, not laminated, soluble in acids and alkaline solutions, and emitting under the blow-pipe a fetid odour.

Sixth. There is also the *fusible calculus*, composed of a mixture of the triple phosphate of magnesia and ammonia, and of the phosphate of lime; of a white colour, and fusible by the blow-pipe. This kind of calculous deposit is occasionally seen between the foreskin and glans-penis in old cases of phymosis.

Seventh. The constituents of the different kinds of calculi are sometimes deposited in distinct alternate layers in the same stone, when it is called the *alternating calculus.*

Other varieties have been described, like the *compound calculi*, the *carbonate of lime calculus*, the *lithate of ammonia calculus*, &c.

The presence in the bladder or kidneys of any solid substance, whether introduced artificially, or formed naturally from lithic acid concretions, or clots of blood, favours the formation of calculi. Whether the cause of these deposits in the urinary organs, is attributable to the peculiar composition, or the compact structure, or the comparative temperature of the nuclei, we are unable to determine: but all are aware of the fact, that catheters, bullets, splinters, or other solid substances, accidentally introduced into the bladder, become speedily coated over with the urinary sediments, which are converted into hard crusts.

Calculi are more frequently observed in the male, than in the female sex; but this circumstance has been attributed to the difference in the structure of the urethra in the two sexes, rather than to a difference in the original diathesis. The urethra of the female being short and easily dilated, gives passage without difficulty to gravel and small calculi, which in the long and contracted male organs would be obstructed either by causing spasmodic contractions, or from an actual want of room to pass.

It is said that the *right* kidney is far more commonly the seat of these formations than the *left*, that their form is generally spheroidical, and that their average weight is from one to two ounces. Sir Astley Cooper, however, expresses the opinion that a majority of urinary calculi weigh less than one ounce each.

Calculi may originate in the kidneys, the bladder, or the prostate gland, but the first organ is the primary seat of a large majority of cases, as is evident from the fact that the pains are almost always confined to the region of one of the kidneys in the first instance. It is probable that the *nuclei* of most stones found in the bladder, are first formed in the kidneys, and then conveyed through the ureters into this viscus, to serve as the foundation of still farther deposits from the urine.

Diagnosis.—A calculus may remain in the kidney or bladder for a long time, without exciting much pain or uneasiness. The patient experiences perhaps a more frequent inclination to urinate than natural, and after violent exercise on horseback or in a carriage, has temporary pains in the region of the organ affected, but in other respects he feels well. This state of things may exist for an indefinite length of time, when, if the stone is situated in the kidney, some exciting cause may operate, and give rise to what is denominated a "fit of the stone." In these instances the patient is usually attacked suddenly, with severe cutting pains in the region of the kidney, which increases as the stone passes along the ureter to the bladder, sometimes extending to the groin, the cremaster muscle, or along the crural nerve, as it passes over the nerves connected with these parts. During the paroxysm, the pain is often of the most violent and intolerable character, and is accompanied with continual nausea, vomiting, inability to retain any thing upon the stomach, frequent desire to urinate, high coloured and sometimes bloody urine, bent position of the body, with the muscles flexed as much as possible, heartburn, painful retraction of the testicle, irritable bladder, and febrile symptoms. There is often a remission of these symptoms for a longer or shorter period, during the descent of the stone through the ureters, and the paroxysm now and then comes on, and subsides suddenly and permanently, the stone not having effected an entrance into the ureter.

After the stone has passed into the bladder, we have the following train of symptoms: frequent inclination to urinate, "the patient making the first portion with ease, and complaining of great pain coming on when the last drops are expelled."—(*Earle.*) Sudden stoppage of the current of urine, in consequence of the stone moving in front of the urethra, itching and tingling at the extremity of the penis, difficulty or absolute inability of retaining the fæces when urinating, on account of the sympathetic irritation of the rectum, "sense of weight and pressure at the lower part of the pelvis," dull pain at the neck of the bladder, bloody, mucous, or purulent urine, pains in the region of the bladder increased by exercise, especially riding on horseback or in a jolting carriage, febrile symptoms, irritability, loss of appetite, emaciation, inability to sleep or rest quietly, night or day. In boys, the prepuce generally becomes much elongated, from their constant habit of pulling at it, to relieve the itching in the glans. After the stone has continued in the bladder for a considerable time, this organ becomes very much contracted, its coats become thickened and diseased, and the patient sinks under the constitutional derangement consequent upon the protracted irritation of the foreign body.

It will be observed that all of the symptoms which we have enumerated, are similated by the affections of the urinary organs. Thus, simple *nephritis* gives rise to the symptoms of calculus in the kidneys; and inflammation of the prostate gland and bladder, to those of stone in the bladder. But in some instances the patient can actually feel the motion of the calculus, as he turns over from one side to the other. This circumstance, taken in connection with the abrupt stoppage of the stream when urinating, in consequence of the stone getting before the urethra, and the occurrence of severe pain after the urine has been mostly evacuated, in consequence of the stone coming into more direct contact with the walls of the bladder, will enable us to decide with much certainty respecting the presence of a stone.

But the only *positive* indication of a calculus is our ability to *strike it* with a *sound* introduced into the bladder, and a prudent surgeon will never cut for the stone unless he can *feel* it with his sound immediately before he commences his operation.

Therapeutics.—Our therapeutical measures may be classed under four heads.

First. To correct the diathesis on which the morbid sediments depend.

Second. To relieve the distress and suffering attendant on the presence in the urinary organs of gravel or stone.

Third. To dissolve the stone.

Fourth. To extract it, either by lithotomy, or by the aid of Civiale's lithotriptor.

The first object may be attained by removing the causes upon which the diathesis depends. Some of the more prominent of these causes are, errors in diet, including quality and quantity of food, and irregularity in hours of taking meals, abuse of stimulants, use of water abounding in lime, excessive mental or bodily fatigue, undue exposure to atmospheric vicissitudes, insufficient nutriment, the depressing passions, tendency to gout and rheumatism, dyspepsia, and disease of the urinary organs.

When the depositions depend upon a *lithic acid diathesis*, every thing of an acid nature should be avoided; a large quantity of animal food should be enjoined, and baths, frictions, and abundant exercise taken, to ensure a healthy action of the skin.

The *phosphatic diathesis* may depend upon a loss of tone in the digestive organs, too free use of animal food, profuse sweats, use of lime water, and over-exertion, mental or physical. Here a farinaceous and vegetable diet, and a free use of fruit and acids, should be advised. If the depositions arise from gout attacking the mucous membrane of the bladder, the suitable medicines will speedily dissipate the morbid condition, When the diathesis appears to proceed from general debility, or derangement in the digestive or assimilative functions, our dietetic regulations, as well as our medicines, should be prescribed with reference to these conditions.

In all calculous affections, a cheerful state of mind, with country air, or a sea-voyage to a hot or cold latitude, will prove serviceable.

To fulfil the second and third indications as far as possible, we shall, farther on, point out those remedies which we deem most suitable. But it is matter of much doubt whether there are at present any remedies known, capable of dissolving a calculus in the urinary organs after it has attained a considerable size. We may be able to correct the diathesis upon which the morbid sediments depend, and to enable the urinary organs to expel calculi of small size; but the dissolution of a large stone in the bladder has never yet been effected. Such can only be removed by crushing them according to the method of Civiale, &c., so that the fragments will pass off by the urine, or by the operation of lithotomy. For the details concerning these important operations, we refer the reader to the standard works on Surgery.

The principal medicines in the treatment of urinary concretions, are *cannabis, uva ursi, nux vomica, sarsaparilla, lycopodium, calcarea carb., phosphorus, aspara-*

gine, monarda punctata, alchemilla arveusis, chininum sulph., alisma plantago.

Cannabis and *uva ursi* are excellent remedies during a fit of the gravel, accompanied with painful micturition ; discharge of slimy, purulent or bloody urine ; burning in the bladder and urethra during and after micturition ; and itching at the extremity of the glans penis.

Dr. Gross has highly commended the employment of *nux vomica* and *sarsaparilla* for the cure of gravel and calculous affections. So far as the former remedy is concerned, my own experience coincides with that of Dr. Gross. I have in several instances prescribed *nux vomica* with unequivocal benefit, in calculous affections which apparently originated from chronic derangement of the digestive organs. In one case, likewise, where the patient experienced the most severe spasmodic pains from the passage of a calculus from the kidney to the bladder, with constant nausea, vomiting, painful and bloody micturition, and high-coloured urine, the most prompt and happy results followed the use of *nux.*

This remedy is decidedly indicated when lithiasis arises from dyspeptic symptoms, sedentary occupations, abuse of stimulants, excesses in eating, and also for the acute constrictive and spasmodic pains which proceed from the irritation of a calculus when passing from one point to another.

Lycopodium is adapted to patients of a lymphatic temperament, and who have been subject to chronic affections of the mucous membranes. The lycopodium pains occur mostly in the urethra and perineum, and are of a burning, smarting, or cutting character during micturition. The urine is of a dark colour, very fœtid and deposites a red or yellowish sand.

Calcarea carb. is suitable for the calculous affections of scrofulous or chlorotic children. It is indicated when the pains in the urinary organs, and the desire to pass water, are worse during the night, and the urine is of a dark colour, fœtid, and deposites a white sediment. *Calcarea* is also indicated in debility of the assimilative functions, emaciation, and great weakness and exhaustion of the whole system.

Phosphorus may be given in lithiasis occurring in broken down constitutions from loss of fluids, and in old and debilitated subjects. The phosphorus symptoms are characterized by loss of power over the urinary organs, involuntary passing of urine and fæces at the same time, sudden interruptions of the course of the urine, desire to urinate, with dull pains in the hypogastrium, emission by the urine of an ammoniacal odour, and deposites of a whitish or brick-dust sediment.

We have exhibited *asparagus* in two cases of lithiasis dependent upon a gouty diathesis with marked success. In one of these cases the calculous symptoms all disappeared in a few weeks after commencing the medicine, and the morbid character which the urine had presented for several years, was entirely changed to a healthy condition. We are inclined to believe that asparagus is a remedy of much greater power in urinary affections and in dropsies, than has ever been attributed to it. Our experience with it in those maladies has been somewhat extensive, and generally of a most satisfactory character. It is especially called for when there is frequent inclination to urinate; burning and cutting in the urethra and kidneys; dull drawing pains in the groin; tenderness and pain in the perineum; sensation as if urine was passing off, after all has been discharged; urine straw-coloured or brown, with a very offensive smell, and a whitish sediment; palpitation of the heart; rapid and oppressed respiration on the slightest exertion.

Monarda punctata, alchemilla arveusis, and *alisma plantago*, also cover most of the symptoms enumerated under *asparagus*, and may sometimes succeed this remedy with advantage.

Chininum sulph. is recommended when there are minute crystallized grains in the urine, of a reddish or yellowish colour; increased flow of acrid and offensive urine; emaciation; irritability and much constitutional disturbance.

Administration.—During the violent paroxysms which occur in calculous diseases, we may employ the medicines from the first to the third attenuation, and repeat every hour until the desired impression is produced. But under ordinary circumstances, a dose once in twelve or twenty-four hours will suffice.

SECTION VIII.

URETHRITIS.—INFLAMMATION OF THE URETHRA.

The term *gonorrhœa*, derived from two Greek words, γονὴ, semen, and ῥεω, to flow, is very generally used by American and English physicians to designate this malady. Dr. Swediaur, perceiving the erroneous impression which this definition might convey, substituted another term no less etymologically inaccurate, *blennorrhœa*, or *blennorrhagia*, derived from two other Greek words, βλέννα, mucus, and ῥεω, to flow. But as modern researches have demonstrated that the involuntary discharge which is a characteristic of this disease, does not consist of semen or mucus, but of a purulent and infectious matter, we think the erroneous terms commonly employed to designate the complaint, should be abolished. Many reasons may be adduced against naming the affection from the supposed character of the discharge ; for, notwithstanding as a general rule it is decidedly *purulent*, cases occasionally occur where, from the intensity of the inflammation, there is no discharge at all, and constituting that form of the disease denominated by French writers, "*blennorrhagie sèche*." The matter is likewise sometimes composed of a mixture of pus, mucus, semen and blood. For these reasons we prefer to make use of the more general term, *urethritis*. Inflammation of the urethra may indeed arise from other causes than the application of infectious matter during an impure connection, and present all of the symptoms peculiar to the venereal inflammation, but the malady is none the less urethritis on this account, although the secretion accompanying the inflammation is not infectious. So may an inflammation of the eye owe its origin to the application of venereal matter, external irritants, atmospheric changes, injuries, scrofula, and abuse of stimulants, and yet notwithstanding these different causes, the disease is none the less *ophthalmia*.

All secreting surfaces are liable to be irritated when

operated on by certain unnatural stimuli. The mucous membrane of the throat, the bronchia, the lungs, the nostrils, the frontal sinuses, and the conjunctiva of the eye, are all subject to different grades and kinds of inflammation, and their secretions to become changed in quality and quantity, according to the morbid cause which has been in operation. The lining membrane of the urethra is also subject to the same laws : it may become inflamed and pour out a purulent discharge from the presence of calculi in the bladder, from gout and rheumatism, from acrid urine, from the absorption of certain diuretics, from ulcers, from mechanical injuries, and finally from the application of infectious matter during an impure coition. In a very large majority of cases, *urethritis* arises from the cause last enumerated. This morbid virus induces a specific inflammation in the urethra, of so troublesome and inveterate a character as often to baffle all the remedial measures of the most skilful and experienced medical men. The inflammation is supposed by some to be of the erysipelatous kind, and generally attacks the lacunæ of the urethra.

All who have had much experience in this disease, will agree with me that it is one of the most intractable with which we have to deal: Mackintosh assures us "that he has been more annoyed and disgusted in conducting the treatment of gonorrhœa than of any other affection."

We are at present in ignorance respecting the primary source of infectious urethritis, but the doctrine entertained by the ancients, and so strenuously advocated by John Hunter, and his cotemporaries, in regard to the identity of the gonorrhœal and syphilitic virus, is now universally abandoned. The disease under consideration, is one of a purely local character, and if left to itself, under favourable circumstances, will ultimately terminate in spontaneous recovery. It is a matter of doubt whether ulcers of the urethra ever proceed from this inflammation, when entirely uncomplicated, but it is probable that the few cases which have been reported by Sir Astley Cooper and others, in which the malady was connected with ulcerations, were attributable to the application of the virus of both affections.

We have, in several instances, inoculated individuals with the matter of infectious urethritis, but have never been able to produce a chancre or any well-marked constitutional symptoms. We have, in one instance, also witnessed the introduction of the gonorrhœal virus into the blood, but without giving rise to any appreciable effects. While on the other hand, it is well known, that if syphilitic virus be inoculated or introduced directly into the mass of the blood, the symptoms of syphilis speedily result. The application of gonorrhœal matter to the eye, gives rise to a very violent and dangerous purulent *ophthalmia ;* while the application of syphilitic virus to this organ, causes an ulcer generally circumscribed, and unaccompanied by violent or dangerous inflammation of the surrounding parts. The application of the former to the anus, causes inflammation, with augmented secretion, and change in its character from mucus to pus ; the application of the syphilitic poison, causes chancre and its concomitants.

Urethritis is often suspended during attacks of acute disease, but it invariably reappears again after the subsidence of the febrile symptoms.

From these facts it may be fairly inferred, that gonorrhœal matter contains a specific morbid principle, capable of producing a peculiar inflammation and discharge, when brought in contact with mucous surfaces. This inflammation and discharge present a uniform appearance quite unlike what occurs in leucorrhœa, in several particulars. The matter of the former is infectious, while that of the latter is non-infectious ; the inflammation of the former is of the *erysipelatous* kind, while the condition of the mucous membrane in the latter is more allied to *relaxation* and *debility* than to inflammation ; the former can only arise from the contact of gonorrhœal matter with a mucous surface, while the latter never proceeds from any cause of this kind, but from constitutional weakness, confinements, excesses in venery, want of exercise, and other debilitating habits.

We may also infer, from what has been observed,

that the syphilitic matter likewise contains a specific morbid virus, *sui generis*, and only capable of exciting chancre, when applied to abraded or delicate surfaces.

It should always be remembered, that every morbid substance capable of impressing the organism, contains a certain *specific morbid principle*, which usually operates in a definite manner, causing a uniform train of symptoms, and requiring a certain *specific medicinal agent* to effect a prompt cure. These morbid principles only exist in infinitesimal quantities in their media, and on this account we are unable to detect or analyze them, but we ought none the less to acknowledge their presence, appreciate their influence, and endeavour, if possible, to discover their specific antidotes.

Diagnosis.—The ordinary period at which infectious urethritis makes its appearance after an impure connection, is from two to four days. We have known it to commence in a few instances, in eight or ten hours after exposure, and we have likewise occasionally observed an interval of six weeks to elapse before its onset. Some constitutions possess the power of resisting the action of the poison to such a degree as to constitute an almost entire exemption from the disease. Other individuals are so little susceptible, that if pains be taken to urinate and perform thorough ablution soon after the sin, no ill consequences result. Others again are so highly susceptible, either from natural organization, or from abuse of stimulants, that almost the very touch of a contaminated female speedily communicates the inflammation.

The disease commences by a tingling or itching sensation at the orifice of the urethra, which is noticed especially when urinating. In a short time, the lips of the urethra become red and swollen; the blood-vessels of the organ distended; the inflammation increases and extends up the passage for an inch or two; there is a burning or scalding pain on passing water; an increased secretion takes place from the part affected, at first of a mucous character, but as the inflammation increases presenting a purulent appearance, of a yellow colour, or if the disease is violent, green and sanious. The urine, which often contains some thread-like substances, arising from the inflammatory action, flows from the urethra in a diminished, spiral or divided stream.

In a *first* attack, the inflammation does not usually confine itself to the extremity of the urethra, but extends along the canal to the prostate gland, and even to the bladder itself. Not unfrequently it attacks the glans penis and the frænum, in which case it often occasions an effusion between the foreskin and glans, and *phymosis*.

When the inflammation is intense, and extends up as far as the neck of the bladder, there is a frequent and urgent desire to urinate, the *ardor urinæ* becomes more extensive and painful, involuntary and painful erections occur, chiefly during the night, and sometimes cause distressing emissions of semen ; sympathetic irritation is communicated to the perineum, occasioning painful sensations when evacuating the bowels, or the bladder ; there is more or less inflammation and effusion of lymph into the corpora spongiosa, giving rise to those adhesions and painful contractions termed *chordee ;* the glands of the groin become irritated and enlarged, and there is a partial or even total suppression of the discharge, in which latter case the disease is termed *dry urethritis*, or the "*blenorrhagie sèche*" of the French.

In old sinners, the inflammation is quite prone to attack the prostate gland, and give rise to those unpleasant symptoms which we have enumerated when alluding to affections of this structure.

As we have before remarked, if the disease be left to itself, and the patient is strictly prudent and temperate, a spontaneous recovery will eventually take place ; but from improper medical treatment, undue exposure, or excesses of different kinds, the disease often terminates in gleet, strictures, abscesses, diseased prostate, irritable bladder, hernia humoralis, inflammation of the testicle and epididymis, or bubo.

The acute stage of urethritis, under ordinary circumstances, terminates in from one to three weeks, when, if suitable remedies have been employed, the discharge ceases, and the parts speedily recover their tone ; but in the majority of instances, the acute stage runs into a *chronic* inflammation, when it receives the name of

GLEET.

In this stage of the disorder, the painful symptoms peculiar to the first period, *ardor urinæ,* frequent inclination to urinate, chordee, spasmodic pains in the region of the perineum, and the heat and swelling of the penis, subside, and we observe little else than an increase and alteration in the character of the secretion from the urethra. This discharge, which during the acute symptoms was purulent, and of a yellow or greenish colour, now presents a light mucous appearance, sometimes transparent and ropy. The character of this discharge, however, is often temporarily changed again to a purulent matter of a yellow or even green colour, sometimes sanious, from over-exercise, excesses in drinking or eating, sexual intercourse, and exposure to protracted heat or cold. The discharge of a simple gleet usually proceeds from the lacunæ of the urethra. Some writers have promulgated the dangerous doctrine, that the matter of a gleet is not infectious; but this is an error, for we have known many well authenticated instances where virulent urethritis has arisen from the application of gleety matter.

When a gleet has been permitted to continue for a long time, and particularly if the case has been injudiciously treated by inordinate doses of copaibæ, cubebs, turpentine, and the endless train of irritating injections, there often supervenes a

STRICTURE OF THE URETHRA.

A stricture may occur during the height of acute urethritis, from tumefaction of the mucous membrane of the canal, or from the irritation caused by improper or unskilful introduction of bougies, and by strong injections. The obstruction in some cases of this description is so complete, that very painful retentions of urine, with its accompanying symptoms, supervene, requiring the most prompt remedial measures in order to ward off the necessity of puncturing the bladder. This variety of stricture may be removed in a short time by proper medicines, without the aid of a surgeon.

There is a second variety of stricture not necessarily connected with infectious urethritis, termed *spasmodic stricture.* The disease consists in a sudden spasmodic contraction of some portion of the urinary canal, which impedes the flow of urine, and sometimes causes a partial retention. These spasmodic contractions may arise from mechanical injuries, diseased prostate, or stimulating diuretics, but they are for the most part connected with permanent stricture.

The third variety of stricture, which is by far the most common and serious, is termed the *permanent stricture.* Its approach is so gradual and imperceptible, that individuals rarely suspect anything of the kind, until it has made considerable progress. The disease arises from a gradual thickening of the mucous membrane of the urethra, from badly treated or long continued inflammation.

The first symptoms observable in this stricture are, a sensation after urinating as if a few drops remained behind; stream diminished in size, and issuing from the urethra in a spiral form, or split in several parts; straining to pass the water more rapidly through the obstructed canal; aggravation of all the symptoms on wetting the feet, taking cold, over-exercise, fatigue, and venereal excesses. In this stricture, there is always more or less discharge of a ropy kind of mucus, which is often temporarily changed by excesses, into a purulent or bloody matter. This complaint is quite apt to induce inguinal hernia, from the straining efforts employed in urinating.

It is probable that two-thirds of the cases treated as simple gleets, and which so frequently baffle the physician, are, in reality, dependent solely on this kind of stricture.

In bad cases of permanent stricture, the urine is passed drop by drop, the distention and pain in the region of the bladder become very severe, much constitutional irritation occurs, and the patient is unable to rest day or night. Whenever this state of things obtains, immediate recourse should be had to bougies.

The removal of a permanent stricture can only be

accomplished by means of the knife, or the application of caustic, or by gradual dilation by means of bougies. The cure by the latter means is, at the present time, almost universally recommended.

Almost all strictures are located far up the canal of the urethra, behind its bulb, but they may occur near the extremity of the penis, or three, four, or five inches above this point.

An occasional consequence of stricture is,

FISTULA IN PERINEO.

When the contraction is so great as to cause considerable obstruction to the passage of the urine, this fluid is forced by the frequent and violent efforts at expulsion, into the parts back of the stricture, in such a manner as to form a kind of *cul de sac*, which, from constant distention, eventually ulcerates an opening externally, and a *perineal fistula* is formed.

Abscesses also arise sometimes from inflammation and tumefaction of the lymphatic glands in other parts of the urethra. These little swellings may open into the urethra, or discharge themselves externally. The most common seat of these abscesses is near the frænum, or opposite the scrotum.

DISEASED PROSTATE,

May also be ranked amongst the occasional consequences of repeated attacks of urethritis. During the continuance of the latter affection, not only the urethra, but the prostate, the bladder, and the testicles, receive an unusual supply of blood, in consequence of which they become irritated, and often enlarged, from depositions of coagulable lymph. This condition of things may exist without attracting much attention until the individual is advanced in years, when a scirrhous degeneration, or an abscess, is exceedingly apt to result. Either lobe of the prostate may become enlarged separately, or the whole three may be involved ; but the most troublesome symptoms arise from an enlargement of the middle lobe, on account of its proximity to the orifice of the urinary canal.

Sir Astley Cooper was of opinion, that enlargement

of this gland is attributable to advanced age, rather than disease; but from the fact, that persons who have been afflicted in this manner have almost invariably been subject to repeated venereal attacks in early life, we may fairly infer, that a predisposition is always established in the structure, which renders it liable to take on diseased action when the powers of the organism have become impaired by age.

Enlargement of the lateral lobes of the prostate may be readily detected by introducing the finger into the rectum. The middle lobe may always be felt by the catheter when much enlarged, and it will generally be found exceedingly difficult to pass it by the gland into the bladder. By directing the point of the instrument, (which should be of medium size,) slightly upwards, and depressing the handle at the proper time, the object may usually be accomplished. But of all others, these cases require great delicacy of touch and practical tact, to enable the operator to succeed facilely, and without doing injury to the irritated parts.

Diseases of the prostate are quite liable to become aggravated by over-exertion, riding, acrid urine, exposure to wet and cold, and stimulating drinks.

Another exceedingly unpleasant consequence of neglected or badly treated urethritis, is the disease termed

IRRITABLE BLADDER.

This affection arises from long continued inflammation, which in the end so impairs the function of the bladder, that the presence of a very small quantity of urine forces it to contract, and thus forms an incontinence of urine. Although this condition of the bladder may arise from numerous causes which have already been enumerated, it not unfrequently proceeds from extension of urethritic inflammation to this organ, and from protracted use of diuretics. The malady is readily distinguished from stone, by the *relief* which always follows the evacuation of the bladder, while this operation aggravates the painful sensations in the latter affection.

This disease generally baffles all the resources of

allopathy, but we take pleasure in appealing to the philosophic practice whether the same remark is just with reference to *homœopathy*.

The next malady to which we shall allude in connection with urethritis, is

HERNIA HUMORALIS.

During the acute stage of urethritis, the inflammation sometimes extends even to the spermatic chord, the epididymis, and the testicle. This is very apt to occur when the discharge is suddenly arrested by irritating injections, especially when the inflammation pervades the whole extent of the canal. When the substance of the testicle becomes involved, the pain is very severe, and febrile symptoms more or less grave, set in. This inflammation may terminate in resolution, suppuration, or chronic enlargement and induration. In those instances where suppuration occurs, the abscesses usually break externally, and form fistulous passages which are difficult to cure, on account of the continual irritation kept up by the secretion of semen, a portion of which is constantly being discharged through these ulcerated openings.

Chronic enlargements of the testicles should command our early attention, on account of their strong tendency to terminate in scirrhous degenerations.

In urethritis, and other affections of the urino-genital apparatus, the prudent physician will always advise the use of the suspensory bandage, as a precautionary measure.

When the urethritis is so severe as to affect the lymphatic glands of the penis, the disease may be propagated to several of the glands of the groin, when we have a

BUBO.

These buboes are called *sympathetic*, in contradistinction to those which proceed from syphilitic infection. The frequent occurrence of such tumours during the course of urethritis, probably first led medical men to confound this disease with syphilis. But, on close examination, the sympathetic bubo will be found to be composed of *several* enlarged glands, while that of syphilis is an enlargement of a *single gland.*

The sympathetic bubo is not usually attended with great pain, nor does it run on to suppuration, unless the patient is decidedly scrofulous; while syphilitic bubo is attended with much inflammation and pain, and is very prone to advance to the suppurative stage. A very large majority of sympathetic buboes subside spontaneously, and require no medicinal treatment.

In *females*, all of the symptoms of the disease are lighter than in the male sex. Indeed, the similarity between this affection and *leucorrhœa* is so great, that it is sometimes a matter of great difficulty to distinguish them.

Mr. Travers asserts, that the urethra itself is rarely affected in females, but that the inflammation attacks the clitoris, the inferior commissure of the labia and rapha, the nymphæ, and the parts (Cowper's glands) around the orifice of the urethra.

In the worst form of the complaint, as it occurs in women, the labia, the nymphæ, and the clitoris, become swollen and painful, the inflammation extends to the womb and bladder, and there will be frequent inclination to urinate, severe scalding by the water, and a purulent, irritating discharge. But all of these symptoms are often met with in inflammatory leucorrhœa, and the discharge itself even acquires so acrid a character as to become capable of propagating a similar discharge by contact with the male organ. We have, in more than one instance, been consulted by parties of the highest respectability, in relation to purulent discharges, and scalding of the urine, which have been contracted from the wife, but by explaining the circumstance just alluded to, have been able to dissipate the most unjust suspicions, and to restore confidence and harmony which must have been utterly destroyed without such explanation.

The following are the surest diagnostic marks, with which we are acquainted, between the two diseases: leucorrhœa is gradual in its progress, and may be generally traced to constitutional debility, or to difficult and protracted labours, or mechanical injuries during accouchement. It is usually accompanied also by prolapsus uteri, or dragging pain, or tired feeling in the left side, bearing down pains, and general feelings of relaxation and debility.

Gonorrhœal inflammation is sudden and rapid in its approach, and attacks individuals in the soundest health: the symptoms acquire their greatest severity in one or two weeks, and the discharge causes a deep-coloured (yellow or greenish) stain upon the linen, surrounded by a palish yellow border.

A careful attention to the history of each individual case, will aid us materially in forming a correct diagnosis.

Therapeutics.—Infectious urethritis is at the present time almost universally looked upon as a purely *local* disease,—confined in its first stages to a small portion of the mucous membrane of the urethra. It is true that the inflammation often extends up the urinary canal to the prostate gland, and to the bladder; but it is highly probable that these secondary symptoms are owing to bad treatment, or imprudence on the part of patients, rather than to the natural and legitimate tendency of the malady. We adopt this opinion from having often observed spontaneous cures occur in six or eight weeks without medicine of any kind, and without any structure but the urethra becoming affected,—the patients having simply placed themselves under a rigid dietetic regimen.

It may be questioned whether any internal remedy is now known, which can be considered a true and certain specific for the cure of this local inflammation. Many medicines have been brought forward by both schools as worthy of our entire confidence, but *not one of them* has yet stood the test of practical experiment, —not one has been able to control the symptoms, or remove the complaint with any degree of certainty. On the contrary, many of them have repeatedly been observed to aggravate the inflammation, causing it to extend to the neighbouring structures, and thus seriously to complicate this naturally simple disease.

The ordinary plan of treatment, according to the old-school method, is in the *first* stage to bleed, leech, foment, physic with mercurials, or the neutral salts, and to nauseate, sweat, and prostrate the system with antimonials. In other words, it is deemed necessary to punish the whole organism;—to inflame the bowels with cathartics,—to impair the tone of the stomach by nauseating doses of antimony,—to debilitate the capillaries by profuse sweats,—to abstract the life-giving principle from the veins,—and to reduce the patient to a state of prostration and positive illness, in order to reach a little circumscribed inflammation in the urethra! After the patient has been reduced *secundem artem*, the custom is then to administer enormous doses of *balsam copaibæ, cubebs, turpentine, lyttæ, iodine*, and *nitre, internally*, and to make use of stimulating injections of zinc, lead, copper, mercury, nitrate of silver, oil of vitriol, chloride of lime, and diluted sulphuric acid, *ad libitum. Balsam copaibæ* is the medicine employed in most instances, and as it operates specifically upon the stomach and the respiratory organs, we often observe the most serious affections of these organs arise in consequence of its free and protracted use. Who that has made use of this remedy to any great extent, has not witnessed the occurrence of troublesome dyspeptic symptoms, of hæmoptysis, of cough, and other indications of dangerous pulmonary disorder, from it?

Cases however occur, in which the symptoms of urethritis cease under the use of this, and the other diuretics alluded to, but such instances are rare, and the remark of the celebrated Dr. Forbes respecting allopathic remedies in general, will hold good here, viz.: that "the patient gets well *in spite* of the doctor."

We shall not discuss the propriety of the antiphlogistic course adopted during the acute stage, for we believe that all whose prejudices will permit them to exercise that admirable requisite, *common sense*, will perceive at a glance the folly of tormenting and prostrating the *whole body* for the sake of acting upon a *simple local inflammation*, which, when left to itself, never terminates in ulceration or disorganization of the tissue affected, but in *spontaneous recovery*.

And what shall we say of the homœopathic remedies which are usually employed in the treatment of this complaint? Why, simply that the true specific has not yet been discovered. We have tested these medicines in numerous instances, both the high and low attenuations, and we regret to announce as the result of our observations, that they have proved but little more successful than the pernicious applications of the old school.

We are quite aware that it is much easier to find fault with prevailing methods of practice, than to propose and introduce better new ones. But if we succeed in attracting the attention of physicians more particularly to the subject, and putting them on the *qui vive* to find out a positive specific, our object will be accomplished. In the mean time we shall point out the course of treatment which we have found most successful in the different stages of the malady.

For therapeutical purposes the disease may be classified as follows:

First. The *preventive period,*—or that which intervenes between the exposure and the first symptoms of the malady. The average duration of this period is about three days.

Second. The *forming stage,*—or the period which elapses from the commencement of the prickling, tingling, or itching sensation, with slight redness and swelling of the lips of the urethra, and a slight oozing of mucus or limpid matter, up to the period when the inflammation has extended to the *fossa navicularis*, and become strongly pronounced, with a purulent discharge of a yellow or greenish colour. This stage usually lasts from twelve to forty-eight hours.

Third. The *acute* or *inflammatory* stage,—including the period which commences at the termination of the last stage, and the subsidence of the *ardor urinæ*, the acute inflammation of the urethra, the swelling and tenderness of the penis, and the change of the yellow or greenish secretion, to one of a light transparent and ropy, or a muco-purulent character. The natural duration of this stage, when proper restrictions are used as to diet, stimulants, and exercise, is from one to two weeks.

Fourth. The *chronic stage*, or that form of the malady termed *gleet.*

Now, as our object, in accordance with the homœpathic doctrine of cure, is to próduce in the tissue morbidly affected, a new and healthy medicinal action, which shall supersede the morbid inflammation, we apply our remedies *directly* to the diseased part, instead of bringing them in contact with it through the stomach, blood, and kidneys. The malady is not constitutional,—there is no other structure of the economy affected, or upon which we wish to act,—but our sole object is to prevent or to remove a simple *local* inflammation.

Our remedies then, during the first or *preventive period*, are the occasional injections into the urethra, of a solution of nitrate of silver, (in the proportion of two or three grains to the ounce of distilled water,) or of sulphate of zinc, in the proportion of four grains to the ounce of water. The occasional use of these injections after an impure coition, with strict temperance and quiet, will usually prevent the occurrence of the disease. These remedies neutralize the absorbed virus before it has time to impair the function of the membrane with which it is in contact, and thus its power to do injury is summarily destroyed.

There is also a certain and speedy cure for the *second* or *forming stage*. The symptoms of this stage, as we have seen, are a tingling or itching at the end of the urethra, with a slight redness, and a slightly increased secretion of mucus. The remedy for this stage, is a *saturated solution of nitrate of silver*, a small quantity of which is to be applied, by means of a small glass syringe, or by a small bit of sponge, to the urethra for an inch in extent. The solution should be delicately and rapidly applied, and a quantity used just sufficient to give the portion of the membrane touched, a *white* cast. This causes a smart but healthy medicinal inflammation which subsides in about 24 hours, leaving the structure cured. This course is strictly homœopathic, for we impress directly the tissue affected, produce a powerful *medicinal aggravation* of the symptoms, and overwhelm the disease by substituting temporarily, another inflammatory action. No unpleasant consequences ever result from the use of this remedy, when it is employed before the commencement of the *third* or *acute stage*. Our experience with this solution has been extensive, and we therefore confidently recommend it as a perfectly safe and sure remedy in this stage of the complaint.

During the *third* or *acute stage*, it is a question whether any remedies, either general or topical, can be employed with any material advantage, with the exception of the internal use of *aconite*, which may be given to shorten the inflammatory stage. This medicine is particulary applicable when febrile symptoms are present. Throughout this stage, the patient should be restricted to the most rigid vegetable or farinaceous diet, to cold water, and prohibited from taking much exercise. Ablutions with cold water, should be often employed, in order to keep the parts as free as possible from the irritating discharge. After the urgent symptoms have subsided under the use of *aconite*, and the other means we have just pointed out, and the *fourth* or *chronic stage* has commenced, we may resort to injections composed of one grain of sulphate of zinci to ℥ viii. of water. These injections, in order to be efficient, must be repeated every half-hour during the day, until the discharge ceases. It will be of no service to use this solution three or four times in the day, for the chief object is to wash out the urethra as fast as the matter forms, and thus prevent the constant reabsorption which would otherwise take place.

The principal reason why urethritis is so difficult to cure, when once fully established, is, that the matter itself being infectious, and liable to be constantly reabsorbed, thus operates as a continual exciting cause. If at any given instant the whole urethra could be restored to perfect health, a single drop of the morbid secretion which it had been pouring out, applied to the part, would be sufficient to re-excite the disease in all its violence. It is evident, then, that the discharge must be arrested abruptly by the remedy employed, or we must use our injections sufficiently often to dilute and remove the virus as fast as formed, *and at the same time to change the morbid action of the membrane to a healthy medicinal action.*

In regard to the plan of making an application to the urethra, of a medicine so powerful as to arrest the discharge suddenly, like the solution mentioned under our *second* head, it is attended in this stage of the affection with many dangers. The canal of the urethra is generally affected so high up as to render the certain application of this or any other sufficiently powerful solution entirely impracticable.

But the other method, to which we have alluded, is one of entire feasibility and safety, and is for the most part attended with success, when the discharge is entirely unconnected with a stricture. It is proper to observe that, in all cases, the patient should urinate previous to the use of injections. Another injection which we have sometimes used with marked success in this stage, is a mixture of *calomel* and *olive oil*, in the proportion of a drachm to the ounce, once or twice a day, until the cessation of the diseased action.

If, however, notwithstanding the thorough and persevering employment of the *zinc* solution and the mixture of *calomel* and *oil*, the discharge still continues, recourse should be had to the introduction of bougies, either plain or smeared with a cerate containing a sufficient quantity of pulverized *nitrate of silver*. These should be carefully introduced two or three times a week, until we have stimulated the diseased membrane to a natural and healthy action.

The above plan of treatment, we believe to be more efficient, safe, and consonant with the true principle of cure, than any other which has yet been promulgated: yet, we do not claim for it infallibility. We can only assure our readers that we have thoroughly tested every theory and process which has been proposed by either school, and that after all of this practical experience, we have presented them with what we deem the best method of treatment in this disgusting malady.

For the information of those who desire to make use of internal remedies either alone or in combination with injections, we name the following medicines as the best with which we are at present acquainted: *cannabis, cantharides, tussilago pertus., cubebæ, mercurius sol., petroselinum, aconite, acid nit., sepia, terebinth., copaibæ, pulsatilla, nux vomica, sulphur, ferrum.*

The remedies which should be consulted in *irritable bladder*, are, *cantharides, cannabis, lycopodium, mercu-*

rius, uva ursa, terebinthina, pulsatilla, copaibæ, cubebæ, sulphur, iodine, and *camphor*.

Inflammation of the testicles and epydidimis :—

Our first care in this complaint, should be to suspend the inflamed organ by means of a suitable apparatus, in such a manner as to afford complete support in all positions, and thus prevent the enlarged gland from dragging upon the spermatic chord. The recumbent posture should be strictly enjoined, and we should have constantly applied to the parts, cloths wet with cold water. As soon as the cloths are warmed by contact with the inflamed testicle, they should be again dipped and reapplied until the heat and inflammation have disappeared.

If the disease has arisen from sudden suppression of urethritis, or from the use of powerful injections during the *acute stage*, we may give *mercurius, aconite, nux vomica, spongia, clematis*, or *iodine*.

When it has been caused by the injudicious introduction of bougies, *arnica, aconite*, and *pulsatilla*, will be found applicable.

In cases where the inflammation has degenerated into a *chronic induration of the testicles*, our best remedies are, *aurum, acid nitric, rhododendron, sulphur, mercurius, spigelia, iodine*, and *cicuta*.

SECTION IX.

SYPHILIS.

Much discussion has taken place respecting the first introduction of this disease into Europe. Some maintain that the followers of Columbus brought it with them from America ; others that it was communicated by the Spaniards to the French, during the siege of Naples, by Charles VIII., in 1495. It appears, however, that occasional allusion is made in different parts of the scriptures, to a disease of the sexual organs, capable of being propagated by coition, contact, &c. In Leviticus, Moses mentions such an affection, and speaks of those afflicted as being polluted and unfit to associate with the healthy. David also describes one variety of syphilis in the thirty-fourth psalm. Heroditus, too, speaks of an affection of the sexual organs which the Scythians contracted from the women with whom they had connection, after profaning the temple of Venus Urania. Later writers, Salicetus, Gordoneus, and Valereus, who flourished about the year 1250, allude to an infectious disorder of the genitals, proceeding from the copulation of men with unclean prostitutes. Many reputable authors have entertained the opinion that the ancient leprosy was nothing more than syphilis, rendered severe by exposure, hardship, insufficient nourishment, and improper medical treatment. But an objection has been urged against this view, from the supposition that leprosy could be communicated by contact with an infected person,—by drinking from the same cup, by inhaling his breath, or even sitting at the same table with him. It is no less true that syphilis occasionally presents a character equally virulent and diffusible. During a great portion of the sixteenth century, it was so contagious in some parts of Europe, that it was communicated by lying in the same bed, by the clothes, gloves, money, or breath of the patient. A variety of syphilis also prevailed in Canada some years ago, of so virulent a nature, that it was communicated by the breath, and by contact.

We fully concur with Dr. Thompson, who "thinks it probable that the disease has existed, more or less, and under different grades of severity, in all ages, and that it has been thousands of times generated *de novo* by impure sexual intercourse."

The causes which may have conduced to vary its character at different periods, are numerous; and we suggest the following as a few of them.

It has been observed that exposure of the body to a cold, humid atmosphere, excessive fatigue, changes of diet and of climate, unwholesome food and neglect of cleanliness, favour the rapid progress and destructiveness of the malady; while a dry, warm and equable temperature, cleanliness, nutritious food, and comfortable lodgings, are circumstances which conduce to render it comparatively mild. These facts go far to explain the reason of its great violence amongst those ancient tribes who were accustomed to dwell in tents, and to move about from place to place; and who were so negligent in their habits of living, their food and their persons, that Moses deemed it necessary to make rigid laws in regard to the selection of food and the habit of personal ablutions. When we reflect that persons who were supposed to be leprous, were immediately driven out of the camp — away from all intercourse with the healthy—and thus forced to undergo every exposure in respect to raiment, shelter and food, we cannot be surprised that the disease, supposing it to have been syphilis, should so often have assumed a frightful aspect.

Its violence during the siege of Naples in 1495, may also be explained, when we bear in mind the forced marches, the changes of climate and of diet, and the constant excitement and fatigue to which the soldiers were exposed. The same severity marked its prevalence in the British army in Portugal, while the natives themselves were but slightly affected, although exposed to similar contamination.

One of our army surgeons recently informed me that the same difficulty was experienced among our soldiers during the Mexican campaign in 1847 and 1848: they contracted the disorder, while the Mexicans experienced but slight inconvenience, although exposed to the same virus. The argument also holds good with respect to sailors who are so constantly subjected to the vicissitudes of temperature, the noxious air of vessels, and the stale, salt regimen which is used at sea.

May it not, then, be fairly inferred, that whatever causes impair the forces of the organism, serve also to render it less able to resist the deleterious influence of the syphilitic poison?

In regard to the doctrine of Hahnemann respecting the identity of syphilis and sycosis, we agree with Hartmann, that the mass of evidence upon the subject renders it almost conclusive that the two diseases are distinct in their nature. The origin of each is in a specific morbid poison capable of impressing the organism in a distinct and peculiar manner.

Diagnosis.—There are unquestionably a great variety of ulcers which make their appearance upon the genitals after impure connections, which are not syphilitic, and which will heal over without causing constitutional symptoms, simply by the aid of mild dressings. The true syphilitic chancre is now of rare occurrence, but the great majority of those intractable ulcers which are looked upon as real venereal chancres, are nothing more, primarily, than simple non-infectious sores, which have been converted into an unhealthy condition by the use of mercury. Who can doubt this fact when he contemplates the dreadful effects which a course of mercury often produces on the healthy organism? Who could be tempted, in health, to take the enormous quantities of this drug which are deemed necessary for the cure of syphilis? Let the provings of it—let the horrible consequences which its accidental absorption sometimes occasions upon the surface,—in the mucous membranes, —the bones,—the glands and the nervous system, answer. For our part, we would prefer the foul syphilitic poison itself, rather than the uncontrollable ravages of such an enemy as mercury, in allopathic administrations, is admitted to be by the fair-minded of those even who most earnestly defend its use.

In order to be fully convinced that many of the effects of *mercury* are improperly attributed to the action of the syphilitic virus, it is only necessary to regard carefully the symptoms which are constantly presented to our observation in what are called venereal affections, and to notice the opinions of many of the most eminent medical observers.

Thus, Sir Astley Cooper,* in his lectures, used to observe, "do not think that it is a rare occurrence for the penis to be destroyed by *mercury;* no, a chancre that has remained weeks in a healthy state, shall become irritable, and, by maltreatment, by the injudicious and improper use of *mercury*, shall slough, and end in the destruction of the penis; this is not a rare case, and is attributed to the venereal disease, but in reality is an effect of the improper use of *mercury*." The great Hahnemann, in his remarks upon syphilis and sycosis, constantly alludes to the

*Castle's Manual of Surg., p. 280.

pernicious results of the abuse of this drug in the hands of the allopathist.

There can be no question that those dreadful mutilations of the penis, of the nose, the palate, the eyes, of the surface of the body, and the nodes and caries of the bones, which we occasionally observe, are all effects of *mercury* and not of *syphilis;* and it is in the highest degree probable that the immunity enjoyed by the Portuguese, the Mexicans, and certain other nations, from the severe forms of this malady, is attributable solely to the fact that they use no mercury in its treatment.

Chancre.—The primary chancre usually presents itself on some part of the genital organs, in from three to seven days after contamination, in the form of a darkish red pimple, attended with slight itching, and surrounded with an erysipelatous blush. In a short time matter forms in the centre of the pimple, and an excavated ulcer, with a yellowish surface, hard and ragged edges, and an indurated base, makes its appearance, marking the sore as a true chancre. The most common seat of primary chancre is on the inside of the foreskin and the corona glandis, but it occasionally occurs on the glands and the external parts of the genitals.

Many varieties of venereal chancre have been described by authors, as the *simple*, the *indolent*, the *irritable*, the *sloughing*, the *indurated*, the *phagedenic* of Carmichael, the *superficial* of Mr. Evans, the *Hunterian*, &c.; but as these diversities in the appearance of the chancre are not owing to any difference in the character of the virus, but to the condition of the patient as regards constitution, temperament, and mode of life, at the period of contamination, we should abstain from making those minute classifications which some writers have attempted.

The circumstances which may operate to modify the character and appearance of a simple chancre, or which may conduce to develop primarily an intractable and destructive one, are numerous.

Individuals whose constitutions have been impaired by abuse of stimulants, undue exposure, hardship and fatigue, and insufficient nourishment, are liable to be attacked from the first with that variety which is denominated the *indurated sloughing chancre.*

Those whose systems have been loaded with mercury, and enfeebled by previous disease, are peculiarly subject to that description which is termed *irritable* and *sloughing*. Persons who go from temperate to tropical climates, are especially in danger of the *phagedenic* variety. Scrofula and scurvy also predispose the system to this form of it.

The *simple* chancre is by far the most common, particularly in temperate latitudes, and usually occurs to individuals of a sound constitution. Some have supposed the cause of this variety to consist in "gonorrhœal matter, and other morbid vaginal secretions," brought in contact with the penis during coition ; but of this there is no proof. The simple ulcer very often becomes converted into an *irritable*, *sloughing*, or *erysipelatous* one, by some excess or imprudence which impairs the vigour of the body, or by the abuse of mercury. On the other hand, so long as the constitution remains sound and unimpaired, resistance is offered to the action of the virus, and the secondary impression which it makes will be very slight, and in some instances imperceptible. It is in cases of this description that we sometimes witness spontaneous cures of what was originally true syphilitic contamination.

The most certain marks of a true syphilitic chancre are, the excavated surface, the hard, ragged edges, and the indurated base. These appearances, taken in connection with the previous history of the case, will generally enable us to decide with sufficient certainty respecting the character of the sore ; but where any doubt exists, we would most strongly commend the practice discovered and successfully adopted by Ricord of Paris, of inoculating a sound part with the matter from the suspected ulcer. In case a second chancre is produced by this operation, there will no longer remain a question in regard to the true nature of the malady.

After the syphilitic poison has passed from the chancre through the absorbent glands of the groin, into the blood, it possesses a specific affinity for only three parts of the body, viz., "the mucous membrane of the throat and nose; the skin, or surface of the body; and the bones, with their periosteal coverings."* Thus, it will be remarked, that the *internal* organs are never impressed by this virus; and this fact should induce the allopath to pause before he loads the system with a poison which spares scarcely a single structure during its operation.

The secondary, or specific effects of the syphilitic virus, after its entrance into the blood, are:

First. Upon the mucous membrane of the mouth and throat, which becomes red and inflamed, and covered in some parts with pimples, which soon degenerate into ulcers, resembling in many respects the primary simple chancre. These ulcerations extend into the nostrils, and sometimes even into the larynx itself, giving rise to loss of voice, severe cough, violent constitutional disturbance, and death. In cases which have been improperly treated, the bony palate and the nasal bones become affected, and exfoliate, and thus cause those disgusting mutilations of the nose and face which so often stare the old school physician in the face.

Second. Another part of the body acted on by the absorbed virus is the skin. Its manifestations in this case are, *slightly elevated copper-coloured eruptions* of different sizes, attended with uneasy or itching sensations, sometimes covered with a kind of scurf or scale, or, in other instances, with incrustations and ulcerations. These eruptions make their appearance on the face, head, breast, palms of the hands, and arms. Eruptions which are called *tubercular*, often appear on the scalp, the eyebrows, the breast, back, and arms, and ultimately form very troublesome ulcers. In healthy subjects these secondary eruptions are not very troublesome, being simply copper-coloured blotches, covered with a thin scurf; but in irritable and impaired constitutions they often assume the character of foul and sloughing ulcers. The particular variety of these secondary eruptions will be

* Sir A. Cooper's Lectures.

determined by the peculiarities of constitution in each individual case, and not from any original difference in the virus itself.

Third. Another, and the last portion of the organism capable of being impressed by the absorbed venereal poison, is the osseous structure, with its periosteal covering. The morbid inflammation in the first instance seizes upon the periosteum, causing severe nocturnal pains, and some tumefaction in the affected region. If the malady continues to increase, an osseous deposit will be formed between the periosteum and the bone, constituting what is termed the *venereal node.* This node, in its early stages, does not usually give rise to much inflammation of the surrounding skin, nor is it attended with a great amount of pain, but after it has existed for a considerable time, and particularly if the patient has been drugged with mercurial preparations, it becomes quite painful, especially during the night. The ordinary location of venereal nodes is on the anterior portion of the tibia, or on the surface of the cranial bones.

We believe that the above-enumerated symptoms constitute all of the legitimate effects resulting from the action of the absorbed syphilitic virus. The great variety of eruptions and ulcerations described by Hartmann and others, are attributable to other causes, operating either by themselves, or in conjunction with the venereal poison. It is of vast importance in affections of this description, to distinguish with all possible accuracy between the syphilitic action and that of mercury, scrofula, and other causes. Farther on we shall endeavour to make this distinction as clear as possible.

Bubo.—Another primary manifestation of syphilis consists in an enlargement of one or more of the absorbent glands of the groin, termed *bubo.* This enlargement usually succeeds the chancre, and is caused by the absorption of the virus of the latter. It is rare in real syphilis that more than one gland in each groin becomes affected with the virus, although some of the other glands now and then become slightly swollen from sympathy. The swelling ordinarily partakes of an inflammatory character, and if not opposed by appropriate remedies, runs on to suppuration, and sometimes to sloughing.

The disease has been supposed to be purely local, until after the swelling in the groin has proceeded to the suppurative stage; but this is evidently erroneous, from the fact that secondary symptoms not unfrequently occur, without there having been any previous enlargement of the gland in the groin.

Bubo sometimes makes its appearance without the previous existence of a chancre, but such instances are by no means common. Swellings of a non-venereal character may likewise occur in the groin from a strain, or from too great violence during the indulgence of sexual passion. But as chancre for the most part precedes the bubo, there will rarely occur any difficulty in our diagnosis.

Therapeutics.—Hahnemann, Gross, Hartmann, Hunter, Abernethy, and many other distinguished members of the profession, entertained the opinion that the constitutional symptoms of syphilis are always progressive, and never disappear, unless opposed by medicine; but the fact is now completely established, not only that *mercury* is not necessary for the cure of either the primary or secondary symptoms, but that they often terminate in a spontaneous cure *without any medicine.* We are assured by Dr. Fergusson and other surgeons who have observed the disease in Portugal, that the natives cure themselves permanently of the primary symptoms by simple topical applications; and of the secondary effects, by decoctions of sarsaparilla and sudorifics. They remark, that "the virulence of the disease has there been so much mitigated, that, after running a certain course (commonly a mild one) through the respective order of parts, according to the known laws of its progress, *it exhausts itself, and ceases spontaneously.*"—(*Med. and Chir. Trans.*, vol. iv. pp. 2–5). This is still further corroborated by the numerous cures of the primary and constitutional symptoms recorded by Messrs. Rose, Dease, Hennen, Guthrie, Good, and Whympor, without mercury, or any other means than simple dressings. In the cases which they describe, *no caries of the bones* occurred, as is so commonly observed when mercury is used, " and in no instance was there that uniform progress, with unrelenting fury, from one order of symptoms, and parts affected, to another, which is considered as an essential characteristic of true syphilis."—(*Med. and Chir. Trans.*, vol. viii., p. 422).

Hahnemann, and most of his disciples, as well as Hunter and other eminent allopathists, entertained an opinion that the chancre is simply the *vicarious* symptom of the *internal* disease, and that by removing this ulcer by *external applications*, "the disease is forced to embody itself externally, in the more troublesome and speedily suppurating bubo. And after this, too, has been removed, as is foolishly done, by external treatment, the disease is forced to manifest itself throughout the organism with all the secondary symptoms of a fully developed syphilis. This *unavoidable* development of the internal syphilitic disease generally takes place after the lapse of two or three months."—(*Hahnemann's Chronic Diseases*, p. 116).

We speak advisedly when we pronounce this last assumption altogether erroneous; for we have repeatedly seen true venereal chancres cured by topical treatment alone, while the patients have remained entirely free from any secondary manifestations for years afterwards. When a student of medicine, the author passed some time at the United States Marine Hospital, Chelsea, then under the superintendence of the able and accomplished Dr. Stedman. In this institution, the internal use of mercury had been dispensed with in the cure of syphilis, for several years previous to my entrance; and I ascertained that it was a very rare occurrence to observe secondary symptoms in those who had been cured at this hospital, although patients were constantly returning with other complaints, who had been cured of chancre years previous. The treatment chiefly relied on consisted of topical applications of a mild and simple character, the internal use of decoctions of sarsaparilla, and a rigid regimen. The ordinary period for the cure of primary chancre, was from three to four weeks; and for bubo, from six to eight weeks.

So long as a chancre exists, the matter generated in the contaminated part continues to be re-absorbed, and thus to supply new fuel to the mass of the blood; it is therefore important to change the morbid action of the ulcer, and heal it up as soon as possible. The matter formed in ulcers of the mucous membrane of the throat, which have arisen from the constitutional effects of syphilis, is also capable of propagating the disease by contact with abraded surfaces, or by being directly re-absorbed into the blood. There is reason to believe, therefore, if all these ulcers be speedily healed by topical treatment, so that the blood shall only contain a given quantity of the virus, this limited amount will gradually become diluted, by the constant addition of new and healthy blood, and by its frequent circulation through the lungs, so that its power to impress the structures is finally lost, and the parts which have already been affected, gradually recover their health and tone.

In advocating the practice of topical applications, however, we by no means wish to be understood as placing entire reliance upon them, to the exclusion of internal remedies. We only assert that local applications are capable of effecting speedy cures of chancres, thus of destroying these sources of contamination, and placing the blood in the most favourable condition to be purified by the inspired oxygen, by the newly formed blood, and by remedial agents. A morbid action is set up in the chancre, which causes it to generate matter of a virulent quality. This is evident from the fact that the matter of buboes and other venereal abscesses, as well as the blood of syphilitic persons, is incapable of causing contamination in the healthy. We repeat, then, heal the chancres as soon as possible, by destroying their *morbid* action, with some local application which shall induce a *healthy medicinal* action, and we have already done much towards abridging the power of the disease. Our admirable specifics will, then, readily accomplish what remains to be done in perfecting a cure.

The remedial agents which we have found most useful in the management of syphilis are, (*topical,*) *nit. argenti., acid nit., zinc chlorid., hydrg., præcip., rub. creosote,* and (*internal,*) the preparations of *mercury, aurum mur., thuya, acid nit., sulphur, hepar sulph.. sarsaparilla, silicea, mezereum, hyd. potassæ.*

In the treatment of chancre, our attention should be directed in the first instance to the cauterization of the sore, in order to change as speedily as possible the morbid action. For this purpose, either of the first named medicines may be employed, although in most cases we prefer the nitrate of silver in substance. After a healthy action has been excited in the ulcer, by these applications, lotions of simple water may be employed until the cure is established. It will be well to keep a dossil of lint moistened with water constantly upon the ulcer. This course, in conjunction with the remedies advised below, will generally effect speedy and permanent restoration.

Of the internal remedies, *mercury* is the most important. By comparing the pure effects of the different preparations of this drug upon the healthy human organization, with the constitutional effects of the syphilitic virus, it will be observed that the former are capable of causing all the symptoms of the latter, as well as many others which are peculiar to the drug. According to *Pereira*, the following are the effects of mercury in large doses:

First. On the mucous membrane of the nose and throat: *ulcerations* of the mouth, gums, throat, tonsils, and nose, which are often followed by extensive *sloughing* of the parts.

Second. On the skin or surface of the body: *eczema mercuriale, erythema mercuriale, lepra mercurialis, erysipelas mercuriale, spilosis mercurialis, miliaria mercurialis,* and other cutaneous eruptions which bear a close resemblance to *herpes, impetigo, psydrasia,* and the copper-coloured eruptions of syphilis.

Third. On the bones and their periosteal coverings: "inflammation of the bones or periosteum, and the consequent production of nodes (*symphoresis periostei mercurialis.*")

By the above it will be seen that all of those parts capable of being impressed by the venereal virus, are also acted on by mercury. That the operation of the latter is often more violent and destructive than the former, will not at this day be questioned.

But in addition to the symptoms just enumerated, mercury, in large doses, causes almost innumerable other symptoms, which have no bearing upon the subject of this chapter, except as indicating its danger in the hands of allopathists.

We have quoted above from an eminent allopathic writer, in order that every reader may be convinced of the analogy between the effects of the venereal poison and of mercury, upon the human constitution, and to show the difficulty of distinguishing between syphilitic and mercurial symptoms, in the old school mode of practice.

For an accurate and complete description of the pure effects of mercury upon the healthy organism, we refer to the provings of Hahnemann and other homœopathists.

Hahnemann preferred the fluid quicksilver, carried up to the decilionth degree, over all other preparations, in the treatment of both primary and secondary syphilis.

For the cure of primary chancre, Hartmann recommends the first or third trituration of *mercurius sol.*, in doses of one grain, night and morning. If no improvement occurs within the first eight days, he gives a lower trituration, or, if necessary, a low trituration of *merc. præcip. rub.*, in doses of one-sixth of a grain, two or three times a day. In the *Hunterian*, *phagedenic*, and the *elevated indurated* chancres, Hartmann employs the *red precipitate*, in its lower attenuations, from the first.

Dr. C. Müller, of Leipsic, is also most decidedly in favour of the *red precipitate* or the *hydr. sulph. rub.*, in the treatment of syphilitic chancres and buboes, in whatever state they may present themselves. He advises a grain of the first trituration, to be given twice a day until the ulcers have nearly healed. For painful nodes and other syphilitic affections of the bones, *hydriodate* of *potash* is advised.

I have also made use of the *precipitate* at the third attenuation, with marked advantage, in uncomplicated syphilis. I have known the best results, also, from the *hydr. mur. cor.*, in both the primary and secondary forms of the malady. For the cure of troublesome secondary symptoms, in the forms of cutaneous eruptions, glandular enlargements, and nodes, the *protiodide* of *mercury* has extraordinary power. Speedy cures have been effected by it after the other mercurial preparations had failed. It may be used at the third attenuation, in doses of a grain, twice a day, until the eruptions disappear.

When syphilis is complicated by psora, scrofula, or any other chronic disease, suitable remedies should be alternated with the mercurials.

Muriate of gold ranks next in importance to *mercury*, as a remedy in secondary syphilis. The late Dr. Taft, of New Orleans, employed it in secondary ulcers and eruptions which would not yield to *mercury*, with the most gratifying results. In syphilitic eruptions of long standing, we have often administered it with entire success. The second or third trituration may be employed, in half grain doses, night and morning, as long as necessary.

Nitric acid will be serviceable in many cases of ill conditioned chancres, which seem to withstand the curative force of mercury. It is also of great value in protracted secondary cases, accompanied with emaciation, debility, caries of the bones, unhealthy ulcers upon the surface, and great derangement of the nervous system. If these symptoms have been aggravated by abuse of mercurials, the indication is still stronger for the acid. The first, second and third dilutions are to be preferred in these cases, a dose to be given twice daily until the disease yields.

Sulphur, *hepar sulph.*, and *hydr. sulph. rub.*, are the proper specifics when the chancre occurs in psoric constitutions. As a general rule, the two first should be alternated with some mercurial preparation.

Hyd. potassæ is eminently worthy of consideration in the indolent glandular swellings which sometimes originate from a combination of syphilis and scrofula. It is also an efficient medicine in the treatment of venereal nodes.

Silicea, *mezereum* and *sarsaparilla* are often valuable auxiliaries in syphilis complicated with scrofula. These medicines should also be given in alternation with some other suitable specific.

In conclusion, we call attention to the following reliable mark of cure, alluded to by Hahnemann in his *Chronic Diseases:* "So long as the original spot upon which the chancre had been developed, exhibits a reddish morbid-looking, red, or bluish scar, we may be sure that the internal disease is not completely cured; whereas, if the chancre has been removed by the internal remedy, the original spot of the chancre can no longer be traced, on account of that spot being covered by as healthy-coloured a skin as the rest of the body."

SECTION X.

LEUCORRHŒA.—FLUOR ALBUS.—WHITES.

Diagnosis.—This disease is characterized by a discharge, from the utero-vaginal structure, of a mucous or purulent character, of a white, yellow, or greenish colour, either thin and watery, or of the consistence of starch or gelatine. This discharge, in contradistinction to that of *gonorrhœa*, arises from a benignant morbid action, and is *non-contagious*. The assertion of Hartmann, respecting the identity of gonorrhœal and leucorrhœal inflammations—the difference, in his view, consisting only in the *location* of the disease—is evidently erroneous. This author defines gonorrhœa to consist of an inflammation of the female urethra, and leucorrhœa of a similar inflammation of the mucous membrane of the vagina or uterus. The opinion falls to the ground when we reflect that the latter disease not unfrequently extends to the urethral mucous membrane, giving rise to ardor urinæ, burning pain on passing water, heat, fulness, and swelling of the part, and a purulent discharge, which is *non-contagious.* Leucorrhœal inflammation always originates from causes which have impaired the healthy tone of the mucous membrane; gonorrhœal inflammation, on the other hand, may arise from the *simple contact* of a drop of gonorrhœal matter with the most sound and healthy membrane. The former is the result of an ordinary inflammation, which is analogous in its character to that of catarrh and chronic bronchitis: the latter proceeds only from the application of a specific infectious matter, which developes a particular morbid inflammation, and a contagious purulent secretion.

The character of the discharge and of the symptoms, will depend upon the location of the disease, its causes, and the amount of inflammation present. Inflammation of the *cervix uteri*, for example, causes a discharge of "white mucus, and when the inflammation is intense, tinged with blood."—(*Hall.*) Acute vaginal or urethral inflammation gives rise to a purulent discharge of a yellow or greenish colour, sometimes tinged with blood. A more chronic affection of the same parts induces a thinner, more glairy, and muco-purulent secretion. *Scirrhus uteri* causes an ichorous, bloody and fœtid discharge. In chlorotics, with deranged menstruation, the secretion is thin, serous, acrid, and of a lightish or straw colour. The discharge which often accompanies pregnancy, is thick, glairy, and white or yellowish ; but in some instances after accouchement, more particularly in scrofulous and cachectic subjects, the matter is ichorous and highly irritating to the parts with which it comes in contact. In *polypi* of the uterus or vagina, the discharge is at first mucous, but when the tumours have attained some size, it becomes tinged with blood, and in some cases of this kind profuse hæmorrhages occur. The signs which denote the existence of these tumours, are, sense of weight and fulness in the uterus, dragging pains in the small of the back, bearing down pains, and turns of profuse hæmorrhage.

In light cases of leucorrhœa, the discharge is usually thin, glairy, transparent, and starchy; but when the disease is thoroughly seated, and the patient is of a delicate or cachectic habit, the fluid may be muco-purulent, serous, sanious, and of a white, yellow, or greenish colour.

As a general rule, the discharge is worse about the period of the monthly sickness, owing probably to the increased determination of blood to the parts during this natural phenomenon.

The diseases which are ordinarily accompanied by leucorrhœa are, amenorrhœa, chlorosis, polypus and scirrhus uteri, dysmenorrhœa, menorrhagia, prolapsus uteri, and chronic inflammations of the uterus, vagina or urethra.

When the affection is inveterate, and attended with

an abundant discharge, the whole system becomes injuriously affected: the face assumes a pale or sallow colour; the eyes are surrounded with dark or leaden-coloured circles; the functions of the stomach and bowels are impaired; the patient experiences a weary and dragging sensation in the left side; there are also dull pains in the back, loins, and abdomen; cold extremities; nausea; palpitation and dyspnœa after exercising; lassitude; debility; feeble pulse; loss of physical and mental energy; partial or total suppression of the menses; increase or diminution of the sexual propensity.

These are the symptoms to which protracted and severe attacks of leucorrhœa give rise; but the malady may exist for years, in a mild form, without the development of any of these consequences.

This disease is far more common in cities amongst the rich, indolent, luxurious, and dissipated, than in the country. Indeed, the small number of births, and the frequent miscarriages occurring in large towns, are attributable in a great measure to the very common prevalence of this weakness.

Leucorrhœa has been considered as one of the symptoms of *prolapsus uteri;* but we are of opinion that in very many instances, the latter is a *consequence*, rather than a cause of the former. This opinion derives support from the fact that fluor albus often exists for years before the signs of prolapsus manifest themselves: and it is probably from this circumstance that the tone of the uterus becomes impaired, and the muscles and ligaments gradually lose their strength and contractility.

Leucorrhœa occurs at all periods of life, but is most common after puberty, and previous to the "change of life," when so many causes are constantly conspiring to induce free determinations of blood to the utero-genital organs.

Causes.—The conditions which predispose to attacks of leucorrhœa, may be enumerated as follows: a lymphatic temperament; a scrofulous dyscrasia; general debility and relaxation of the muscular and membranous structures, whether from natural organization, or previous disease.

Amongst the more immediate causes may be mentioned, an inactive and luxurious mode of life; immoderate sexual indulgence; abortions; congestions and inflammations of the uterus and vagina; menstrual derangements; want of cleanliness; a humid atmosphere; scirrhus uteri; polypi and other abnormal growths in the uterus; metastases of rheumatism; herpes; hœmorrhoidal, catarrhal, and bronchial inflammations; the uterine debility and relaxation consequent on parturition, and too early exercise after confinement; neglect of mothers to exercise the office of nursing; and finally, according to Marshall Hall, *undue lactation.*

All of these causes doubtless exercise an influence in the production of fluor albus, but in the vast majority of cases the disease may be justly attributed to the combined operation of several of these influences, rather than to any single one. We may almost predict beforehand, that the child, born of parents who have always lived in compactly populous cities, and have indulged in their artificial habits, will sooner or later be afflicted with leucorrhœa. This is but one of the signs which indicate the gradual but sure progress of degeneration to which the luxurious and dissolute habits of large towns inevitably lead. In the first instance, indolence, stimulating drinks, overheated apartments, exciting theatrical exhibitions, romances, pictures, statuary, etc., all tend to divert the mind towards *sensual enjoyments.* Deprived in a great measure of those pure and sublime pictures which nature has so lavishly scattered throughout the country, to please the sight, to elevate the mind, and to ennoble and purify the whole being; and of the thousand sources of happiness which pertain to country life; they turn to artificial pleasures, and reap the fruits which are ever entailed by a violation of natural laws.

Is it strange then that fluor albus is so common in cities? that the degenerate offspring of these *artificial* human beings should grow up so puny, so weak, mentally and physically; so prone to disease, and so incapable of performing properly those functions for which nature has designed them? If any one doubts the inferences which these remarks suggest, let him but observe the families of the wealthy and luxurious, who have inhabited large cities for two or three generations, and he will doubt no longer.

Prognosis.—Leucorrhœa often leads to prolapsus uteri, amenorrhœa, menorrhagia, abortion, anasarca, hysteria, and general debility, but it very rarely terminates fatally. By impairing in a gradual manner the energies of the system, it predisposes it to take on serious disordered action from slight causes, and thus becomes indirectly an important morbid agent. When the complaint is recent, and occurs in females of a robust constitution, from some temporary congestion, difficult parturition, or mechanical injury, we may expect to remove it, by the aid of suitable remedies, in a short period; but if the patient be of a lymphatic temperament, of a delicate, lax and scrofulous constitution, and subject to irregular menstruation, the disease will most probably baffle our best curative efforts, and persist, with a greater or less degree of severity, during life. In individuals of this description, the most insignificant causes are capable of inciting and perpetuating the weakening discharge, so that, in many cases, it will prove a hopeless task to attempt to remove all the influences which exercise an injurious bearing upon the case. Even when the affection exists as a mere symptom of some other disease, it seldom subsides with the other symptoms, but is quite prone to degenerate into a chronic fluor albus.

Therapeutics.—There are several conditions which are absolutely essential to the successful treatment of "whites," the most important of which are, abundant active exercise in the open air; an avoidance of all excesses in venery, and in the pleasures of the table; a withdrawal of the thoughts and affections from exciting spectacles, from crowded balls and parties, from lascivious imaginings, from romances, and intrigues; and lastly, frequent daily ablutions, in order to ensure the most perfect cleanliness of the utero-genital organs.

The vast importance of this last point cannot be too strongly insisted upon, for without a rigid attention to cleanliness, all our efforts will prove futile. The morbid secretion is at best sufficiently irritating, but when it is permitted to accumulate and remain for a long time in contact with the mucous membrane, it becomes partially decomposed, fetid, and highly pernicious to the well-being of the parts. On this account, the constant and thorough use of local applications of tepid or cold water, as circumstances require, should be strictly enjoined. We may then carry out our remedial measures in all their details, with a reasonable prospect of success.

We call attention to the following remedies: *Calcarea carb.*, *sulphur*, *stannum*, *sepia*, *iodine*, *pulsatilla*, *alumina*, *lycopodium*, *phosphorus*, *cocculus*, *sabinæ*, *secale cor.*, *china*, *arnica*, *bovista*, *aconite*, *mercurius*, *nux vom.*, *silicea*, *psoricum*, *copaibæ*, *mezereum*, and *manganum.*

Calcarea carb. is suitable in chronic leucorrhœa, affecting weak, scrofulous and cachectic females, and particularly indicated when the menses are too frequent and too profuse. The discharge is milky, transparent, mucilaginous, starchy, unirritating, and accompanied with itching of the parts, especially the pudendum; also lassitude; depression of spirits; pains in the chest and back; cough; and general debility.

When the complaint arises from a scrofulous, or psoric taint, antipsorics, like *sulphur*, *stannum*, and *iodine*, will be required. The discharge in these cases is thin or yellowish, and highly irritating to the parts with which it comes in contact. The strength is also much impaired, and there are indications of pulmonary and scrofulous disorder, such as hectic fever; emaciation; loss of appetite; wandering pains in the chest; cough; profuse mucous or purulent expectoration; feeble and rapid pulse; night-sweats.

Sepia is suitable for females who are naturally delicate and sensitive, with clear and transparent complexions. The discharge is mucous, white, yellowish, or watery, mild or acrid in its nature, most abundant just before or just subsequent to the menses, and attended with itching and stitching pains in the genital organs.

Pulsatilla is an admirable remedy in leucorrhœa accompanying pregnancy. It is also useful when the disease occurs about the period of the monthly courses.

The discharge may be thin, acrid, and burning, or thick, white, and tenacious, like the white of eggs. Shifting flatulent pains in the abdomen still farther point to *pulsatilla*.

Alumina has proved successful in several varieties of fluor albus ; but is particularly indicated when the discharge is very profuse and acrid, most abundant during the day when walking, and previous to the menstrual periods, and attended with a burning and itching sensation in the genital organs and rectum.

Fluor albus brought on by masturbation, and occurring at intervals, with a milky, serous, ichorous, or reddish discharge, will be best covered by *lycopodium*, *phosphorus*, or *cocculus*. These remedies are suitable to lymphatic temperaments, to those who are highly sensitive to cold, and subject to catarrhal affections, and whose nervous systems have been morbidly excited.

Sabinæ and *secale cornutum* are proper in fluor albus depending upon weakness of the utero-vaginal structure ; also when arising from suppression of the menses ; from miscarriage ; from severe and protracted labours ; polypi, and prolapsus uteri. The discharge is attended with itching of the pudendum. and inordinate sexual propensity.

China will serve our purpose when the complaint originates from excessive loss of blood, or other animal fluids, extreme debility from fevers, acute inflammations, abuse of drugs, insufficient nutriment, and respiration of foul air.

Bovista is applicable in fluor albus occurring *after* the catamenia, with discharge of a thick, glairy, and tenacious matter, of a yellow or greenish colour, and highly corrosive.

Arnica is indispensable in leucorrhœa originating from mechanical injuries during accouchement, from polypi, hydatids, and other morbid growths in the uterus or vagina, prolapsus uteri, and undue mechanical pressure from without.

Aconite corresponds to plethoric and sanguine constitutions, and to females who are subject to congestions and hæmorrhages from different organs. The discharge is purulent, yellow or greenish, and attended with ardor urinæ, heat, pain, and fulness in the genital organs, quick and full pulse, hot skin, and other febrile symptoms.

When there is reason to suspect that the discharge is from a syphilitic origin, whether it be mucous, watery, or purulent, mild or corrosive, *mercurius* is our best remedy.

Nux vom. is recommended when the disease arises from irregular menstruation, abuse of stimulants, rich and indigestible food, with a very profuse sanguineous or yellowish and fetid mucous discharge, and attended with cramplike pains in the abdomen, constipation, sinking at the stomach, and palpitation of the heart.

Cases may occur which will require the use of *silicea, psoricum, copaibæ, mezereum, manganum, nitric acid,* to which the reader is referred.

Administration.—We advise the employment of the first, second, and third attenuations, the dose to be repeated once in twenty-four hours until primary or secondary medicinal symptoms appear, when we may await the result for some days, or so long as the amendment continues. When the symptoms become stationary, we may again resort to the remedy.

SECTION XI.

AMENORRHŒA.

General description.—Many of the symptoms of this complaint bear a close resemblance to those of chlorosis, and it is on this account, probably, that some authors have confounded the two maladies. As retention or suppression of the menses is a very common and prominent symptom of chlorosis, it is not surprising that it has been deemed a *cause* of chlorotic symptoms, rather than as a mere *symptom.* But the fallacy of this doctrine will be evident, when we reflect that chlorosis occurs in males, in young children, and in females whose catamenial functions are regular through the whole course of the disease.

Two kinds of menstrual irregularity are generally included under the above head: first, *retention* of the catamenial flux beyond the natural period, from constitutional causes or mechanical obstruction; and second, partial or total *suppression* of already established courses, from phthisis, chronic hepatitis, general debility, chlorosis, fevers, and exposure to cold and dampness.

It is not improbable that the same causes which contribute to the development of chlorosis, also operate to prevent the usual menstrual flux at the period of puberty, and thus to establish one variety of *amenorrhœa.* Natural delicacy of constitution, a highly impressible nervous system, and a lymphatic temperament, are general conditions which precede and accompany both maladies, although amenorrhœa sometimes occurs in the most robust females.

The revolution which nature causes in the female organism at the period of puberty, ought always to become manifest in the menstrual flux; but the causes which often operate to retard it, and thus to thwart the kind efforts of nature, are numerous and diversified.

Singular phenomena are sometimes observed at the period of puberty in relation to this periodical evacuation; for, in the place of the usual uterine secretion, fluxes now and then take place from the top of the head, the ends of the fingers, the soles of the feet, the stomach, intestines, nose, and other parts of the body, and apparently assuming the place of the monthly periods. Occasionally the supplementary secretion occurs in the form of ulcers, enlargement and irritation of certain veins, and eruptions.

The menstrual discharge varies much in its quantity and character. In hot climates, puberty arrives earlier, and the discharge is more abundant, than in temperate latitudes.

When the discharge comes on at the proper period, but is deficient in quantity, or is composed of serum, mucus, or pus, other parts of the economy suffer, as by pains in the back, pelvis, limbs, and head, until the period has passed, after which the sufferings abate until the succeeding epoch, and are then renewed. This deficient secretion may continue for months and even years, without giving rise to any structural lesion, or any other symptoms than those enumerated, when some new circumstance, like marriage, a sea-voyage, or change of climate, may restore the function to its natural condition.

Puberty, with its usual accompaniment, the menstrual flux, does not occur in cold regions until the age of fifteen or sixteen years, while in tropical countries, it arrives at the age of eight, nine, and ten years. Frank* records cases where the courses appeared in children of one, three, and four years. This physician also treated, at Pavia, a woman who had given birth to three children without ever having had a menstrual or lochial discharge. Many cases of this kind are mentioned by other writers, who also allude to the masculine organization and characteristics of these women, such as firmness of muscle, harshness of voice, and smallness of the breasts.

From these facts we infer with Frank and others, that the menstrual function is not absolutely essential to the occurrence of conception, and that a woman may go through her whole term of pregnancy, and finally give birth to a healthy child, without any development whatever of the catamenial function.

Frank, in his Practice of Medicine, expresses the same opinion: "Nous concluons de ces observations que l'apparition des menstrues est, à la vérité, un des principaux signes qui annoncent le dévelopment de l'organe utérin et l'abord du sang dans ses vaisseaux, mais que la conception et la nutrition du fœtus peuvent également s'opérer, quoique cette fonction périodique ne soit pas encore établie; que la fécondité depend d'une autre cause, d'un principe analogue à celui dont elle dérive chez les femelles des animaux; que la nature a soumis en général toutes les femmes bien organisées au tribut menstruel, mais qu'elle ne l'exige pas toujours avec la même rigueur sous peine de stérilité."

In regard to the natural duration of the catamenial discharge, nothing definite can be advanced, since so much depends upon the constitution, the climate, and the habits of life; but the average duration is about three or four days.

Diagnosis.—As the period approaches when the *girl*

* Traité de Med. Practique, vol. ii., p. 253.

is to become a *woman*, new ideas, new thoughts, and new desires take possession of her mind. Instead of amusing herself with her doll, she prefers to enjoy, although with much coyness and timidity, the society of an attractive young friend of the other sex; instead of the romping freedom of the child, we now observe the retiring manners and the burning blushes of the maiden. Her physical developments, also, become more symmetrical, perfect, and pleasing to the eye, and she looks forward into the dim vista of life with deeper interest, higher aspirations, and a more proper appreciation of the responsible duties she may be called upon to fulfil.

If, in conjunction with these physical and moral changes, the catamenial discharge makes its appearance naturally and regularly, the girl retains her health and vigour; but if the period passes by without the usual development of the monthly tribute, we are presented with the following symptoms of

RETENTION OF THE MENSES.

Pale, waxlike, or sullen and sickly countenance; furred tongue, and foul breath in the morning; variable and sometimes morbid appetite; nausea, general debility, lassitude, and sense of fatigue; pains in the small of the back, pelvis, abdomen, head, side, and limbs; disinclination to mental or physical exertion; coldness of the feet; constipation; leucorrhœa; depression of spirits; sad and weeping mood; distress in the stomach after eating; distention of the abdomen; faintness; palpitation of the heart after exercise; rapid pulse; headache; vertigo; roaring in the ears; nightly wakefulness; hysteric symptoms; peevishness and irritability; hæmorrhages from the nose, stomach, lungs, and rectum; supplementary discharges from certain parts of the body.

SUPPRESSION OF THE MENSES,

May arise from a natural cause, like pregnancy, or from general debility resulting from excessive loss of blood, chronic and acute diseases, inordinate mucus, purulent and seminal discharges, polypi, venereal excesses, constant and severe muscular exertion, and mechanical obstructions; or it may occur suddenly during the flux from violent emotions of the mind, exposure to cold and dampness, cold baths, or any other cause which abruptly shocks the system.

The symptoms which follow suppression are usually more acute and dangerous than those of retention of the courses. It is not uncommon for the former to induce serious hæmorrhages from the lungs and stomach, also inflammations and congestions of the brain, lungs, uterus, and liver; while in the latter, the symptoms arise so gradually, that the organism in some measure adapts itself to the morbid condition, and thus escapes the inflammatory and febrile attacks which are so common in suppression.

Suppression occurs in the most sound and robust constitutions, as well as in those that are weakly: *retention* but rarely happens in healthy and vigorous subjects, but follows usually as a consequence of original delicacy of constitution, or of some long standing chronic affection. The symptoms of the former are more violent than those of the latter, but upon the whole, less dangerous to life, and more readily controlled by medicines.

In cases where the monthly secretion takes place, but is retained in the uterus from some mechanical obstruction, the blood often preserves its fluidity and freshness for a long period. This is owing to the exclusion of the oxygen of the air, the presence of which is essential to the process of decomposition.

Causes.—Natural or acquired delicacy of constitution, combined with a lymphatic temperament, and a highly sensitive nervous system, is by far the most common cause of retarded menstruation. A certain amount of stamina, of physical and nervous energy, is essential to the healthy performance of the functions, and so long as the organism is without the proper supply of this force, all of the functions must be imperfectly executed.

Structural lesions which give rise to profuse purulent, mucous, or sanguineous discharges, operate both as causes of retention and suppression. In this class may be included, tuberculous ulcerations of the lungs, chronic bronchitis, abscesses of the liver, and lumbar abscess.

Other causes of retention, are, malformations of the uterine organs, or the vagina, like imperforate os tincæ, imperforate hymen, malorganization of the ovaries or fallopian tubes, unnatural growths in the uterus or vagina which oppose an obstruction to the passage of the menstrual secretion.

Dr. McIntosh divides the mechanical obstructions to the discharge of the menstrual fluid, into two classes, viz.: "those occasioned by cohesion of the sides of the vagina and labia, and an imperforate hymen, and those caused by an imperfect or imperforated state of the *os uteri* itself. All these cases are comparatively rare, but few men can have been in extensive practice for twenty years, without meeting with several, and therefore they require some notice in this place. In the first set of cases, in addition to the constitutional symptoms and local pain already mentioned, there is great fulness, distention, and a sense of weight in the passages, accompanied sometimes with severe pain, and a feeling of bursting; straining at stool and micturition, together with enlargement of the abdomen, which excites suspicion of pregnancy. The nature of the case can only be determined by examination, and can be relieved only *by the knife*.

"In the second set of cases, there is greater difficulty in detecting the state of parts, from the natural impediment to an examination which exists at the orifice of the vagina; but I may mention, at least as a curious coincidence, that in the only two cases of imperforated os uteri which have fallen within my observation, there was no hymen, and the passages easily admitted the introduction of two fingers." Dr. M. punctured the os uteri, in one of these cases, and afterwards dilated the passage with bougies, until the discharge found free exit, when all of the unpleasant symptoms subsided, and the patient was restored to perfect regularity and excellent health. The other patient, whose delicacy forbade the operation, gradually sank under her symptoms and died. I have met with one case of retention, from adhesion of the walls of the vagina. The patient was a healthy young married lady whose menstruations had been regular until she became pregnant, after which they ceased, and she advanced as usual until the fifth month, when she had the misfortune to miscarry. During the delivery of the fœtus, so much violence occurred to the parts, that inflammation and sloughing of the vagina followed, adhesions took place between the vaginal walls, and the passage became entirely closed to the escape of the menstrual fluid. The patient experienced for many months most severe pains in the pelvis, abdomen, back, and especially at the monthly periods; many severe constitutional symptoms set in, and she became reduced to a very low state of health. A free incision through the cicatrix, gave vent to a large quantity of fluid blood, exhibiting but slight signs of decomposition, and the patient speedily regained her health.

The most harmless cause of suppression, is that which arises from pregnancy. But although this is a *natural* cause, its constitutional effects are manifested in the form of frequent nausea, morning sickness, ptyalism, &c. These symptoms, although quite troublesome and annoying to the patient, serve the important purpose of guarding the brain, lungs, and other vital parts, from dangerous inflammations and congestions.

One of the most notable causes of suppression during the flow of the courses, is abrupt exposure to cold. This obstruction is apt to arise in going suddenly from a warm room after exercise, and when the pores are open, into the cold air. It is also caused by plunging the limbs or body into cold water during the period. Insufficient clothing and thin shoes may also be mentioned as common causes.

Violent emotions of the mind, vehement anger, terror, sudden joy, intense grief, revolting sights, and electric shocks, may likewise be reckoned as frequent causes of obstruction or suppression of menses during the period.

It has been asserted that severe physical exertion often induces suppression, and the fact that habitual dancers are subject to but slight catamenial discharges, has been adduced as a proof of the assertion. We are inclined to credit this statement, from reflecting that operatives who labour long and hard, have but a very slight seminal secretion, and consequently but little inclination for sexual enjoyment; while he who enjoys his *otium cum dignitate*, abounds in this secretion, and experiences frequent amorous desires. The same result may happen to females, with reference to their monthly secretion, and yet no unpleasant consequences arise from the diminution or suppression of the discharge, since a sufficient amount of the vital stimuli has already been expended in severe muscular exercise.

Prognosis.—Retention proceeding from a natural lack of constitutional vigour, is always difficult to cure; but where no serious organic difficulty exists, we may generally hope for ultimate success. In cases, however, which are complicated with chronic pulmonary disease, dropsical affections, and organic disease of the heart or liver, the prognosis must always be unfavourable. Retention from imperforated os uteri, or hymen, and from vaginal adhesions and polypi, are all readily cured by surgical means.

When suppression arises as a symptom of some chronic disease, especially if it has persisted for several months, we shall, for the most part, find the case incurable; when, on the contrary, it has arisen from an acute disorder, the cure may be easily accomplished.

Obstructions which are consequences of anger, grief, fright, jealousy, or exposure to wet and cold, may also be speedily restored by suitable specifics.

In forming an opinion respecting the probable termination of amenorrhœa, it should always be borne in mind, that it is almost invariably either a symptom of some other disease, or that it owes its origin to a general lack of constitutional vigour. Much, therefore, depends upon the general condition of the system, and upon the curable or incurable nature of the malady which causes the menstrual derangement, as to whether our prognosis be favourable or otherwise.

Therapeutics.—In the management of amenorrhœa, our first attention should always be directed to the removal of the cause upon which it depends. Those cases of retarded menstruation dependent upon a want of constitutional vigour, will derive material benefit from well regulated exercise, nutritious diet, change of scene and of climate, sea air, sea voyages, and bathing. Retention from mechanical obstructions, can only be cured by the aid of the surgeon.

But in suppression or obstruction, unattended with any serious local complication, and originating from exposure to cold, mental emotions, suddenly checked perspiration, cold drinks, fevers, &c., we may afford the most prompt relief by the employment of suitable remedies.

We call attention to the following medicines: *pulsatilla, sabinæ, china, calcarea carb., ferrum, graphites, conium, serpentaria virg., sulphur, sepia.*

Pulsatilla is adapted to females of a mild, timid, and amiable disposition, who are easily excited to tears or to laughter. It may be used in cases where menstruation is delayed a few days beyond the natural period, in abrupt suppression of the courses, from cold bathing, wet feet, sudden suppression of perspiration from cold air, violent passions and emotions, and in fevers, in alternation with other suitable medicines. It is also valuable in partial obstructions, accompanied with dyspeptic and hysteric symptoms. The general indications are, lassitude, weariness of the limbs, unpleasant arterial pulsations in different parts of the body, congestion, anxiety, and oppression of the chest and heart, after exercise, and in the night when in the recumbent posture: variable appetite; coldness of the feet; sleeplessness; pains in the back; weeping mood; vertigo or giddiness; colicky pains in the abdomen.

Sabina is only useful in that irregular variety of amenorrhœa in which the menses appear too soon, and too profusely for a few hours, and are then suppressed either temporarily or permanently. The kind of amenorrhœa in which this medicine is applicable, is for the most part induced by a hyposthenic condition of the uterus.

China and *ferrum* are especially serviceable in retarded menstruation dependent on constitutional debility, whether natural or acquired. The general indications for their use, are, pale, sallow, or cachectic countenance; emaciation; muscles soft and flabby; rapid circulation; rapid and difficult respiration after exercise; palpitation of the heart, excited by mental emotions, exercise, or eating heartily; lassitude, debility, and general indisposition to think or act; transient pains in the chest, back, side, pelvis, and limbs; swelling and pain in the hepatic region; bitter taste; feeble appetite; impaired digestion; nightly restlessness; leucorrhœa.

Calcarea carb., *sulphur*, *graphite*, *conium*, and *sepia*, are indicated in the catamenial irregularities of scrofulous, rickety, and syphilitic subjects. The history of each case will enable us to decide respecting the precise nature of the disease upon which the amenorrhœa is dependent, and thus render it easy to select an antipsoric which shall gradually remove the original cause of disorder, and cure the patient. As a general rule, *calcarea carb.* agrees best with young persons whose menses appear *too soon*, while *sulphur*, *graphite*, *conium* and *sepia* may be exhibited at all ages, but for the most part, in cases of retarded and suppressed menstruation.

Serpentaria virg.—We have often used this medicine in suppressed and obstructed menses, from cold, violent emotions, and the debility consequent on fevers, with marked success. A recent cure of amenorrhœa, verging on chlorosis, has also come under my observation, which, taken in connection with the other examples alluded to, convince me that it is a specific of much value in disorders of this character.

As a majority of the cases of amenorrhœa have their origin in some inherent constitutional vice, and are, in reality, but mere symptoms of some other affection, it is of importance that our attention be directed to all of the remote and slight symptoms which may exercise an influence upon the economy, as well as to the more immediate and visible signs of the malady.

Administration.—When the menstrual derangement has approached gradually, and is evidently a symptom of some general disease, like scrofula, chlorosis, phthisis pulmonalis, dropsy, or chronic hepatitis, the remedies must be selected with reference to these maladies, and the same attenuations and repetitions employed as advised under these different affections.—

As a general rule, in these cases, we employ the first, second, and third attenuations, and repeat the dose but rarely; but in abrupt obstructions, occurring in females of a robust constitution, from undue exposures, or over-excitement, we make use of the first or second attenuations, and repeat every two, three, or four hours until we are satisfied with the effect produced.

SECTION XII.

DYSMENORRHŒA.—PAINFUL MENSTRUATION.

Diagnosis.—Painful menstruation is of most common occurrence in females of sanguineous and robust constitutions, and of ardent and animated temperaments. The monthly flux makes its appearance at the usual period, but generally in small quantity, often becoming entirely suppressed for several hours, and then reappearing to a greater or less extent, perhaps again to be suppressed. Females subject to dysmenorrhœa, are almost invariably troubled with constipation, and frequent headaches, from rush of blood to the brain, in the interval between the catamenial periods.

The usual symptoms attending dysmenorrhœa, are, severe bearing-down pains in the uterine region, similar to the pains of labour, and coming on in paroxysms; constant aching in the small part of the back, the loins, the pelvis, and the limbs; accelerated action of the heart and arteries; flushed cheeks; headache; cutting and pressing pains in the abdomen; flatulence; spasmodic sensation in the region of the stomach; nausea; eructations; oppression in the chest; anxiety and irritability; scanty discharge of blood which is not coagulable, and containing lymph, and shreds of a membranous structure, or clots of dark blood.

Causes.—The chief causes of dysmenorrhœa, are, an inflamed condition of the secretory vessels of the uterus, an unnaturally small *os tincæ*, and inveterate constipation. Of these causes, the first is the most common, and occurs in females of a full plethoric habit, of fancies easily excited to activity, who are fond of

22*

the pleasures of the table, of love, and shows, and who prefer to pass their time in heated parlours, or crowded ball-rooms, rather than in active exercise out of doors. When we reflect upon the habits and the mode of life which the customs of refined society impose upon young females, we shall no longer wonder that this important function of the uterus should so often become disordered. The foolish mother, anxious that her child should grow up according to the laws of a false elegance, with a shape of body moulded to suit the *code of fashion*, rather than in those once approved proportions which the Creator gave her, envelopes her in corsets and stays, pressing the abdominal viscera downward upon the bladder and uterus, and the thoracic organs upwards towards the throat, and thus moulds a waist sufficiently *small* and *wasp-like* to meet the requirements of a sham gentility. In carrying out this wicked whalebone and buckram system, the important functions of circulation, respiration, digestion, and menstruation are of no sort of consequence to the deluded victim or her friends, when compared with the imperative demands of *fashion*. God made the human body of precisely the right proportions for the healthful exercise of all the organs; civilized woman baffles this ordination by mechanical devices, and makes of the form an artificial thing, recognised and known as a specimen of gentility, the functions of which are subject to continual derangements, by consumption, chlorosis, dysmenorrhœa, amenorrhœa, constipation, and organic affections of the heart. After the innocent young girl has been thus cheated, not by "dissembling nature," but by a fashionable mother, "out of her fair proportions," it is deemed necessary, in order to complete her education, to prim her up within the crowded walls of a boarding-school; to cram her mind with some ten or twelve studies at a time, including, of course, music, and the current literature; and to neglect active exercise, wit, fun, mirth, and other health-promoters, as *vulgar*. In this manner the countenance acquires that pale and distingué cast so much coveted, and the body that frail and enfeebled state so common in cities.

Another cause which occasionally gives rise to painful menstruation, is an unnaturally small *os tincæ*, Dr. Mackintosh supposes this to be a very common cause of dysmenorrhœa, and details numerous cases of the kind which have come under his own observation. When the painful symptoms do not yield readily to the proper remedies, an examination should be made, and if the fault is in the *os tincæ*, our efforts should be immediately directed to the dilatation of the part with bougies.

The other causes which should be particularly noticed, are collections of indurated fæcal matter in the colon and rectum, uterine polypi, exposure to cold, and rheumatic affections of the uterus.

Therapeutics.—Abundant active exercise in the open air, regular hours, a plain regimen, abstinence from wine, coffee, and green tea, and a temperature not exceeding 68° Fahr., within doors, are prime conditions to the successful treatment of dysmenorrhœa. By attending rigidly to these important points, constipation will be obviated, the circulation of the blood equalized, the animal heat uniformly diffused, and all undue determinations of blood prevented. If, however, obstinate congestions have already set in, a few doses of a suitable specific will soon restore the organism to its normal condition.

The medicines to which we call attention, are *aconite, pulsatilla, secale cornut., belladonna, nux vom., platina, ferrum, cocculus, sabinæ, conium, graphite.*

Dysmenorrhœa arising from an inflammatory condition of the uterus, and attended with marked febrile symptoms, quick pulse, hot skin, thirst, rapid respiration, headache and general restlessness, demands the employment of *aconite*.

If the menses are scanty, and accompanied with cutting pains in the uterine region, abdomen, back, and loins, vertigo, loss of appetite, chilliness, nausea, and discharge of thick, black blood, alternating with short discharges of bright red blood, we may resort to *pulsatilla*. If the pains shift about from one point to another, the indications are still stronger. *Pulsatilla* also operates best when the derangement has arisen from fright, grief, mortification, or from exposure to wet and cold.

When the menstrual irregularity proceeds from uterine congestion, and presents us with the following tableau of symptoms, viz., violent spasmodic, or bearing-down pains from the small of the back to the uterus, with tenesmus and pressure on the bladder and rectum, coldness of the extremities, rapid and feeble pulse, frequent and severe contractions of the uterus, *secale cornutum* should be employed.

Belladonna is an admirable remedy when the patient is of a plethoric habit and sanguine temperament, and the disorder has originated from some violent mental emotion, and is attended with serious determination to the brain. It may sometimes be employed with advantage in alternation with *aconite.*

Nux vomica is valuable in scanty and painful menstruation, from uterine congestion, arising from scybalous accumulations in the colon and rectum. The pains are of a spasmodic character, and extend from the uterus to the neck of the bladder, and into the abdomen. Considerable gastric derangement usually attends this variety of dysmenorrhœa.

Platina, ferrum, or *sabinæ,* are applicable in that variety in which the menstrual discharge is sufficient, or even inordinate in quantity, but is attended with severe bearing-down pains in the uterine region, cutting pains in the back, loins, and thighs, pressure in the groins, cramps in the abdomen, blood dark, and containing membraneous shreds, and too frequent appearance of the menses.

For uterine and abdominal spasms, nausea, faintness, impeded respiration, and a scanty discharge of coagulated blood, mixed with mucus, we may give *cocculus* or *conium.*

Graphite is an important remedy when the menses appear too late, and are too scanty. The uterine discharge is thick and dark, there are severe labour-like pains in the pelvis, also cutting pains in the abdomen, small of the back and hips, vertigo, constipation, chilliness, cold hands and feet, flatulence, and general lassitude and debility.

Administration.—The medicines may be employed at the first, second and third attenuations, and repeated every two hours during the more severe symptoms.

The remedy should also be given once in two or three days during the intervals between the monthly epochs.

SECTION XIII.

MENORRHAGIA.—UTERINE HÆMORRHAGE.

Diagnosis.—Profuse uterine hæmorrhages may take place at any period of life from puberty to extreme old age, and in every variety of constitution. But the most common kind of menorrhagia to which the attention of the physician is called, is that which happens during the monthly periods, from a congestion or relaxation of the uterine secretory vessels. A certain amount of menstrual fluid is secreted each month, and this natural quantity is determined by the temperament, constitution, and habits of life of each particular subject. Thus, robust and plethoric females, who live richly and drink wine, may lose a large quantity of blood at each period, and suffer no inconvenience from it; while individuals of delicate and relaxed constitutions, would immediately experience ill effects from so profuse a flow. It is when this healthy, natural flux becomes morbidly augmented, that we apply to it the designation of *uterine hæmorrhage*, and deem it necessary to employ medicinal means.

Dangerous uterine hæmorrhages often occur during pregnancy, from disturbance or rupture of the membranes or of the placenta, and also from concussions, blows, violent exercise, fright, anger, cathartics, and emmenagogues.

The symptoms which precede menorrhagia, occurring at the menstrual periods, are, general uneasiness and dissatisfaction, petulancy, lassitude, sense of fulness and oppression in the head, weariness and wandering pains in the back, loins, and inferior extremities, sense of weight and pressure in the pelvis, chilliness, unnatural determinations of blood, cold feet, rapid pulse, and impaired appetite.

The symptoms attendant on the flux, will depend entirely upon the nature of the case, the constitution, and the amount of blood lost in each instance. In light cases of menorrhagia, the patient only experiences a general sense of lassitude, debility, and weariness, faintness, tired and uneasy sensations in the back and limbs, indisposition to exercise, a faint and deathlike feeling at the pit of the stomach, paleness of the face, cold extremities, and feeble and unsatisfactory respiration.

In more serious cases the patient becomes almost exsanguineous; the face, lips, and surface become blanched; the muscular strength entirely prostrated; every attempt to move or converse induces immediate syncope; there is more or less determination of blood to the brain, as is evinced by sharp pains, delirium, ringing in the ears, and throbbings of the carotid and temporal arteries; the vision is impaired, floats circulate before the eyes, respiration is oppressed, palpitation of the heart ensues from exercise or emotions; pulse rapid and extremely feeble; general coldness of the surface; great and undefinable uneasiness and nervous irritation. The blood gushes upon every exertion to change position, and on coughing, sneezing, or vomiting. After the patient has become reduced by its loss to a very low state, frequent and protracted fainting turns come on; respiration and circulation become almost suspended; the blood clots at the mouths of the uterine vessels, and thus the flooding is temporarily arrested. As soon, however, as the organism reacts, these clots are liable to be expelled by the contractile efforts of the uterus, and the flowing to re-appear. These different conditions may occur several times during the progress of the disorder, until finally the patient is so completely prostrate, that there is no re-action, the clots are not expelled, and time is allowed for the uterine vessels to recover themselves sufficiently to resist any further morbid secretion. Cases of this description are not uncommon, and the cures are often erroneously attributed to monstrous doses of opium and sugar of lead, rather than to the kind offices of nature in inducing syncope, and a consequent coagulation of the blood in the uterus.

We have enumerated amongst the symptoms of the complaint, *determination of blood to the head, and inflammation of the brain.* These symptoms have been so often observed in connection with profuse hæmorrhages, and the question has been so often discussed, in regard to the propriety of *blood-letting* for the cure of a cerebral inflammation which has been *caused by excessive loss of blood,* that no one will deny the fact, that these symptoms actually occur as a direct consequence of menorrhagia. Examples of this kind should teach the important truth, *that excessive loss of blood is always a powerful predisposing cause, and in very many instances a direct exciting cause of inflammations of the brain, lungs, and other structures.* It ought also to induce the exercise of a little reason in therapeutical measures, rather than a persistence in the empirical routine of the old school, of venesection, opiates, and astringents.

Menorrhagia originating in organic derangements of the uterus, like indurations, cancers, tumours, and ulcers, will be accompanied with the symptoms peculiar to these different maladies, in addition to their ordinary signs. Cases of this description will require careful attention, both in a diagnostic and in a therapeutical point of view. Thus, if the disease be dependent on a scrofulous or psoric diathesis, or a syphilitic taint, our remedies must be directed as well to these original and general causes, as to those which are more immediate and local. By this means we may strike the silent and invisible enemy, while subduing others which are manifest to our senses.

Causes.—We include among the *remote* causes of this affection, improper physical and moral education, excesses in eating and drinking; insufficient nutriment; scrofulous, syphilitic, or psoric taints; pressure of the abdominal viscera downwards upon the uterus, by mechanical contrivances; an ardent sanguine temperament, and a plethoric habit, or a lymphatic, venous temperament, and a relaxed habit.

The *proximate* causes are, irritation, congestion, or inflammation of the secretory vessels of the uterus; the various disturbances and injuries occurring during pregnancy, and from *accouchement,* cancers, ulcers, tumours, indulgence in the pleasures of love, and of stimulating drinks during the catamenial period.

Prognosis.—A favourable termination may be expected when no organic affection exists, if the patient is moderately robust, and the disease depends upon simple local inflammation, or the accidents arising from pregnancy and accouchement. Many of the floodings, however, which proceed from miscarriage, from abnormal positions of the fœtus and placenta, and from accidents during delivery, require prompt, bold, and judicious efforts on the part of the accoucheur to rescue the patient from fatal prostration. But no woman need bleed to death under any of these circumstances, if there is proper knowledge and decision on the part of the physician.

The circumstances which must render our prognosis unfavourable are, chronic induration or softening of the uterus, cancerous and other incurable ulcerations and tumours, and morbid growths within the viscus. But even in these apparently hopeless cases, we should never despair, for the resources of homœopathy sometimes surpass our most sanguine expectations.

Therapeutics.—After having removed, as far as possible, all disturbing causes, a suitable remedy may be selected from *platina, pulsatilla, belladonna, ipecacuanha, sabina, secale cor., ferrum met., arnica, china, chamomela, sepia, bryonia, nux vom., carbo animal., acid phos., hyoscyamus, crocus sat., creosote.*

Platina is particularly suited to females of a sensitive and impressible organization, and who suffer from too frequent and too profuse catemenia. The flow is accompanied, and occasionally preceded, by cutting and pressing pains in the abdomen, back, and pelvis; dull pains in the groin and thighs; sensation of fulness in the uterus; chills alternating with flushes of heat; unusual sensitiveness of the genital organs; headache; sadness; debility; restlessness; leucorrhœa; menstrual discharge red and fluid, or dark, thick, and coming away in clots. This remedy is applicable in menorrhagia arising from *induration* or *cancer* of the womb.

Pulsatilla is useful in menorrhagia occurring in females at the "turn of life," or from *schirrus uteri*, or from simple passive congestion of the uterus, or during pregnancy and accouchement. The blood is generally dark and coagulated, and is expelled only at intervals, but in large quantities. In profuse hæmorrhages after delivery, when the uterus does not contract, and the patient is much prostrated from pain and loss of blood, *pulsatilla* is an excellent remedy. It may also be given in menorrhagia characterized by inconstant and shifting pains in the back, loins, abdomen and pelvis.

Belladonna is our best remedy in superabundant menstruation proceeding from irritation and active congestion of the uterine vessels, and also in uterine inflammations consequent upon abortions, violent passions, or protracted continence. It is an invaluable remedy in cerebral inflammations arising from excessive uterine hæmorrhage.

The general indications for *belladonna* are, a plethoric habit; ardent, sanguine temperament; frequent determination of blood to the head; strong passions; pressing pains in the small of the back and the abdomen; sense of fulness in the uterus; full and rather rapid pulse; vertigo and pains in the head; nausea; ringing in the ears; partial loss of consciousness; inflammation of the womb; profuse discharge of bright red blood; flushed cheeks; brilliant and congested eyes; *schirrus uteri*. *Belladonna* has been advised in alternation with *arnica* or *platina*, when the pains resemble those of labour, and there is a profuse discharge of bright red blood.

Ipecacuanha may be exhibited when the catamenia appear every two or three weeks, attended with pressure in the uterine region, and profuse discharge of fresh blood.

Sabina is indicated in menorrhagia during and after miscarriage, and at the menstrual period. The flooding is accompanied with bearing down pains in the abdomen and pelvis; abdominal spasms; pain in the uterus; ardor urinæ, and profuse discharges of dark and coagulated blood, or of fluid red blood. *Sabina* is especially useful in protracted uterine hæmorrhages arising from a loss of tone in the vessels of the uterus, whether from previous disease or the weight and pressure of the *fœtus in utero*.

Secale cornutum is recommended in hæmorrhages

arising from passive congestion of the uterus, cachectic habit, and debility, and want of tone in the uterus, from difficult parturition or disease. The general indications are, pale face ; cold surface ; feeble pulse ; white lips ; pains and tenesmus in the rectum and bladder ; discharge of dark and offensive blood, increased on motion, coughing, or sneezing ; great prostration ; numbness ; spasms ; humming in the ears ; obscuration of vision ; loss of contractive power in the uterus.

Ferrum met. is indicated in profuse hæmorrhages after parturition and at the monthly epochs. The discharge is attended with spasmodic and labour-like pains in the loins and uterine region ; flushed cheeks ; hard and full pulse ; hot skin ; headache ; hot and scanty urine ; constipation ; shudderings.

Arnica is our remedy in menorrhagia, originating from mechanical injuries during pregnancy or delivery, or from blows, falls, contusions, strains, etc.

China is applicable in hæmorrhage proceeding from an asthenic condition of the uterus. It is especially useful in enfeebled and cachectic females, who flow too profusely after parturition, from an atonic condition of the uterus and its non-contraction. A general appearance of debility and exhaustion ; blanched countenance ; discharge of serous or thick, dark, and clotted blood ; pale, sunken countenance ; restlessness ; constant fainting turns ; soft and flabby muscles ; coldness of the extremities ; and rapid and feeble pulse, point to this remedy.

Chamomela is adapted to bilious and nervous constitutions, and may be employed in menorrhagia, attended with pains and pressure in the pelvis ; ardor urinæ ; tearing pains in the small of the back, uterus, and legs, with frequent discharges of coagulated blood. It has also been highly commended in uterine hæmorrhages occurring at the change of life. Females of an angry, violent and quarrelsome disposition derive most benefit from this drug.

Sepia may be used in cases proceeding from scrofulous and schirrous affections of the uterine organs. It is likewise advised in protracted chronic cases where the system has become much exhausted from previous disease and suffering.

Bryonia agrees with bilious and choleric females, and is commended in menorrhagia attended with stitching pains in the head, back, and pit of the stomach, when stooping, or stepping.

Nux vom. will apply in cases of menorrhagia from uterine congestion, accompanied with spasmodic pains in the uterus, and a discharge of clots of dark red blood.

Carbo animal. has been successfully used in a few cases of moderate uterine hæmorrhage, from chronic induration of the uterus.

Acid phosph. is specific in too profuse menstruation, attended with swelling and pain in the liver.

Hyoscyamus is specific in superabundant menstruation of hysterical females, who experience before and during the continuance of the flow, general spasms, convulsive laughing or weeping, twitching or trembling of the limbs, headache, and occasional delirium. The discharge is bright red.

Crocus sat. corresponds to active or passive uterine hæmorrhages. It is useful after miscarriage, when the discharge is very profuse, dark, and viscid, and the patient is anxious, feeble, chilly, faint, sick at stomach, restless, thirsty, and annoyed with palpitation of the heart, vertigo, impaired vision, vague pains in the back and pelvis, and unpleasant dreams. Movement and coughing increase the hæmorrhage.

Kreosote is advised in passive uterine hæmorrhages originating in scirrhous degenerations of the uterus, or in general laxity of the uterine vessels. The menses appear too early, are too profuse, and accompanied with a leucorrhœal or ichorous discharge, which irritate the parts with which it comes in contact.

Administration.—In urgent cases of uterine hæmorrhage, we give the first attenuations, and repeat every half-hour until medicinal symptoms appear, or the flooding abates. In less dangerous cases, we repeat every two, three, or four hours, so long as is necessary. With the internal remedies, cold water may be applied to the pelvic region by means of cloths. The hips must be elevated and supported, while the head and shoulders are lowered, and the patient be kept cool, quiet, and free from excitement.

CHAPTER XXVII.

DISEASES OF THE FIBROUS AND MUSCULAR SYSTEM.

SECTION I.

ACUTE RHEUMATISM.

Diagnosis.—Acute rheumatism usually commences after an abrupt suppression of perspiration, in consequence of exposure to wet, cold, or to a highly variable temperature. It first manifests itself in the form of slight chills, lassitude, and general uneasiness, which are soon succeeded by swelling, redness, pain, and augmented heat in the part affected. The pains vary much in character, being sometimes aching and gnawing, at others, lancinating and darting, or dull and throbbing, or numb, pungent, and prickling, and aggravated by movement, by exposure to drafts of cold air, and by the pressure, or touch of the hand. In the first instance, rheumatism seizes upon the fibrous textures, but as the inflammatory action becomes developed, other tissues become involved, the capillaries of the neighbouring parts become distended with red blood, and the usual phenomena are present. The larger joints are more subject to rheumatic inflammation than other parts of the body, although it is not uncommon for the inflammation to commence in the head, neck, chest, arms, or legs, and gradually extend into the neighbouring joints. The more common accompanying symptoms of acute rheumatism are, bitter taste in the mouth, coated tongue, rapid and full pulse, moderately hot skin, thirst, scanty, high-coloured and sedimentitious urine, intense pain on moving the affected part, anxious and distressed expression of countenance, and occasional perspiration.

Rheumatic inflammations are liable to shift from joint to joint, and sometimes to fix upon important internal organs, like the brain and its membranes, the pulmonary structures, and the heart and its appendages. So long as the malady confines itself to the joints, or to the external parts of the body, it is unattended with danger to life; but when metastases occur to important internal organs, the disease becomes in an eminent degree perilous.

Acute rheumatism occurs for the most part, in young, healthy, and robust subjects, and can be generally traced to undue exposure to cold, or to a wet and variable atmosphere.

Chronic rheumatism differs from the acute form in many respects; as for example, absence of febrile symptoms; the fixed character of the pains; no perceptible swelling or redness in the affected parts; the pains sometimes aggravated, and at other times ameliorated by walking, and other exercises; great sensibility of the diseased tissues to changes of temperature, to humidity, and to cold; dryness and inactivity of the skin; rigidity in the parts, most apparent when attempting to move, or to walk, after having been quiet for a considerable period; sedimentitious urine; weakness, trembling, or numbness of the disordered parts.

Therapeutics.—We enumerate as the principal remedies, *rhus, bryonia, aconite, colchicum, belladonna, pulsatilla, dulcamara, mercurius, nux vomica, phosphorus, calcarea carbonica, veratrum, hepar sulphur, arnica, colocynth, lycopodium, sulphur.*

Rhus tox.—External indications.—The integuments about the joints swollen and red; surface of the body hot and moist; tongue dry and red; pulse frequent, and hard; urine dark, or red, and turbid.

Physical sensations.—Drawing and tearing, or tensive stinging and dragging pains in the affected parts, increased by exposure to cold, by rest, and by movement after having been for some time quiet; rigidity, lameness, and weakness of the muscles in the vicinity of the diseased textures; increase of the febrile symptoms, and of the pains, at night, in bed; perspiration, especially during the pains; pains alleviated by exercise; throbbing, and burning in the knees, or ancles; painful involuntary contractions of the muscles of the calves of the legs; chronic rheumatic pains occurring early in the morning, and disappearing on moving about.

Mental and moral symptoms.—Intellect unimpaired; disposition irritable and impatient.

Administration.—One drop of the first dilution may be given in a dessert spoonful of water, every two or three hours, until the pains begin to subside, or until a medicinal action is produced upon the inflamed tissue.

Bryonia.—External indications.—Swelling and redness of the inflamed textures; countenance pale or sallow, or flushed and hot; tongue covered with a white or yellow fur; hot and dry surface, or perspiration of an acid character after exercise; considerable thirst, frequent and soft pulse; red or yellowish urine; position such as to relax the muscles bearing upon the diseased parts.

Physical sensations.—Pains of a tearing, throbbing, or lancinating character, aggravated by movement, by the touch, by the contact of cold air, and by eating; a relaxed state of the muscles, and perfect rest, affords almost entire relief from suffering; bitter taste, or dryness of the mouth, with thirst; nausea; bilious vomiting; severe pulsating headache; morbid sensibility of the whole surface to the touch; stitching pains in the region of the liver, and in the intercostal muscles; symptoms worse during the night.

Mental and moral symptoms.—General uneasiness, anxiety, and irritability; sleeplessness.

Administration.—The second or third dilution may be employed—a dose every two, three, or four hours, as the symptoms appear to require. For the active febrile symptoms which occasionally accompany the affection, we are in the habit of prescribing *aconite* and *bryonia* in alternation, with satisfactory results.

Colchicum is a valuable remedy in both acute and chronic rheumatism. The pains are lancinating, jerking, or tearing, worse in the night, and increased by care, anxiety, or movement: or, there may be only stiffness and lameness in the joints, when attempting to walk, with œdematous swellings of the parts in the vicinity of the inflammation. Dr. Schroen commends *colchicum* in those cases which resist the clearly indicated medicines, provided the skin is moist, and the urine is turbid. Dr. S. advises it to be given in the form of *vini seminis colchici*, and in doses of twelve drops daily. We have found a single drop of the first dilution, repeated once in from three to six hours, according to the acute or chronic nature of the case, very efficacious, in several obstinate cases which had resisted the action of other medicines.

Belladonna will prove an excellent remedy, in rheumatic attacks accompanied with a high degree of nervous irritability, and a morbid activity of the cerebral organs. The pains are very severe, especially at night, increased by touch, or by remaining too long in one position.

Pulsatilla is indicated when the pains shift rapidly from one part to another, and are unattended with any great swelling or redness of the integuments ; also, in chronic rheumatism characterized by weakness, rigidity, coldness, and sensation of weight in the disordered structures.

Dulcamara often proves speedily curative in rheumatic inflammations which have been caused by exposure to cold and dampness. The affected parts usually feel as if bruised or beaten, and after remaining for some time in one position, are attacked with severe pains which do not subside until the patient moves about. The pains are most common in the back, and in the joints of the arms and legs.

In cases of frequently recurring rheumatism, of scrofulous or psoric subjects, we must use one or more of the following medicines: *calcarea carbonica, sulphur, lycopodium, mercurius.*

When the disease has become chronic and inveterate, and abnormal depositions occur about the joints, with thickening of the membraneous tissues, and permanent rigidity, weakness, and tenderness on motion, a persevering employment of *rhus*, or *hepar sulphur*, or *nux*, or *phosphorus*, or *veratrum*, or *lachesis*, will induce curative results of the most satisfactory character.

Other medicines which have occasionally proved successful in rheumatic affections, are, *colocynth, iodine, ferrum, china, arsenicum, arnica, carbo vegetabilis*, and *hyoscyamus.*

Administration.—In the acute form of the malady,

we employ from the third to the sixth attenuations, and repeat the doses every two hours until a medicinal impression is evident. In chronic rheumatism, we prefer the first attenuation, and prescribe a dose once or twice daily.

SECTION II.

ARTHRITIS.—GOUT.

Although rheumatism and gout are described by authors as different diseases, it is altogether probable that the nature of the inflammatory action is the same in both instances. When this peculiar inflammation seizes upon the young and robust, and pervades the larger joints and the muscular structures, it receives the name of rheumatism; but when individuals advanced in life, are the subjects of attack, and it appears in the small joints, it is recognised as gout.

A fit of the gout is almost always preceded by some gastric or intestinal derangement, like impaired appetite, furred tongue, bitter taste, acid or bitter eructations, flatulent distention of the stomach and intestines, and occasionally diarrhœa. The inflammation is, for the most part, situated in the ball of the great toe, but it may attack any of the smaller joints, and as the disease advances, the veins in the vicinity of the pain become distended; the integuments swollen, œdematous, and of a bright scarlet colour; the pains become severe, of a darting, throbbing, or a persistent aching and burning character, increased by contact or by movement; there is an almost entire loss of muscular power of the affected parts; the pains are worse during the night, and accompanied during this period by active febrile symptoms; nearly all the functions of the organism are sympathetically deranged; the urine is small in quantity, high coloured, and becomes turbid on standing; the patient is restless, irritable, and morbidly sensitive to moral and physical impressions. The disorder usually arrives at its maximum of intensity, in two or three days from the commencement of the inflammation. At this period, the whole toe, and sometimes the foot itself, become œdematous, and the numbness and prickling are frequently experienced in the swollen textures, especially during the day: the pains and the nightly febrile exacerbations, now commence subsiding, until at the end of from seven to ten days, the active inflammatory symptoms have disappeared and left the patient with a debilitated and œdematous limb.

When the paroxysms of acute gout occur very frequently, they serve, after a time, to impair the constitution, to cause permanent thickenings of the articular membranes, or cretaceous deposits about the joints, and to induce that condition of the parts which leads to *chronic* gout. This form of the complaint is characterized by dull, burning, or tensive pains, œdema, thickening of the membranes of the affected joint, with rigidity, weakness, and partial loss of muscular power; more or less gastric derangement, augmented sensibility of the mind and body to external impressions, depression of spirits, and general restlessness and irritability.

Causes.—Gout is generally supposed to be hereditary, although cases are constantly occurring in which no natural predisposition can be traced. There is no doubt, however, that in the majority of instances, an hereditary predisposition exists. The exciting causes of gout, are, high-living, want of sufficient exercise, abuse of stimulants, especially wines, and general irritability of the nervous system, from loss of rest, and irregularity in eating.

Therapeutics.—The principal remedies for acute gout, are, *bryonia, nux vomica, colchicum, bell., aconite, rhus, pulsatilla, actæa spicata, actæa racemosa, guaiacum, arnica, arsenicum, china, ledum, sabinæ, cantharides.* For chronic gout, the best remedies are, *calcarea carbonica, sulphur, phosphoric acid, aurum muriate, iodine, hepar sulphur, phosphorus, mercurius, sepia, silicea.*

It will very commonly happen that several of these medicines will cover most of the manifest symptoms which are usually present in gout, but in making our selection, the strictest regard should be had to all remote and exciting causes which may have exercised an influence in originating the malady, in order that we may strike deeply at the foundation of the disturbance, as well as at the more immediate and visible phenomena.

In prescribing for gout, we may be governed by the general indications for the different medicines, as pointed out in the last section.

CHAPTER XXVIII.

HYDROPS.—DROPSY.

SECTION I.

General description.—Dropsy is generally but a mere symptom of some other affection. Its proximate cause consists in an inflammation, congestion, or exalted action of the capillary extremities of the arterial vessels of the serous and cellular membranes, and a torpor or inactivity of the venous absorbents of the same parts.

The remote and general causes of dropsy are, excessive loss of blood, and other animal fluids; general debility resulting from disease, mechanical injuries, obstructions of the liver, spleen, kidneys, veins, lungs; abuse of drugs and stimulating drinks. At first view, an inflammation or congestion of the serous exhalents, would seem to be incompatible with general debility, arising from excessive loss of blood, and diseases of the liver, kidneys, lungs, spleen, &c., but the fact is now well established, that these circumstances actually favour the formation of these very capillary inflammations and congestions.

Some writers maintain that serous effusions do not occur until the active inflammatory symptoms are passing off, and a state of sub-acute inflammation obtains; while others, like Laennec, and Johnson, lay it down as a fundamental law of serous membranes, "that they begin to effuse the moment they become inflamed." It is true that acute inflammations of serous membranes often occur and subside without leaving any traces of effusion, but this is owing to the fact, that, during the general febrile excitement, the venous absorbents of the affected cavities, being equally irritated with the exhalents, exercise their functions with preternatural activity, thus conveying off the fluid as fast as exhaled, and securing the equilibrium between exhalation and absorption. After the inflammatory symptoms have subsided, if the exhalents and absorbents both recover their tone, health returns; but, as frequently happens, if the latter remain feeble, while the former return to their normal state, the healthy balance is lost, and dropsy is the result.

In health, " the cellular tissue and all of those cavities lined by serous membranes, are continually lubricated by a fluid which exhales from the capillary extremities of the arterial vessels."—(*Frank.*) This fluid serves to render the parts soft, pliable, and mobile, and to prevent the adhesive inflammation which would otherwise occur from friction during the movements of the body. These exhalents give out nearly a given quantity of vapour, and a due equilibrium is established between the amount secreted for the use of the organism, and that which is afterwards taken up by the venous extremities, and thrown off by the skin, kidneys, salivary glands and intestines. So long as this proportion is maintained, all goes on well ; but whenever any of the serous membranes, like the peritoneum, the pleura, the pericardium, or the arachnoid, secrete more fluid than is required for the wants of the economy, or than can be absorbed by the venous extremities, then drafts are made upon other and healthy parts to supply the increased demand. On this account the perspiration becomes suppressed, and the skin dry and husky, the saliva scanty and viscid, the urinary secretions small, high-coloured, fetid, and sedimentitious, the stools scanty and difficult, and the functions generally deranged.

In cases of dropsy arising from excessive loss of blood or starvation, the normal physical condition of this fluid is changed,—the impression it produces upon the structures is altered, and a superabundance of serum is poured out into the cavities and the cellular tissue. This increased exhalation may be due either to the greater affinity which the serous membranes exert upon the altered blood, or to an irritation of the capillary extremities which induces an exaltation of their exhaling function. The experiments of Matteucci teach us, that different fluids pass through the animal membranes in definite quantities and with certain degrees of rapidity, according to the character of the fluids used and the condition of the tissue operated upon. These different phenomena are termed *endosmose* and *exosmose*, and it is by no means improbable that some varieties of dropsy may be partially dependent upon this peculiar action.

Another very important circumstance connected with the formation of dropsies, is alluded to by Eberle, in his Practice of Medicine, viz., "I have already observed, that immediately after a profuse loss of blood, absorption goes on with unusual activity. The blood-vessels are rapidly replenished with crude fluids; for the absorbents being extremely active, nearly all the aqueous fluids, received into the stomach, are speedily absorbed into the circulation; and this is especially favoured by the very great thirst which almost always occurs after excessive sanguineous losses. The blood being thus inordinately supplied with a crude and watery fluid, becomes more irritating to the heart and capillaries, and diluted to such a degree as to pass off more rapidly by the exhalents." Direct experiments on animals have proved that artificial dropsies may be produced, by abstracting blood, and drenching them with water. On the other hand, Majendie and Matteucci have equally demonstrated, that a *fulness* of the blood-vessels very materially *retards*, and in some instances, entirely suppresses the function of absorption.

We think, then, it may be safely concluded, that in every case of dropsy, there are two simultaneous morbid conditions present, namely, *increased exhalation*, and *decreased absorption*, and that, although *irritation* and *congestion* of the *exhalents* are generally indispensable conditions to this morbid action, yet that effusion may result in certain cases simply from an alteration in the character and quantity of the blood, by *endosmose*.

Dropsies are acute or chronic, primitive or secondary, simple or complicated; and the character of the effusion is dependent upon the age, sex, and constitution of the patient, and the nature of each particular case. Generally, however, the fluid is composed of albuminous matter dissolved in more or less water, with different phosphates and carbonates and a little sulphur, (*Frank,*) of an oily character, of a citron, orange, or straw colour, and of a consistency semi-gelatinous, or like the white of eggs. But these appearances are sometimes subject to variations, as cases are reported in which the liquid was brown, white, green, purulent, bloody, saccharine, urinous, and in some instances containing substances like hydatids, and bits of membrane.

Much light is sometimes thrown upon the nature and causes of dropsy, by an examination of the urine. In certain cases of anasarca, for example, it is found that the urine coagulates on the application of heat, and from this circumstance we may suspect the existence of the disease so ably described by Dr. Bright, under the name of *granulated kidney*. The application of heat in these cases, first causes the urine to become milky, and afterwards to present a curdled, or flaky appearance. "In hydrothorax following scarlatina, the urine is mixed with cruorine; in hydrothorax depending upon degeneration of the spleen and liver, the urine contains a large quanity of urea and uric acid, rosic acid and purpurate."—(*Hartmann.*) In other instances we find the urine loaded with albumen.

In acute dropsies the effusion does not occur until the active inflammatory symptoms are passing off, and a condition of sub-acute inflammation supervenes. In these cases, also, the exhalation takes place with more rapidity, and is attended with more painful symptoms, than in the chronic varieties. Now and then slight accumulations take place, which remain stationary for years, when they entirely disappear, or the morbid condition of the exhalants returns, and the disease advances to its full development. Instances of this description are often observed in hydrocele, and in ovarian dropsy.

An excellent diagnostic arrangement of the dropsies

has been made by Marshall Hall, founded upon their *causes*, viz:

"1.—INFLAMMATORY DROPSY.

"First. *The history.*—This form of dropsy generally takes place rather suddenly, and is to be traced to exposure to wet and cold."

"Second. *The symptoms* consist in the appearance of diffuse, tense anasarca, generally with dyspnœa, and frequently with the signs of effusion into the head, thorax, or abdomen, and with a coagulable and occasionally a sanguineous condition of the urine."

"Third. *The morbid anatomy* varies according as the dropsy is confined to the cellular membrane, or extended to the serous membranes; in the latter case there is frequently the effusion of coagulable lymph, as well as of serum, from the serous surfaces. The kidney, in protracted cases, becomes disorganized, granular, scabrous, etc."

"2.—EXANTHEMATOUS DROPSY.

"First. *The history.*—This form of dropsy succeeds to some exanthematous diseases, but by far most frequently to *scarlatina.*"

"Second. *The symptoms* are similar to those just detailed as designating *inflammatory dropsy;* there is the same disposition to effusions into the brain, thorax and abdomen."

"3.—DROPSY FROM EXHAUSTION.

"First. *The history and symptoms.*—This form of dropsy is known by being traced to the loss of blood. It occurs in the form of anasarca, and of effusion into the cavities. I do not know whether the urine be coagulable."

"Second. A similar form of dropsy is induced in cases of neglected *chlorosis.*"

"4.—DROPSY FROM DEBILITY.

"First. *The history and symptoms* sufficiently establish and distinguish this form of dropsy. The patient has frequently had returns of dropsical affection, and has a pale and cachectic appearance. The urine coagulates into brownish flakes by exposure to heat."

"5.—DROPSY FROM OBSTRUCTION IN THE FLOW OF VENOUS BLOOD.

"This form of dropsy arises from—

"First. *Disease of the heart, especially of the valves.*"

"Second. *Disease of the lungs.*"

"Third. *Disease of the liver, especially the 'cirrhose.'*"

"Fourth. *Pressure, or disease, of the veins themselves.*"

"*The history and symptoms.*—This kind of dropsy is distinguished by ascertaining the seat and nature of the original disease. Like the rest, it assumes the form of anasarca, and of effusion into the serous cavities, and into the cellular membrane of the internal organs, as *the lungs, intestines,* &c. *The urine is not coagulable.*"

"6.—DROPSY FROM DISEASE OF THE KIDNEYS.

"For the detection of this species of dropsy, the profession and mankind are indebted to Dr. Bright."

"First. *The symptoms.*—It is distinguished by the coagulable condition of the urine. The urine is apt sometimes to be sanguineous."

"Second. *The complications.*—There is, in this kind of dropsy, occasionally—

"First. *An attack of apoplexy;* and frequently,

"Second. *Inflammation of the serous membranes, and especially of the pleura.*"

"The *liver* is usually found free from disease.

"*The morbid anatomy.*—Dr. Bright describes three kinds of this disease of the kidney. In the *first*, the kidney loses its usual firmness, and becomes of a yellow mottled appearance externally. The size of the kidney is not materially altered. In the *second*, the whole cortical part is converted into a granulated texture, and there appears to be a copious morbid interstitial deposit of an opaque white substance. The kidney is generally rather larger than natural. In the *third*, the kidney is rough and scabrous externally, and rises in numerous projections not much exceeding a large pin's head, yellow, red, and purplish; it is hard and inclined to be lobulated, and its texture approaches to a semi-cartilaginous firmness; there appears, in short, a contraction of every part of the organ, with less interstitial deposite than in the last variety."

General diagnosis.—The symptoms most commonly observed in dropsy are, sensation of weight, oppression, fulness, and uneasiness in the part affected, with more or less disturbance of the neighbouring tissues; dyspnœa and sense of suffocation after attaining the horizontal posture, and after active exercise; general feeling of debility, and disinclination to bodily or mental exertion; partial, and in some instances, almost total suppression of the urinary, salivary, and perspiratory secretions; impaired appetite; feeble digestion; rare and scanty alvine discharges; thirst; countenance pale, sallow, or cachectic; emaciation; "diminution of animal heat, sensation, and motion," (*Frank,*) general derangement of nearly all the functions.

In cellular dropsy, the affected part is swollen, the skin presents a smooth and shining appearance, with blue veins traversing it in different directions, and pressure with the finger causes a deep indentation or pit, which remains for a considerable time. There is also an apparent diminution in the temperature of the part, and a sensation of weight and tension is experienced, rather than of acute pain. The accumulation of serum becomes so great in some instances as to burst through the integuments, and thus partially discharge itself.

In acute dropsies of the serous membranes, the symptoms are more active. Here we have general febrile disturbance; acute tenderness and pain in the disordered part, especially on pressure, or contact of light clothing; urgent thirst; hot and dry skin; urine very scanty and high-coloured; saliva viscid, tenacious, and small in quantity; loss of appetite; furred tongue; rapid sinking of the physical energies. These acute symptoms often subside, and leave the inflamed membrane in a state of sub-acute inflammation, thus developing a well-pronounced chronic dropsy.

It will be observed in our previous description of symptoms, that we have included a diminution of the urinary, salivary, and intestinal secretions, as characteristic of this malady; but these signs are not invariably present, for in a few instances we have witnessed an abundant and natural urinary and salivary secretion during the continuance of the complaint. So, also, one or more of the other symptoms described may be wanting, and yet the dropsical affection proceed to a fatal termination; but these circumstances are rather to be looked upon in the light of exceptions, than as general occurrences.

Prognosis.—Our prognosis must depend much upon the cause and nature of each particular case. Simple cellular or serous dropsies, uncomplicated with disorganization of any of the important organs, are, for the most part, curable. In this class we may rank exanthematous dropsies, and those which have arisen from loss of blood, from acute diseases in which no serious organic derangement has occurred, and from abuse of mercury and other drugs. In these cases, a speedy removal of the causes which have conduced to the disease, with pure air, a generous diet, and a judicious course of homœopathic medicines, will generally enable us to remove permanently the morbid accumulation.

On the contrary, if the effusion has arisen from an organic affection of a vital organ, like the heart, the liver, the lungs, the kidney, or from incurable obstruction in the veins, our prognosis must be unfavourable. In these cases of complicated dropsy, our remedial efforts must be adapted to the remote general disease, as well as to the immediate symptoms of the malady. Although the chances of cure are small in cases of this description, yet, as recoveries do occasionally take place in individuals of naturally vigorous constitutions, and in those who are tenacious of life, we should never prostrate our patients by discouragement and a grim visage, but constantly point them to a beacon of hope in the dim distance. By this means, we secure a powerful auxiliary to co-operate with us in our efforts to bring about those changes in the organism which may lead to a cure.

We come now to treat of the different species of dropsy, viz.:

First. *Anasarca.* Second. *Ascites.*
Third. *Hydrothorax.* Fourth. *Hydrocephalus.*
Fifth. *Ovarian dropsy.* Sixth. *Hydrocele.*

1.—ANASARCA.—CELLULAR DROPSY.

Diagnosis.—The term anasarca is used to designate that variety of dropsical effusion which takes place from the exhalents of the sub-cutaneous cellular tissue. The malady first manifests itself in the inferior extremities, particularly after standing or walking for some time, and it gradually extends upwards until the whole sub-cutaneous cellular tissue of the organism becomes involved. The tumefaction is usually soft, doughy, and inelastic, pitting on pressure, and the skin is white, shining, and below the medium temperature. The swelling disappears, in a great measure, after the patient has been for some time in the recumbent position, but returns again when he has resumed the erect posture. Cellular dropsy may exist for years without causing serious inconvenience, when confined to the inferior extremities, but it is rare that the whole cellular surface becomes involved, unless some vital disorganization exists, or the energies of the system have become dangerously impaired.

The cases of anasarca attended with the least danger, are those arising from scarlatina, pregnancy, loss of blood, debility consequent upon convalescence from acute diseases, abuse of arsenic and mercury, enlarged inguinal glands, the pressure of tumours, or any other curable cause which operates to prevent the free return of the venous blood.

Effusions of this kind may very properly be termed *passive* dropsies, for we agree with Dewees, "that there are both active and passive dropsies, or rather dropsies that depend upon an increase of action or of inflammation, and others where there may be a mere loss of balance between the exhalation and absorption."

In cases of dropsy arising from venous obstruction, for example, the venous absorbents below the seat of the obstruction, are preternaturally distended with blood, and, as a consequence, their powers of absorption proportionably diminished, while the arterial exhalents exercise their function with the usual activity. In this manner the equilibrium between exhalation and absorption is destroyed, and dropsical accumulations obtain. So in phthisis pulmonalis, and affections of the heart, the blood being but imperfectly decarbonized in its passage through these diseased organs, becomes congested in the venous absorbents, and thus gives rise to diminished absorption, and consequent serous accumulations.

Anasarca is not usually attended with much constitutional disturbance, or with symptoms that are painful. There are present, however, coldness of the surface, and diminished secretion of urine and sweat. The countenance is also pale and sallow, and the general appearance indicates ill-health. Not unfrequently the effusion continues to increase until the affected parts become enormously distended, and finally crack and give issue to the accumulated serum. When this happens in erysipelatous or syphilitic subjects, sloughing and gangrenous ulcers sometimes supervene, which prove highly troublesome and dangerous.

Causes.—The peculiar condition consequent upon scarlatina, measles, phthisis pulmonalis, chlorosis, and diseases of the heart; venous obstructions caused by the gravid uterus, by the pressure of tumours, enlarged glands, ligatures, and mechanical injuries, sudden and excessive loss of blood, abuse of stimulants, arsenic and mercury.

2.—ASCITES, OR ABDOMINAL DROPSY.

Diagnosis.—Dropsy of the belly may arise suddenly in consequence of acute peritoneal inflammation, and be attended with the ordinary symptoms of other febrile diseases, or it may make its appearance in a gradual and imperceptible manner, unattended by any notable constitutional disturbance. During attacks of peritonitis, there is an increased exhalation from the inflamed serous vessels, from the very commencement of the disease, and so long as the whole organism labours under the exalted action incident upon the fever, the venous absorbents dispose of this superabundance of serum; but after the active symptoms have subsided, a corresponding depression obtains in all parts of the economy, except, perhaps, the affected membrane, in which there still may remain a sub-acute inflammation and its consequence, a preternatural effusion of serum. In vigorous constitutions, the absorbents continue to remove the exhalation as fast as formed; but in feeble, delicate, or scrofulous subjects, the function of absorption often languishes, the equilibrium between the exhaling and absorbing functions is destroyed, and an ascites is the result.

The signs which characterize abdominal dropsy are, gradual enlargement of the abdomen, first observed in the epigastric region, and afterwards extending over the whole abdomen; tenderness on pressure; difficulty of breathing on taking exercise, and some time after lying down; distinct fluctuation on percussion; sallow and unhealthy complexion; dry skin; scanty secretion of high-coloured and sedimentitious urine; foul tongue, with a small secretion of viscid saliva; impaired appetite; constipation, or relax; sensation of weight and stiffness, particularly when attempting to move about, or bend the body; general feeling of languor and debility.

The only diseases which are liable to be confounded with ascites, are pregnancy and tympanitis; but the history and circumstances of each case will enable us to distinguish with sufficient facility and certainty between the different maladies. In ascites, the situation of the swelling, the fluctuation on percussion, the suppression of urine, dry skin, and the previous history of the case, will mark the nature of the complaint; and in pregnancy, the gradual swelling at the lower part of the abdomen, the suppression of the menses, nausea and vomiting; the absence of fluctuation on percussion, and the motion of the child, will render our diagnosis accurate. Nor will the acute physician ever mistake tympanitic distention for ascites: for percussion, auscultation, and an absence of the characteristic symptoms of dropsy, will enable him to decide at once in regard to the real nature of the case. Indeed, we can hardly conceive how certain eminent surgeons should have been led to perform the operation of what they have afterwards facetiously termed "*dry tapping*," when the distinguishing marks between tympanitic and aqueous distention are so easily recognised.

Authors have described several distinct varieties of abdominal dropsy, and have named each according to its precise location; thus, *sub-cutaneous ascites*, in which the effusion takes place in a circumscribed cavity or sac in front of the abdominal muscles; *vaginal ascites*, arising from a puncture or other injury to the aponeurosis of the muscles, and causing effusion into the sheath of the muscle; *peritoneal ascites*, or effusion within the serous cavity, and in some rare instances, on the outside of the membrane; *hydatid ascites*, in which the water is enclosed in one or more thin vesicles; also dropsy of the *epiploon*, of the *mesentery*, of the *intestines*, of the *liver*, of the *spleen*, of the *gall-bladder*, and *encysted ascites*. This minute classification is, however, quite unnecessary for practical purposes, since ascites is often complicated not only with several of these varieties, but with hydrothorax, anasarca, and general dropsy. It is so very rare that we find the above-named organs affected separately, that we question the propriety of recognising in them distinct species of dropsy, although it is of some importance to be aware of the fact that these distinct effusions may occur.

Causes.—The most common causes of ascites are peritoneal inflammation, affections ofthe liver, and abuse of stimulating drinks. It may also proceed from venous obstruction, general debility in consequence of disease, loss of blood, and abuse of drugs.

Prognosis.—Our opinion respecting the probable termination of ascites will be determined by the following circumstances: old age, and a constitution impaired by previous disease or by excesses, must always render our prognosis unfavourable. Dropsies complicated with incurable functional derangement of the liver, or other vital organs, and venous obstructions, are for the most part beyond the reach of medicine. On the other hand, ascites consequent upon acute inflammation of the peritoneum, loss of blood, abuse of stimulants and drugs, and the debility arising from fevers and other acute diseases, may generally be set down as curable. When the malady occurs in young and naturally robust constitutions, our prognosis will be still more favourable, and in some instances, may afford grounds of encouragement in highly complicated cases.

Paracentesis abdominis, or *tapping*.—This operation should always be deferred as long as possible, in order to allow a reasonable time for the action of medicines. If, however, the accumulation becomes very great, and the symptoms are so urgent as to prevent all exercise, destroy rest in a sitting or recumbent posture, and thus serve to wear out the energies of the system, the operation should not longer be delayed. At the same time, the most judicious medicinal treatment should be perseveringly directed to both the proximate and remote symptoms of the malady. The operation of tapping is of itself simple, and entirely unattended with danger when proper precautions are used; but as the effusion usually takes place with much more rapidity, after the serum has been evacuated, than before, it will be apparent that *paracentesis abdominis* should only be had recourse to when the symptoms are particularly urgent.

3.—HYDROTHORAX, OR DROPSY OF THE CHEST.

Hydrothorax is either idiopathic, or symptomatic of some other organic disease. By far the most common source of the affection, and one which constitutes a serious complication, is organic disease of the heart. Another frequent cause of dropsy of the chest, is protracted pleuritic inflammation. Dropsy of the heart generally co-exists with hydrothorax, and it is for this reason that we so often find the pulse very irregular. The symptoms are most urgent during the night, after the patient has remained some time in the recumbent posture. The breathing becomes rapid, laborious, and grunting, with frequent sighing, sudden starting during sleep, anxious and distressed expression of countenance, face pallid and wax-like; small secretion of high-coloured urine; puffiness of the face and extremities; fulness of the chest; dull sound on percussion. Dyspnœa occurring from the slightest exercise, or from lying down, sudden starting up with fright, during sleep, dull sound on percussion, and irregular pulsations of the heart, will enable us to recognise the affection without difficulty.

Laennec assures us that hydrothorax accompanies many acute and chronic diseases, and that "its presence announces the approach of death, which it often precedes only a few moments." That these effusions do sometimes occur but a short period before death, from organic affections of the heart, and possibly of other organs, we entertain no doubt, for several cases have come under our observation, strongly corroborative of this fact.

As dropsy of the heart is so constant an attendant on hydrothorax, and the symptoms of each so constantly similate each other, it is unnecessary to enter into a separate description of this malady. When the effusion originates from an affection of the heart, or the pericardium, there will always be a predominance of those symptoms which characterize cardaic disease, and afford us a sure guide in forming our diagnosis.

Paracentesis thoracis may, in some instances, be resorted to with unequivocal advantage, for the relief of purulent collections within the thorax, but very rarely in hydrothorax. We have in two instances saved life by a prompt resort to this operation, where matter had accumulated in the chest, and the patients were at the point of death from suffocation ; but in thoracic dropsies, very slight encouragement can be offered from its performance, although in extreme cases it is not to be lost sight of, since recoveries have now and then taken place after the operation.

4.—OVARIAN DROPSY.

In this species of dropsy, the effusion takes place from the internal face of the membrane which encloses the ovarium. The swelling is first observed in the iliac region, in the form of a small elastic tumour, and unattended with pain, uneasiness, or constitutional disturbance. The enlargement generally progresses very slowly, extending upwards towards the kidney of the affected side, then crossing the abdomen to the opposite side, until ultimately it comes to occupy the whole of the abdomen. No serious inconvenience is experienced, until the tumour has attained such a size as to encroach upon the bladder, stomach, diaphragm, intestines, and the larger blood-vessels, thus giving rise to difficulty in urinating, sense of weight and uneasiness in the stomach, dyspnœa, colicky pains in the bowels, pains in the side and chest, diminution of the secretions, and œdema of the feet and ankles.

The tumour often remains stationary, and almost unnoticed for twenty or thirty years, when some sudden exciting cause will operate, and the swelling rapidly attain an enormous size.

The contents of ovarian tumours vary much in their character, being sometimes serous, sometimes albuminous, or purulent, or sebaceous, or fatty, or composed in part of organized structures. Dr. Clapp, Surgeon to Exeter Hospital, has recently reported a case in which the contents of the tumour "consisted of teeth, hair, bony deposit, some transparent masses of a cellular structure, (as examined by the microscope,) serum, sebaceous matter, and granular fat, which were contained in numerous small cysts. Teeth were found in all parts of the tumour, and were counted to the number of forty-three; some were contained in cysts, others were imbedded in the semi-transparent masses, and two or three were growing from the walls of the parent cyst. In one part, a few were imbedded in a mass of bone, bearing a strong resemblance to an upper jaw united in the mesial line."

Fluctuation can rarely be perceived in the swelling until it has attained a considerable size, but the location of the tumour, and the absence of pain or other unpleasant symptoms, will enable us to form a correct opinion in the early stage of the complaint.

5.—HYDROCELE, OR DROPSY OF THE TESTICLE.

A description of this disease is appropriate to surgery rather than to medicine, but as the usual method of cure serves to corroborate the truth of *similia similibus*, we make some allusion to the subject in this place.

The fluid of hydrocele is situated within the *tunica vaginalis testis*, commencing at the lower part of the scrotum, and gradually extending upwards until it reaches the external abdominal ring. The tumour is pyriform in shape, firm and elastic to the touch, and unattended with pain. It is only troublesome from its bulk and weight.

Much difficulty is sometimes experienced in distinguishing this disease from enlargements of the testicle, and in more than one instance, we have seen this gland destroyed by injudicious attempts to draw off water from chronic enlargements of the substance of the gland. Generally, dropsy of the testicle may be recognised by its peculiar elasticity, its lightness, form, its origin at the lower part of the scrotum, and its gradual extension upwards, and, lastly, by its transparency. By placing the swelling in front of a lighted lamp in a dark room, its character will be apparent from its transparency. But in some cases, from the great thickness of the *tunica vaginalis*, or the dark colour and density of the enclosed fluid, no transparency can be perceived. In these instances, we must be guided by the fluctuation, lightness, form, painlessness, and general history of the case.

Accumulations of fluid also occur within the membrane of the spermatic chord, constituting the disease known as *spermatocele*. This is a local affection, analogous in its nature to hydrocele.

Hydrocele occasionally occurs as a congenital disease, arising from an imperfect closure of the tunica vaginalis, and thus permitting the fluids of the abdomen to descend into its cavity.

Operation.—The most successful means of treating hydrocele is to evacuate the serum by means of the trochar and canula, and then to create a healthy medicinal action in the tunica vaginalis, with suitable injections. Merely drawing off the fluid is of no avail in effecting a cure, for the morbid condition of the membrane still remains, and the exhalents again fill up the cavity. Change then the morbid condition of the structure, and supersede it by a new and different action, and you will cure the disease. But it will be said, that by applying our remedies directly to the structure, we are obliged to create more inflammation than is necessary in order to effect a cure. Show us, then, how it can be effected by internal remedies, with any kind of certainty,—point us to a specific which will reach the case, and we will be of the first to adopt it.

The most reliable medicine we have ever used as an injection, is a mixture of one part of *tincture of iodine* to two parts of water. Let this be injected within the tunic, and remain for five or ten minutes, or until sharp pains are experienced in the gland and the spermatic chord, after which, carefully permit the fluid to escape from the canula. The use of *iodine* is not apt to be followed by sloughing, or undue inflammation, yet it almost invariably suffices to effect a permanent cure.

Other injections have been highly extolled by surgeons, as solutions of alum, zinc and lead, port-wine, &c., but they have too often failed in my hands to inspire me with confidence in their virtues, while uniform success has given me every reason to be satisfied with the *iodine.*

For an account of *hydrocephalus,* we refer to page 381 of this work.

Therapeutics.—It has been already observed, that dropsy is usually but a symptom of some other malady. Some of the causes which induce it, operate for a certain length of time, and then subside spontaneously, together with its symptoms of effusion. Amongst this class of causes may be placed, pregnancy, temporary pressure of tumours, intermittent fevers, and inordinate doses of arsenic.

Another class of causes which demands the gravest attention of the physician, consists of functional derangements of important organs, impaired constitutions, protracted debility from excessive loss of animal fluids, habitual intemperance, general cachectic habit of body, chlorosis.

The first indication of cure consists in removing, as far as is practicable, the cause of the dropsy. To do this successfully, it is necessary to enter into a minute investigation respecting the private habits of the patient, as well as the present symptoms. By this means, abuse of stimulants, of drugs, and excesses of all kinds, may be guarded against, which otherwise would have operated unfavourably during our curative efforts.

As a general rule, pure air, moderate exercise, an agreeable state of mind, a light and nutritious diet, and a sufficient quantity of warm clothing, should be enjoined. A change of location, or a sea-voyage, are often powerful auxiliaries in the treatment.

When dropsy depends upon incurable organic affections of the heart or liver, much may be done towards palliating the symptoms and protracting the patient's life, by an avoidance of all those causes which tend to aggravate the primary source of the disease, such as undue physical exertion, violent emotions and passions, &c.

Our efforts should also be directed, without cessation, towards changing the morbid condition of the membrane upon which the dropsy is dependent. Our remedies, therefore, must cover the remote as well as the proximate symptoms of the malady.

The remedies which we deem most valuable in the treatment of dropsical effusions, are, *apis mel., arsenicum alb., digitalis, china, hellebore, colchicum, dulcamara, asparagus, cantharides, scillæ, hyd. potassæ, mercurius, uva ursa, elaterium.*

In *ascites* and *hydrothorax*, the first trituration of the common honey-bee has proved astonishingly efficacious in our hands. The influence which this remedy exercises upon the urinary organs, as well as upon the peritoneum and pleura, is of the most prompt and decided character. In large doses, it causes a sense of fulness, constriction, or of suffocation in the thorax; difficult and anxious respiration; pain and tenderness of the abdomen, increased on pressure or by contact; symptoms worse in the horizontal posture; great secretion of urine, which is pale or of a straw colour, and deposites a reddish or brick-coloured sediment; frequent desire to urinate, and strangury.

Our method of preparing the medicine is as follows: Enclose the bees in a close vessel, and expose them to a temperature of 90° (Fahr.), until all moisture has escaped from them, and they are sufficiently dry to pulverize readily; we then triturate five grains of this powder with one hundred grains of sugar of milk for the usual period, and administer the trituration in grain doses from two to four times in twenty-four hours. Whether the *active principle* of this substance consists solely of the virus connected with the sting of the insect, or whether other parts possess active properties, we know not: our opinion, however, inclines to the former view.

We quote the following case, which occurred in the practice of Dr. Taft, of Hartford. The patient, a boy of twelve years of age, was attacked in July, 1849, with dysentery. After several weeks of medication under an allopathic physician, the acute symptoms subsided, and the evacuations gradually assumed their natural state, but there remained an unnatural fulness and tenderness of the abdomen, some difficulty of respiration, especially on assuming the recumbent position, a dry and harsh skin, and a materially diminished secretion of urine. Notwithstanding the persevering employment of the usual allopathic routine of cathartics, mercurials, and diuretics, the patient continued to grow worse, his abdomen became very much distended with serum, and very tender to the touch, or from even the pressure of the bed-clothes; the respiration became exceedingly laborious and difficult, obliging the sufferer to remain for a good portion of the nights in his chair; impaired appetite, an almost entire suppression of urine, emaciation, debility, small and rapid pulse, anxious expression, and other signs accumulated.

In this condition he came under the care of Dr. Taft, who administered *digitalis, arsenicum, dulcamara, mercurius, china, sulphur, hellebore*, as the symptoms appeared to indicate, but without any amelioration of the symptoms. In the meantime, the increasing difficulty of respiration, loss of rest, of appetite, and pain, had reduced the patient to so serious a condition, that I was called in council with Dr. Taft, in order to decide respecting the propriety of *paracentecis abdominis*. In consideration of the urgency of the symptoms, and the inefficiency of the remedies which had been used, I evacuated the effused fluid, amounting to sixteen pounds, and advised a second trial of *arsenicum* and *digitalis*. No effects, however, resulted from their use: the secretion of urine remained the same, the skin dry and husky, the abdominal effusion continued, the oppression of the chest, sense of suffocation and difficulty of breathing gradually increased, and signs of thoracic effusion began to be exhibited. Recourse was now had to the powder above alluded to, and with the most speedy and marked results. After two or three doses, a large quantity of urine was passed, and the symptoms were all ameliorated. After the remedy had been continued for two weeks, all traces of effusion disappeared, the appetite and strength began to improve, and the respiration became natural and easy. The patient continued to convalesce without any further unfavourable indication, until perfect health was restored. We have witnessed the effects of this remedy in two other cases of ascites, in one case of protracted general dropsy, and in one case of hydrothorax, and with the same favourable results. The powder of dried honey-bees has long been used as a remedy in dropsies by the aborigines of our country.

Arsenicum.—External indications.—General appearance of exhaustion and debility; pallid, waxen, and sickly countenance; cheeks, lips, and eyelids bloated and puffy, causing a marked alteration in the expression; dropsical swellings of the extremities and abdomen; mouth and tongue dry; tongue tremulous, red, bluish, or covered with a white coat; urine scanty, dark, and turbid or slimy; general coldness and dryness of the skin; general anasarca, with discharging vesicles on different parts of the affected surface; emaciation; dark coloured spots or blisters on different parts of the body; pulse small, feeble, and intermittent.

Physical sensations.—General sense of prostration; great nervous sensibility; paralytic feeling in the swollen parts; palpitation of the heart; turns of faintness; great difficulty of breathing when exercising, and after lying down; restlessness; anguish and oppression in the thorax and epigastric region; humming and roaring in the ears and head; bad taste in the mouth; loss of appetite; dryness of the mouth and tongue; thirst; tenderness of the abdomen on pressure; difficult and scanty alvine discharges, or slight diarrhœa; frequent desire to urinate, although but a small quantity is secreted; anxious, difficult, and rapid respiration while in the recumbent posture; heaviness and stiffness of the limbs and body; disturbed sleep, from impeded respiration, dreams; chilliness, alternating now and then with flushes of heat; diminution of sensation and power in the swollen parts; symptoms worse after eating, exercise, and lying down.

Mental and moral symptoms.—General mental uneasiness; fits of anguish and discouragement; disinclination to remain long in one position; apprehension that it is impossible to recover.

Digitalis.—External indications.—This remedy has been found curative in general anasarca, ascites, and hydrothorax originating in organic disease of the heart; also, paleness of the face; blue lips; swelling of the eyelids; coated tongue; scanty secretion of high-coloured urine; strong and visible pulsations of the heart; irregularity of the pulse; general paleness of the skin.

Physical sensations.—Vertigo; pressure in the forehead and vertex; ringing and hissing in the ears; want of appetite; flat taste in the mouth; thirst; pressure in the stomach; distention of the abdomen, with stitching pains; pressure at the neck of the bladder, with frequent desire to urinate; •throbbing in the chest; sharp stitches in the region of the heart; respiration anxious and difficult on walking or lying down; lassitude and diminished sensation in the inferior extremities; constant inclination to sleep; disturbed sleep; faintness.

Mental and moral symptoms.—Dulness of intellect; vertigo; forgetfulness; gloomy, peevish and indifferent.

Remarks.—Digitalis has proved most advantageous in dropsy consequent on organic disease of the heart, and in anasarca following scarlatina. Dr. Kurtz considers *digitalis* in decoction an excellent remedy in this complaint, and that the dilutions are useless.

Scillæ has been employed successfully in ascites and anasarca, by Hartmann, Currie, Noack and Trinks. Hahnemann did not entertain a high opinion of this substance as a remedy for dropsy, since its *primary* effect was to stimulate the kidneys and cause a copious emission of urine, while its *secondary* effect was always the opposite of this, viz., to suspend almost entirely the urinary secretion.

China.—External indications.—Countenance pale or sallow, sunken and sickly; general appearance of languor and debility; dropsical swellings in one or more parts of the body; enlargement and induration of the liver; emaciation; dryness of the skin, mouth and tongue; urine scanty, pale or dark coloured, and depositing a brick-dust sediment; coldness of the whole surface of the body; skin yellow; tremour in the limbs when attempting to walk.

Physical sensations.—Exhaustion arising from protracted acute diseases, from excessive loss of blood, and from abuse of drugs; pain and tenderness in the region of the liver; heaviness and pressure in the head, from within outwards; humming and ringing in the ears; bitter or flat insipid taste; loss of appetite; thirst for cold water and acids; oppression of the stomach and abdomen, especially after eating or drinking; constipation; respiration short, rapid, and at times suffocative; nights restless, and sleep disturbed by dreams; great sensitiveness to cold; frequent shuddering, when drinking cold water, or when exposed to the air; swelling and stiffness of the limbs; weariness of the limbs, with constant desire to change position; symptoms aggravated by contact, by eating, and at night.

Mental and moral symptoms.—Low spirited, nervous and irritable; sometimes anxious, gloomy and apprehensive of evil, and at other times indifferent, taciturn, and stupid; confusion of ideas; disinclination to physical or mental labour.

Remarks.—China will be found curative in those dropsies which are the result of simple debility which has been caused by loss of animal fluids, protracted illness, and abuse of cathartics. It may also be exhibited in anasarca consequent on attacks of intermittent and other fevers.

Hellebore.—External indications.—Face and lips swollen, and of a pale or yellowish cast; fluctuating swelling of the abdomen; general anasarca; spasmodic or convulsive movements of the head and limbs;

twitching of the eyelids; dulness and stupor; coldness of the surface; suppression of urine.

Physical sensations.—Throbbing or compressive pain in the head; oppression at the chest and stomach; cramplike pains in the abdomen; frequent desire to urinate, with scanty emission; loss of appetite; nausea, and pain in the stomach and bowels, followed by a loose alvine evacuation; short, dry cough; difficulty of breathing; sharp stitches in the head, chest and abdomen; heaviness and rigidity of the limbs; symptoms better in the open air.

Mental and moral symptoms.—Dulness of intellect; weakness of memory; painful stupefaction of the head; frequent sighing and moaning; giddiness on rising up, or walking; confusion of ideas.

Remarks.—Hellebore is particularly commended in dropsies complicated with intermittent fever, after the fever has been cured by *ars.*, also in anasarca and ascites of children, arising from scarlatina. It has effected prompt cures of dropsical effusions upon the brain, attended with convulsive motions of the head and limbs.

Colchicum.—*External indications.*—Face yellow and œdematous; dropsical swelling of the abdomen; œdema of the feet and legs; visible palpitation of the heart; skin dry and cold, or alternating with heat during the night; rapid and difficult respiration; pulse full and hard, or quick and small; urine scanty, and dark coloured.

Physical sensations.—Nausea, burning and icy coldness of the stomach; distention of the abdomen, with pressure and colicky pains; abdomen tender on pressure; loose and painful stools; oppression of the chest; palpitation of the heart; tearing pains and stiffness in the back, side, and limbs; drowsy during the day, but restless nights; symptoms worse during the night; also aggravated by mental labour.

Mental and moral symptoms.—Tendency to exaggerate symptoms; absence of mind; forgetfulness; dissatisfaction from slight causes.

Remarks.—This remedy is useful in dropsical swellings caused by atmospheric vicissitudes, excessive mental labour, sudden suppression of the perspiration, and in anasarca consequent upon scarlatina and measles.

Dulcamara.—External indications.—Face, abdomen, and limbs bloated; urine small in quantity, turbid, and fetid; heat and dryness of the skin; empty eructations.

Physical sensations.—Loss of appetite; dry mouth and tongue; great thirst for cold drinks; empty eructations after meals; nausea; restless, hot and feverish during the night; constipation; catarrhal symptoms; symptoms worse at night, better on motion.

Mental and moral symptoms.—Irritable and angry disposition; also scrofulous and phlegmatic constitutions, and great sensitiveness to cold.

Remarks.—Applicable in dropsies which have arisen from exposure to cold, and general anasarca consequent on fever and ague, scarlatina, and rheumatic fever.

Asparagus.—External indications. — Countenance pale, waxlike, and bloated; general expression of anxiety and distress; unusual fulness of the chest; coldness of the surface; suppression of the perspiration; urine scanty, straw-coloured, and offensive to the smell; visible throbbing of the heart, especially in the night; rapid, laborious, and sighing respiration; pulse feeble and irregular.

Physical sensations.—Feeble appetite; sense of fulness and oppression after eating or drinking; palpitation of the heart; great oppression of the chest, and rapid and difficult breathing, increased after being in bed for some time; sleep uneasy and disturbed by the oppressed respiration; constant inclination to be carried about in the arms by a child; great languor and disinclination to physical or mental exertion; stitching pains in the region of the chest.

Moral symptoms.—Fretful and peevish; disturbed by trifles; constant anxiety and apprehension.

Remarks.—In two cases of hydrothorax following acute attacks of peripneumonia, in children of three and five years of age, I have found *asparagus* of signal service after several other remedies had failed. One of these cases was complicated with an organic affection of the heart, and an almost entire removal of the cardiac symptoms followed the cure of the dropsy. We are quite convinced that this remedy will prove one of great efficiency in the treatment of hydrothorax and general dropsy, and we respectfully urge it upon the attention of practitioners. It should always be advised in dropsies as an article of food.

Cantharides is recommended in dropsy caused by tonic spasm of the neck of the bladder, and by perverted action of the kidneys. It may also be administered in effusion occurring in the last stages of acute and chronic diseases, as a palliative.

Hyd. potassæ is adapted to œdematous swellings resulting from the pressure of enlarged glands upon the veins. It has likewise proved highly beneficial when administered by me for the relief of dropsy arising from Dr. Bright's granulated kidney.

Mercurius has been praised as a valuable remedy in *chronic hydrothorax*, and in *ascites* from diseased liver. It is worthy of attention in ovarian dropsy, and effusions dependent upon enlargement of the spleen.

Uva ursa has cured several cases of *ascites* dependent upon abuse of stimulating drinks, and abuse of drugs. Its influence in restoring the urinary secretions is usually very prompt and satisfactory.

Other remedies which have occasionally been found useful in dropsies are, *elaterium, rhus tox., lycopodium, bryonia, ol. tiglii, potassæ nit., iodine, solanum nig. phosphorus, baccæ juniper.*

Administration.—In the treatment of acute dropsies, we advise the employment of the third to the sixth attenuations, and a repetition of the dose every two or four hours until effects from the medicine are apparent. In chronic dropsies, we employ the first to the third attenuations, and repeat once or twice in twenty-four hours until a suitable impression is produced.

CHAPTER XXIX.

CHLOROSIS.

General description.—Young unmarried females, of delicate lymphatic constitutions, slight figures, and highly impressible nervous systems, are by far most liable to attacks of chlorosis. In a majority of instances, it will be found that chlorotic girls have been remarkable, from birth, for delicacy of organization, daintiness of appetite, feebleness of digestion, and undue sensibility of the whole system. So long as this nervous sensibility is not overtasked, and no important causes operate to derange the delicate equilibrium upon which the proper operation of the functions depends, the individual enjoys passably good health; but when the period of puberty arrives, and nature calls for her monthly tribute from the vital fluid itself,—when new thoughts and new desires powerfully stimulate the system,—when, in fine, the important change of the whole organism, during the establishment of the catamenial function, occurs, then the frail balance is destroyed, the digestive, absorbent, and assimilative functions fail, and those symptoms which mark chlorosis make their appearance.

The disease sometimes attacks married females even when considerably advanced in years; and it has likewise been observed in girls of two or three years of age; but cases of these kinds are of extremely rare occurrence. Men of studious and sedentary habits, especially those who have never taken much exercise, have been occasionally subjected to it.

Chlorosis is more common in cold than in warm climates. This circumstance is attributable, in part, to the pernicious custom at the north, of keeping children a large portion of the year in close rooms, at a temperature of 75 to 80° Fahrenheit, thus preventing that free development of the body which would result from pure air and abundant exercise. Another reason offers itself in the fact, that persons of frail, nervous, and lymphatic constitutions, cannot often withstand the severities of a temperate latitude, without suffering more or less from disorders of the glandular and membranous structures.

Diagnosis.—The symptoms commonly observed during the forming stage of chlorosis are, derangement of the stomach and bowels, manifested by a pale and bloated appearance of the tongue, foul breath, partial or total loss of appetite, morbid craving for certain indigestible articles, like coal, chalk, clay, acids, pencils, etc.; torpid state of the bowels; tympanitic distention of the abdomen, accompanied with occasional griping pains; fæcal discharges, composed of crude and imperfectly digested substances, unnatural in colour and consistence.

Soon after the appearance of these symptoms, if the disease continues, the patient becomes listless, irritable, fond of solitude, and disinclined to bodily or mental exertion; the menstrual function becomes deranged; the face pale and tumid; the lips lose their colour; the eyelids are swollen and surrounded by a dark, greenish, or yellowish circle; emaciation commences; the debility and lassitude become more apparent; many nervous and hysteric symptoms manifest themselves; dyspnœa, and palpitation of the heart, or "fluttering about the præcordia," (*Hall.*) occur from ascending stairs, from rapid walking, or violent mental emotions; the patient is troubled with vertigo, giddiness, and ringing in the ears and head; sleep is disturbed by unpleasant dreams; the spirits become depressed, and the ambition and energy are superseded by apathy and indifference.

As the disease advances, all these symptoms become more strongly pronounced, and confirmed chlorosis is developed. The whole surface of the body now assumes a smooth and puffy appearance; the skin is dry, pale or yellowish, or lead-coloured; the muscles soft and flabby; the feet and ankles œdematous; the countenance very pallid and waxlike; the prolabia of a lilac colour; tongue clean, bloodless, and semi-transparent; conjunctiva of a clear white colour, or slightly tinged with blue; pulse feeble and somewhat rapid; occasional pains in the head, chest, stomach, side and abdomen; throbbing of the carotid arteries, perceptible to the sight and hearing; violent palpitation of the heart; dyspnœa, and "fluttering about the præcordia," after the slightest physical or mental exertion, and often during the night; catamenial secretion, superseded by a profuse leucorrhœal discharge; slight hacking cough on rising in the morning, and after exercise; frequent loose discharges from the bowels of a dark or black colour, and very fetid; extreme prostration of all the energies; marked derangement of the functions of the liver, kidneys, skin, and, indeed, of nearly every part of the body.

It is not an uncommon occurrence for some of these symptoms to assume a serious local aspect during the progress of the complaint, and thus present highly troublesome and dangerous complications. Marshall Hall enumerates these complications as follows:

First, pain in the head; second, cough and dyspnœa; third, palpitation of the heart; fourth, pain and tenderness of the side; fifth, pain and tenderness of the abdomen; sixth, constipation; seventh, diarrhœa; eighth, melœna; ninth, menorrhagia; tenth, tendency to hæmorrhagy; eleventh, purpura; twelfth, leucorrhœa; thirteenth, hysteric affections; fourteenth, œdema, anasarca, erythema nodosum.

It should be borne in mind, that all of these complications are nothing more than *symptoms* of the original malady, and are to be treated only as such. We have deemed it important to direct special attention to these symptoms, to guard the inexperienced physician against mistaking them for distinct and independent affections. When either of them is particularly prominent, the careless diagnostician is apt to form an incorrect opinion of the case. Thus, frequent pains in the chest, violent palpitation of the heart on the slightest exertion, and an irregular or intermittent pulse, have often caused medical men to mistake an ordinary chlorosis for an organic affection of the heart: so have the cough and dyspnœa, and the gastric and abdominal derangements, which accompany chlorosis, been mistaken for *phthisis pulmonalis* and *dyspepsia*.

We have included amongst the signs of chlorosis, suppression of the menses, but this is by no means an invariable symptom, as numerous cases are reported in which the catamenial secretion was perfectly natural and regular during the whole course of the complaint. We may safely infer, therefore, that it is not dependent on retention of the menses, as some writers have supposed.

We have already seen that many of the symptoms of chlorosis strongly resemble those of organic affections of the heart, pulmonary phthisis, dyspepsia, liver complaint, and dropsy, but a minute examination of the history and symptoms of each case, will always enable us to form a correct diagnosis. Thus, disease of the heart is attended with more pain, and more febrile disturbance, than chlorosis: the expression of the eyes, and the appearance of the prolabia and tongue are also widely different. The pure white colour of the conjunctiva, and the bilious and dark colour of the fæces, will sufficiently mark the disease from *chronic hepatitis*. From consumption of the lungs, we may also recognise it, by the absence of febrile exacerbations, the flushed cheek, the copious purulent expectoration, and the more general emaciation which occurs in the former. There are also numerous symptoms by which we may readily distinguish it from dyspepsia and dropsy.

Causes.—There are several points connected with chlorosis worthy of much consideration in a pathological and therapeutical point of view, viz.: first, the prominent gastric and intestinal derangement at the commencement of the malady; second, the small quantity of *crassimentum* in the blood; and third, the peculiar state of the *capillary* system, which gives rise to a hæmorrhagic tendency.

From the history of chlorosis, it appears that the stomach and bowels are the first structures to take on disordered action. For some time previous to the appearance of the pale, waxlike and tumid countenance, the puffiness of the eyelids, the loss of flesh, suppression of the menses, and other signs of confirmed chlorosis, we observe an impaired and delicate appetite, flabby and coated tongue, foul breath, imperfect digestion of the food, unnatural stools, and all those traits which characterize a feeble and imperfect performance of the digestive, absorbent, and assimilative functions. The symptoms which succeed are such as naturally result from such gastric and intestinal derangement.

These facts go far towards explaining the small amount of crassimentum contained in the blood of chlorotic patients. If digestion, absorption, and assimilation were normally executed, would not the blood receive its due proportion of crassimentum, and the muscles and integuments their appropriate supply of the red globules? The organs of the body are dependent for healthy action upon the stimuli of these red globules, which abound in oxygen, and serve to communicate to all parts of the organism its animal heat and consequent vitality. Whenever, therefore, any cause operates upon the digestive and absorbent organs in such a manner as to suspend their functions, the blood must fail of its due supply of red globules, and a derangement of all the organs ensue.

In some chlorotic patients, there is a peculiar tendency to *hæmorrhages* from the nose, the lungs, the stomach, and the uterus. Bloody discharges have been known from the head, the side, palms of the hands, and limbs, in instances assuming a periodical form, and taking the place of the menstrual discharge. On this account, the disease has been attributed by some to a laxity of the capillaries, and a consequent inability to exclude the red globules; but this relaxed condition of these vessels is owing to an absence of their healthy natural stimuli, the "oxygen carriers," rather than to any primary derangement in the capillary vessels themselves.

Other causes which may contribute to the development of chlorosis, in constitutions predisposed to it, are, close confinement in overheated and ill-ventilated apartments; studious and sedentary habits; protracted grief, anxiety, or fatigue; parturition, and its after effects; leucorrhœa; amenorrhœa; unsatisfied love; masturbation; prolonged continence; frequent hæmorrhages; crude and indigestible food; chronic inflammation of the intestinal canal; enlargement and inaction of the mesenteric glands.

Prognosis.—This will depend principally upon the

natural stamina of the patient, and the severity of the local symptoms. A frail and delicate constitution, a highly susceptible nervous system, a decided predisposition to glandular and membranous disease, and an inherent debility of the digestive apparatus, are circumstances calculated to render the prognosis unfavourable. Patients of this description are rarely able to withstand the important changes which the economy undergoes at the period of puberty, without serious local disease, and often organic degenerations of some vital part.

On the other hand, if the patient be of a naturally robust and sound constitution, even if the chlorotic symptoms are quite severe, we may generally predict an ultimate recovery. Here we may trace all the causes of the malady, and bend our efforts to their removal with a prospect of success, and thus restore the system to its original health and vigour; while a body which "has been sent into this breathing world before its time, but half made up," cannot be remodelled into one of "fair proportions" and vigour, by any resources of the physician, although much may be done towards prolonging life, and securing a moderately comfortable state of existence.

Pathology.—In the autopsical examinations of those who have died of chlorosis, the most notable signs of disease are found in the blood, the muscles, and the surface of the body. The blood of chlorotics appears to be deprived, in a great measure, of the red material, and its place supplied by a superabundance of serum. This condition exists to a greater or less degree during the whole course of the disease, and it is on this account that the muscles after death present a peculiarly pale and bloodless appearance, and the skin a palish yellow or waxlike tinge. Unnatural appearances are sometimes found in the chest and alimentary canal, in the form of enlargement and dilation of the ventricles of the heart, chronic inflammation of the lungs, the stomach, and the intestines, flabby and shrunken appearance of the liver and spleen, and unusual accumulations of serous fluid in the cavities, and in the cellular tissue.

Therapeutics.—In the treatment of chlorosis, we

find of especial importance, frequent exercise in the open air, either by gestation or moderate walking, a highly digestible and nutritious regimen, and fresh or salt water baths. It is very desirable that chlorotic patients pass their winters in warm and equable climates, that exercise in the open air may be taken with advantage at all seasons. This is necessary on account of their extreme sensitiveness to the cold, which is often a serious obstacle against exposure to the low temperature of northern winters. The influence of sea air is often very beneficial to patients accustomed to inland districts, and *vice versa.* Short sea-voyages may sometimes be advised in the warm summer months, but caution should be exercised that the changes be not too abrupt.

General bathing is also useful when properly employed. We should commence with tepid baths of fresh or salt water, and gradually diminish the temperature as the strength will admit, until an ordinary cold bath can be advantageously sustained. Sensitiveness to applications of cold water, will frequently deter the patient from a persevering use of this powerful remedy, and rigid directions should therefore be given upon the subject.

A regimen of the most digestible and nutritious meats, as mutton, venison, beef, game, and fowls, with rich animal soups, should be enjoined. Other nutritious food which the stomach will digest may likewise be eaten. Wine, porter, and Scotch ale may be used at meals if agreeable to the invalid. In a word, all of those articles which are calculated to enrich the blood with the red globules, may be resorted to.

The remedies best adapted to meet chlorotic symptoms are, *china, sulphur, nux vomica, pulsatilla, sepia, ferrum carb., platina, calcarea carb., conium, arsenicum, veratrum.*

China.—External indications.—Countenance pale or livid ; lips blackish and shrivelled ; mouth and tongue slimy ; skin yellowish ; œdematous swellings of the limbs ; fæces hard or soft, fœtid, mixed with undigested food, and of a dark or black colour ; offensive breath ; copious leucorrhœal discharge ; menstrual fluid scanty, and possessing but little colour ; suppression of the menses ; hæmorrhages from the nose, mouth and lungs ; pulse feeble and more rapid than natural ; general appearance indicative of an exsanguious and debilitated condition.

Physical sensations.—Vertigo, worse when walking or during motion ; humming in the ears ; disagreeable taste in the mouth, generally bitter or insipid ; unnatural appetite ; canine hunger ; pressure in the stomach after eating ; distention of the abdomen from wind or water ; morbid sexual desire, with nightly pollutions ; difficult and rapid respiration ; throbbing in the sternum ; palpitation of the heart ; constant inclination to move the limbs ; excessive sensitiveness of the whole nervous system, with general feeling of lassitude and debility ; great dread of cold air ; drowsiness during the day, but restlessness at night ; sleep disturbed by frightful dreams.

Mental and moral symptoms.—Nervous, irritable, dissatisfied, taciturn, out of humour ; indisposition to mental exertion ; suspicious of dislike and abuse.

Remarks.—*China* is eminently a specific in chlorosis accompanied or induced by profuse loss of animal fluids, from epistaxis, hæmoptysis, hæmorrhoids, masturbation, involuntary emissions of semen, leucorrhœa, and diarrhœa. It is one of our best remedies when the disease is uncomplicated by any serious local derangement, and where simple debility of the whole organism is its essential characteristic.

Sulphur. — *External indications.*—Face pale and bloated ; eyes surrounded by blue or greenish margins ; swelling of the upper eyelid ; glandular swellings about the neck and lower jaw ; mouth and tongue slimy ; fœtid breath ; distention of the stomach and abdomen ; discharges from the bowels brown, and mixed with undigested food ; acrid leucorrhœal discharge ; profuse expectoration ; short and rapid respiration ; œdema of the feet and ancles ; surface of the body covered with yellowish or brown spots.

Physical sensations.—Vertigo, dizziness and dulness in the head ; humming or roaring in the ears ; putrid or bitter taste in the morning ; loss of appetite ; craving for sweet or sour articles only ; pressure of the stomach and abdomen, and dyspnœa after eating ;

throbbing at the pit of the stomach, with faintness; morbid sexual desire, with feeble power of accomplishment; frequent involuntary emissions; menses too early and too profuse; burning leucorrhœal discharge; weakness of the chest when talking; short and difficult breathing on exercise, and on retiring to bed in the night; frequent palpitation of the heart; stitches and pains in the chest when moving the arms; coldness of the feet; drowsiness in the day time, but wakefulness and restlessness during the night; vivid dreams; night sweats; constant inclination to change position; general nervous irritation; sensitiveness to cold; internal coldness; lassitude and sensations of faintness,—all of which symptoms are without acute pain, and are mitigated by rest, and worse during motion.

Mental and moral symptoms.—Sadness, despondency, and inclination to weep without cause; ill humour, obstinacy, sadness, silence, and frequent moaning.

Remarks.—This medicine is advised for chlorotics of a lymphatic temperament, and those subject to frequent hæmorrhages. Also in chlorosis complicated with tuberculous ulceration of the lungs.

Nux vomica.—External indications.—Pale, yellowish, or clay-coloured complexion; sclerotica natural; cheeks and eyelids swollen; tongue white; fœtid breath; fæces fœtid and dark-coloured; discharges of blood from the rectum; moaning and incoherent muttering during sleep.

Physical sensations.—Vertigo, giddiness, or sense of intoxication; tenderness of the scalp; ringing and hissing in the ears; putrid, or bitter, or sour taste in the mouth; aversion to food of all kinds, and to tea and coffee; distention and oppression of the stomach after eating; nausea; bitter or sour eructations; throbbing sensation in the region of the stomach; flatulent distention of the abdomen, and colicky pains after eating or drinking; bleeding and painful hæmorrhoids; great irritability of the sexual organs, especially after waking in the morning; menses too early, and scanty; frequent turns of nausea and faintness during the menstrual flux; asthmatic respiration when walking, and at night in bed; palpitation of the heart after a generous meal; painful shocks in the præcordial region;

sensitiveness of the whole surface of the body; trembling in the limbs when walking; sleep disturbed by dreams, and so unrefreshing that the patient feels worse in the morning than in the evening; coldness of the feet.

Mental and moral symptoms.—Great sensibility to impressions; noise, bright lights, and strong odours intolerable; sad; anxious; quarrelsome: taciturn; apprehensive of death.

Remarks.—When chlorosis is preceded and accompanied by marked derangement of the alimentary canal, more particularly if the patient is of studious and sedentary habits, and has indulged freely in wines, coffee, or tobacco, *nux vomica* is indicated. Those who are naturally somewhat robust, and of a quarrelsome, ardent and vehement temperament, will be more benefited by it than persons of a mild and phlegmatic temperament.

Pulsatilla.—*External indications.*—Face pale; eyelids puffy; tongue white and covered with viscid mucus; pulsation at the pit of the stomach, perceptible to the pressure of the hand; stools loose, green, slimy, or bloody; acrid, thin leucorrhœa; scanty menstrual discharge; rapid breathing after eating or on lying down; coldness of the hands and feet.

Physical sensations.—Vertigo, resembling intoxication; bad taste in the mouth in the morning; loss of appetite; absence of thirst; nausea; frequent eructations of wind, tasting of the ingesta; beating and fluttering in the stomach; cutting pains in the side and abdomen; suppression of the menses, with general coldness of the body and nausea; asthmatic oppression of the chest after eating, or when lying on the side in the recumbent posture; pain and weakness in the small of the back; disagreeable pulsation of the arteries of the whole body; tremulousness; weariness; restlessness during the night; palpitation of the heart, after eating or talking.

Mental and moral symptoms.—Anxiety; disgust of everything; sullenness; whimsicalness; dissatisfaction.

Remarks.—*Pulsatilla* is adapted to chlorotics who have been irregular in menstruation, and are of a mild, timid, yielding, or sad disposition. When there is a total suppression of the menses, with much pain in the small of the back, frequent turns of chilliness, and absence of thirst, it will be indispensable, either by itself, or in alternation with some other medicine.

Sepia.—External indications.—Swollen and puffy appearance of the whole body; face puffy, pale or yellow; eyes surrounded by blue or greenish margins; tongue coated with a white fur; fœtid breath; menses too early and scanty; yellowish, watery, or mucus leucorrhœa; cold feet and hands when in bed in the evening.

Physical sensations.—Painful beating in the head; roaring in the ears; no appetite, or morbid desire for all kinds of food; absence of thirst; pain in the side and region of the liver; great sexual inclination; frequent dyspnœa; cough with mucus expectoration; stitches in the chest and side; weakness and stiffness in the small of the back; restless sleep, with frequent waking; skin tender and sensitive; sweat on walking; sensitiveness to cold air; weary, faint, and discouraged; symptoms worse at night and when at rest; palpitation of the heart, and intermittent pulse.

Mental and moral symptoms.—Weakness of memory; inability to think or reason; giddiness from walking; melancholy, discouragement, and irritability.

Remarks.—Chlorosis of nervous and delicate females, with a thin and delicate skin, and in whom menstruation has always been irregular, may be cured by *sepia.* If the patient sweats profusely when walking, and is particularly sensitive to cold air, this remedy is still more necessary.

In inveterate cases, attended with extreme prostration, trembling of the limbs, coldness of the surface, entire suppression of the menses, dropsical swellings, great difficulty of breathing, palpitation of the heart, loose state of the bowels, frequent and protracted turns of faintness, we may examine *ferrum arsen.* and *veratrum.* *Carb. calc.* and *platina* are indicated when the menses are too frequent and abundant. These medicines are especially adapted to young female organisms.

Administration.—The remedies should generally be

employed at the first, second and third attenuations, and a dose administered once or twice daily, until there is an apparent effect. No repetition should be allowed so long as the slightest amendment is perceptible.

CHAPTER XXX.

SCROFULA.

This disease was described by the Greeks under the appellation χοίραδες, from χοῖρος, hog, and by the Latins, (*scrophules* from *scropha*, female swine). This name had its origin in the well-known fact, that scrofula was a disease peculiar to the above named animal.

The blood of scrofulous subjects has been found to differ materially from that of healthy individuals. In the former, there is a superabundance of serum and a deficiency of the fibrous portion, and the solids which are generated from this blood are, in consequence, lax, feeble, and incapable of resisting exposure, fatigue and disease.

Scrofula is for the most part *hereditary*, but the physician is frequently presented with well marked cases of the *acquired* disease. The circumstances which favour the formation of an original scrofulous dyscrasia, are, cold and damp habitations, want of healthy and nutritious food, constant confinement at labour in close and ill-ventilated rooms, and finally, the use of *pork* in all its forms as a principal article of food. Respecting this last cause, we submit a few remarks: Since the time of Moses, a large portion of mankind have looked upon the swine as an impure animal, unfit for food. Its impurity consists of a disorder of a purely scrofulous character which is inherent and peculiar to it, and is constantly being developed, especially during confinement and subjection to the ordinary modes of feeding. Probably no animal is more filthy in its habits or more disgusting for its selection of food. Let the pork-eater contemplate an instant, the customary mode of rearing the domestic swine, and observe what offal, filth, putridity, scourings from everything foul and corrupt, constantly swell his diseased carcase. Let him see in the slaughter house, how often the internal organs and the surface of the vile carcases will be studded with tuberculous formations, or scrofula, and then return to pork "like a dog to his vomit," if he chooses.

A strong corroboration of our views is found in the fact, that in all of those countries where the swine is forbidden to be used as food, scrofula is almost unknown. The same law obtains with the Jews, who, abiding by the precepts of their religion, inhabit almost every climate and country, and are scarcely ever afflicted with scrofula.

It is absurd to argue that flesh contaminated with the scrofulous miasm, cannot communicate to the healthy body, after digestion, its morbid particles. The poison pervades every atom of the affected flesh, and no washing or digestion can destroy or banish the noxious quality.

Scrofula is most common in temperate latitudes, where the changes of temperature are abrupt, and where the atmosphere is much of the time loaded with moisture. The miasm operates upon almost every structure: glands, skin, ligaments, membranes, muscles, and bones, all succumb to its attacks.

Diagnosis.—The signs which are supposed to indicate the scrofulous habit, are, precosity of intellect; blonde hair; light complexion; blue eyes; soft and delicate cheeks; lips thick and red; "frequent swelling of the upper lip and nose;" edges of the eyelids red and prone to inflammation; scurf and eruptions on the scalp; large head; sensitiveness to cold; ends of the fingers blunt instead of tapering; muscles soft and flabby; strong inclination for venereal pleasures. These marks are generally supposed to characterize the scrofulous habit, but it has occurred to us to witness far more cases of scrofula in individuals the very opposite of this description; but whether or not this is the result of accident, or whether an erroneous impression has prevailed upon this subject, we know not.

Amongst the most common and simple manifestations of scrofula may be ranked, *glandular swellings of the neck.*

These enlargements occur very frequently during childhood, in the form of what are vulgarly termed, "kernels," on different parts of the neck. They are excited into activity by taking cold, by currents of air upon the neck, by measles, scarlatina, and whooping-cough, and either remain for a long time stationary and inactive, or run on to more violent inflammation and suppuration. These swellings sometimes attain a very large size, involving most of the glands of the neck, and remain in this condition for many years. More frequently, however, owing to injudicious allopathic treatment, the swellings are dispersed by external applications, the malady is forced to embody itself upon the lungs, and a fatal *phthisis pulmonalis* is the result. Another form in which scrofula developes itself, especially in children, is that of

Strumous, or Scrofulous Ophthalmia.

This disease is characterized by extreme sensitiveness of the affected organs to light. Even the slightest ray causes intense pain, and the little patient makes every effort to avoid exposure. During the inflammation an eruption usually makes its appearance on the cheeks, in the vicinity of the eyes, and which often extends to the very organs themselves, thus giving rise to troublesome and dangerous ulcers. These ulcers not unfrequently extend until the structure of the eye becomes so far impaired, that total blindness ensues.

The next form of scrofula to which we shall call attention, is that in which the joints become affected. The most important of these affections are the

White Swelling, (Arthrocace), and the Hip-disease.

The approach of these maladies is commonly gradual and insidious. Occasional pains are complained of in the diseased joint, after exercise; the motions of the limb gradually become impaired, and vague pains are experienced in the neighbouring joints, which sometimes induce the belief that healthy parts are the seat of the inflammation. As the disease advances, the ligaments, cartilages, and other structures composing the joint, become so much thickened by the inflammatory action, that the limb after a time becomes stiff, and the joint immovable. In some instances the inflammation is arrested at this point, the suppurative process is prevented, and a recovery by what is called *anchylosis* takes place. But in the majority of cases the disorder proceeds on to suppuration, the whole structure of the joint becomes involved in this action, a profuse discharge of matter takes place from the part, constitutional disturbance is manifest in the form of emaciation, debility, night-sweats, and other symptoms of hectic fever, and the patient soon succumbs. Scrofulous affections of the joints are very difficult of detection in their early stages. The pains are so vague and indefinite, as scarcely to attract attention; there is little or no swelling or discoloration over the disordered part; and there is no derangement of the general health which indicates that the organism is suffering under a serious malady. It is for this reason that the disease is allowed to make serious progress before its true nature is suspected. Like its near relative, the consumption, it strikes silently, but deeply and fatally.

Another scrofulous disease, common in infancy, is known as

Strumous Disease of the Mesenteric Glands.

The characteristic signs of this malady are, wasting of the limbs, pale and attenuated appearance of the skin, tumefaction and tenderness of the abdomen, sunken eyes, irregular state of the bowels, variable appetite, passage of partially digested food, general irritability. After the disorder is seated, the process of absorption is suspended, so that only a small amount of nutriment arrives at the blood, and the sufferer is soon reduced to that condition which medical men recognise as *marasmus*.

Although the mesenteric glands sometimes suppurate, yet much more frequently the victims to mesenteric disease die from actual starvation. The only hope of cure in these cases is, a detection of the malady at its onset, and the services of a thoroughly competent physician.

In a previous chapter, we have had occasion to treat of another, and perhaps the most dangerous form of scrofula, under the head of *phthisis pulmonalis*, or *tubercular consumption*, to which we refer the reader.

There are numerous other scrofulous affections of the different parts of the organism, as the brain, the liver, the skin, the spleen, and the spinal marrow. The admirable works of Hartmann and Schœnlein may be consulted with advantage with reference to this subject.

Hahnemann has included scrofula as a form of psora, but evidently on insufficient grounds. Psora is contagious, scrofula non-contagious. The matter of a psoric eruption is capable of communicating its similitude by inoculation; that of scrofula is innocuous when inoculated. Psora, in its specific development upon the skin, assumes the appearance of a vesicular eruption; scrofula makes its appearance in the form of extensive ulcers, abscesses, &c. The psoric miasm exercises its specific affinity upon the skin; the scrofulous miasm upon the glandular system. Psora is no respecter of persons, but attacks all constitutions, temperaments, and organizations alike; scrofula is supposed to select its subjects from those who are daintily formed, and possess some peculiarities of organization; psora is readily cured by antipsorics; scrofula always requires much time, and is often absolutely incurable by any course of treatment. Psora cannot be artificially *acquired* by any particular mode of life, or any particular food; with scrofula it is the reverse. Finally, the development of the psoric miasm, when it is clear and apparent, is always specific and uniform, viz., in vesicular eruptions of a peculiar appearance upon the surface, and the malady is unequivocally contagious; while the development of the scrofulous miasm is subject to very great variations, but for the most part attacking the glands, rather than the skin, and decidedly non-contagious.

Causes.—The scrofulous habit is, in most instances, inherited. In its hereditary subjects we may notice from birth a radical unsoundness of constitution, an irritability, sensitiveness to slight exposures, proneness to catarrhal difficulties, and an inability to resist diseases, which is not apparent in healthy children. The *acquired* scrofulous habit is generally amongst the poor, who are ill-fed, clad, and housed. We have before alluded to the causes which especially induce this variety of the disease; they are also the chief *exciting* influences of the *hereditary* dyscrasia. Atmospheric vicissitudes, abuse of stimulants, excesses in venery, onanism, intestinal irritation, excessive mental and physical occupation, scarlatina, measles, abuse of mercury, iodine, and other drugs which unduly stimulate the glandular system, also excite the latent disorder.

Therapeutics.—It has been observed that scrofulous persons are peculiarly sensitive to *cold*, and that abrupt changes from heat to cold, in a moist region, are especially calculated to call into active operation the latent malady. For this reason it behooves those who are liable to the affection, whether by hereditary or acquired predisposition, to dwell, if possible, in a warm and equable climate. When the lungs become affected, this course will often be necessary, in order to save life. In all scrofulous diseases, too much stress cannot well be laid upon the importance of a mild, dry, and uniform temperature.

The food of scrofulous subjects should always be of the most nutritious character, in order that a due proportion of fibrine may be introduced into the blood. Fresh meats, like beef, mutton, venison, fowls, and veal, should constitute the principal articles of food; and bread, rice, and other farinaceous substances, should be made to take the place of watery and succulent vegetables. Porter, ale, and light wines may also be used moderately with advantage.

Much exercise in the open air is also essential. In taking exercise, it is of the utmost importance that the mind should be agreeably occupied, for if we walk or ride as a task, we shall obtain very little benefit.

Bathing, both in fresh and salt water, is also a

means of securing a healthy action of the skin, and of imparting tone and vigour to the whole system.

The clothing should always be adapted to the season, and in temperate and cold latitudes we strongly advise the buckskin wrapper, to be worn over a thin linen, silk, or Canton flannel under-shirt. We commend the use of these garments, during the winter, from personal experience.

The remedies most deserving of confidence in the treatment of scrofula, in its various forms, are, *sulphur, hepar sulph., mercurius, iodine, baryta, dulcamara, conium, belladonna, lycopodium, sepia, calcarea carb., rhus tox., aurum mur., china, ferrum iodid., merc., oleum jecoris aselli.*

Sulphur.—External indications.—Scrofulous ulcers on different parts of the surface; humid eruptions behind the ears; purulent discharges from the ears; scrofulous ophthalmia of children, with eruptions about the eyes, and ulcers on the cornea; chronic enlargement of the tonsils; enlarged ovaria; swelling of the axillary glands; swelled nose; frequent nose-bleed; swelled upper-lip; swelling of the glands under the lower jaw; enlargement and suppuration of the inguinal glands; swelling of the posterior cervical glands; white swelling of the knee; emaciation.

Physical sensations.—Chronic inflammation of the eye-lids; scrofulous ophthalmia, attended with great intolerance of light, and sense of fulness and distention of the lids; pulmonary cough, with sticking pains in the chest, and copious purulent expectoration; inflammation and pain in the knee and hip-joints; itching pimples upon the scalp, and pain at the roots of the hairs; stitching pains in the ears and in the parotid glands; painful swelling of the upper lip and wings of the nose; pain in the region of the liver after exercise; pain in the abdomen on pressure, and in the inguinal glands; sensation of weariness and fatigue in all the limbs; want of vitality; sensitiveness to cold; pains worse during cold weather.

Mental and moral symptoms.—Despondency alternating with gayety; irritable, indolent, and discontented.

Administration.—One grain of the third trituration every twenty-four hours, until a response is manifest.

Rhus tox.—*External indications.*—Tinea capitis; soft tubercles on the hairy scalp; scrofulous ophthalmia, with photophobia, and an eruption about the eyes; chronic swelling and induration of the parotid gland, the axillary, and other glands; enlargement of the bones; herpetic and moist or dry scurfy eruptions in different parts of the body; swelling and other signs of inflammation in the hip and knee joints.

Physical sensations.—Pain in the hip joint, increased on pressing the trochanter major, and attended with shortening of the limb, and alternating pains in the knee; pains of white swelling, and scrofulous affections of the ancle joint; scalp painful to the touch, or from moving the hair backwards; inflammation and tenderness of the edges of the eyelids; eyes sensitive to light; eyelids itch and feel swollen; crusty eruption in the nose, and about the mouth; repugnance to bread and other food; stitches in the side; short, anxious, and painful cough; oppression of the chest; glandular swellings painful when touched; stiffness and lameness of the limbs; very sensitive to the open air; pains worst during inaction, or in the cold air.

Mental and moral symptoms.—Ill humour; languor; disinclination to all mental or bodily exertion.

Administration.—A drop of the third dilution each day, as long as may be deemed necessary.

Iodine.—*External indications.*—Enlargement of the cervical, parotid, thyroid, and tonsil glands; scrofulous inflammation of the knee, with swelling, heat and redness; elongated and enlarged uvula; induration of the os uteri; glandular indurations in different parts of the body; rough and dry skin; general emaciation; with hectic appearance.

Physical sensations.—Catarrhal affections of the mucous membranes depending on scrofula; swelling and pain in the liver; inflammation in the knee, with stitches and burning, and increased pain on motion of the joint or from pressure; contraction of the œsophagus from enlargement and inflammation of the glands and mucous membrane, with stitching pains during deglutition; enlarged mesenteric glands; tumid abdomen, with pains on pressure; swelling and pain in the bronchial glands; glandular swellings about the neck and axilla, painful, especially on pressure; itching pimples on the arms and chest; general debility; hectic fever; pains aggravated by exercise, by contact and by warmth.

Mental and moral symptoms.—Nervous irritability and increased sensitiveness to external impressions.

Administration.—Same as *rhus.*

Baryta mur.—*External indications.*—Chronic induration of the cervical glands; scrofulous eruptions and ulcerations; tinea capitis; enlargement of the liver, of the testes, and of the mammæ; chronic inflammation of the eyelids.

Physical sensations.—Itching eruptions of the scalp; general emaciation and debility; scrofulous disease of the throat, aggravated after every cold; scrofulous affections of the ears, attended with throbbing and itching, and discharge of purulent matter; inflammation and suppuration of the tonsils; pains in the affected joints and in the long bones; liability to sore throat after every cold; disease of the mesenteric glands in children; pains mostly on the left side, when sitting, and relieved by exercise in the open air; adapted to old men and young children.

Mental and moral symptoms.—Imbecility; absence of mind; impaired intellectual powers.

Administration.—The second or third attenuation may be selected—a dose daily—until the requisite impression is produced.

Dulcamara.—*External indications.*—Moist and suppurating herpes, forming crusts, or scurvy, bran-like eruptions; swellings of the cervical and submaxillary, and inguinal glands; swelling of the calf of the leg; emaciation; scrofulous inflammation of the eyelids.

Physical sensations.—Pains in the enlarged glands, particularly on motion; great susceptibility to cold; pains in the joints on exposure to cold; pains worse during rest; paralysis of the upper eyelids; phthisis pulmonalis, before the tubercles commence softening; pulmonary symptoms brought on by repeated colds; pains in the chest; febrile symptoms; lassitude; bruised sensations.

Mental and moral symptoms.—Disposition restless, angry, and quarrelsome.

Administration.—In the same manner as *baryta.*

Conium mac.—*External indications.*—Swelling, induration and suppuration of the external glands; malignant scrofula; caries of the bones; scrofulous photophobia; diseased mesenteric glands in children; enlargement and induration of the liver and pancreas.

Physical sensations.—Scrofulous swellings, which evince a disposition to run into scirrhous degenerations; pains in the bones, and in the malignant ulcerations; inflammation, swelling and pain in the ovaries; painful swellings of the uterus; pain in the region of the liver, when walking; purulent expectoration from softened tubercles; intolerance to light, in consequence of scrofulous opthalmia; dull pain in the knee when stepping; bruised and sore feeling in the calves of the legs; pains worse during rest, and in the night.

Mental and moral symptoms.—Dulness of intellect; want of memory; irritability.

Remarks.—For indurated glands, Dr. Johannsen asserts, that "*conium,* in the second dilution, stands highest as a remedy, and next to it, *mercurius sol.*"

Administration.—We advise the third attenuation—a dose daily until its effects are apparent.

Belladonna. — *External indications.* — Glandular swellings, with suppuration; ulcers; emaciation; inflammation and swelling of the bones; eyelids inflamed; ulcers upon the cornea; photophobia; swelling of the lips, nose, tongue, uvula, tonsils; bleeding at the nose; swollen and spongy gums.

Physical sensations.—Inflammation and pain in the enlarged glands, and in the periosteum and bones; diseased mesenteric glands, with atrophy; inflammation of the eyes, with heat, redness, and great intolerance to light; pain in the ball of the eye; double vision; roaring in the ears; painful swelling of the parotid gland; soreness of the throat; impeded deglutition; lameness of the limbs when moved; smarting and burning pains in the hip joint, increased by contact or motion, and during the night; painful ulcers on the skin; sensitiveness to cold air; adapted to the scrofulous affections of children and females of a mild temper.

Mental and moral symptoms.—irritability; amorous, nervous, excitable, talkative.

Administration.—Same as *conium.*

Lycopodium.—For the scrofulous dyscrasia, and especially where the periosteum, bones, and cervical glands are affected. This remedy is adapted to lymphatic constitutions.

Sepia will be found an efficacious remedy in scrofulous females, who are troubled with irregularities in the menstrual functions. It has been employed successfully in indurations of the uterus, corrosive leucorrhœa, and in pulmonary phthisis with profuse purulent expectoration.

Calcarea carb.—According to Hahnemann, carbonate of lime is indispensable in those cases where the menses appear too early and are too profuse. It is also appropriate in young persons of scrofulous habits. In children presenting the usual marks of the scrofulous dyscrasia, it is one of our most valuable remedies. It is highly recommended likewise in the scrofulous ophthalmiæ of children, particularly after ulcers have formed on the cornea. Also in marasmus arising from diseased mesenteric glands, it is an admirable remedy in alternation with iodine. Scrofulous eruptions and ulcers of children often yield to this remedy, after *sulphur*, *mercurius*, and *hepar sulphuris* have been used in vain.

Hepar sulphuris is adapted to the cure of scrofulous tumours in a state of suppuration, to *scrofulous ophthalmia* with profuse lachrymation, and much mucous discharge from the meibomian glands, and in *coxalgia*, after a purulent discharge has occurred. This medicine is proper for scrofulous and lymphatic constitutions.

Mercurius.—This remedy is advised by Hahnemann in scrofula combined with syphilis. The glandular inflammations will be characterized by a diffused redness, much swelling, and gnawing, stinging or darting pains, worse at night in bed. It should be consulted in affections of the bones, the joints, the eyes, and in eruptions and ulcers upon the surface. The following preparations of *mercurius,* we especially commend in scrofula: *merc. sol., iod. merc.,* and *merc. præcip. rub.*

Aurum mur., ferrum and *china* are worthy of consideration in protracted and obstinate cases, where the strength of the patient has become much impaired, and but little impression has been made by the previous remedies.

Hartmann observes that he has "derived essential benefit from *oleum jecoris aselli* in every form of the disease, especially in the precursory stage, when no particular organ was affected: the patient looked pale, emaciated, the muscles became flabby, the patient showed an aversion to meat and vegetables, and wanted to eat bread and butter all the time. I gave it in teaspoonful doses, morning and evening, almost always with success. In scrofulous affections of bones it likewise proved useful, but less so in other forms of the disease."—(*Hartmann's Chronic Diseases,* vol. iii., p. 54.)

Dr. J. H. Bennett, of London, has found the *cod liver oil* (*oleum jecoris aselli*) of great service in scrofulous cases characterized by general or local atrophy. But in scrofulous affections in which the general health and strength are unimpaired, and the digestive functions are not deranged, Dr. B. advises *iodine.* We have employed the oil in doses of a drachm, three times daily, with eminent success, in almost every form of scrofula.

For scrofulous ulcers with callous edges, and fistulas, *silicea* alone, or in alternation with *phosphorus, acid phos.* and *conium,* was found by Dr. Johannsen most useful.

When the ulcers are *greenish* and *offensive, carbo veg.* or *mercurius dulc.,* is advised.

In scrofulous ophthalmia, indurated glands, and diseases of the bones, *arsenicum, conium, mercurius sol., carbo animal., hepar sulph,* and *aurum,* are the best remedies.

"*Arsenicum* is one of the most important remedies in scrofula, for removing indurations of the glands, and deformities of the bones, for regulating the discharges from the bowels, and for restoring the skin to a healthy state. Also, in scrofulous ophthalmia it is of great service." (*Dr. Johannsen. Homœopathic Journal,* vol. 1, No. 11.)

Administration.—As a general rule, the first to the third attenuations should be selected, and the doses repeated once or twice daily, until a satisfactory impression is produced upon the affected structures.

CHAPTER XXXI.

AFFECTIONS OF THE EYE AND ITS APPENDAGES.

SECTION I.

The eye, in the immediate vicinity of the brain, connected with this organ by the optic nerve, endowed with numerous delicate membranes, nerves and blood-vessels, with its lens, its aqueous and vitreous humours to conduct and modify the luminous rays in their passage to the retina,—all disposed in the most consummate manner to serve the end designed,—may be looked upon as a most complex and perfect optical instrument. It is the mirror in which are reflected the various *tableaux* of external objects, for the satisfaction of the soul within, causing it to respond to such impressions so that the most indifferent spectator may look into its depths, and see the manifestations of the perceptive faculties.

The impressions of external objects, derived through this medium, constitute our principal sources of knowledge and of pleasure. Without this faculty, we learn only by vague comparisons, suggested by touch, taste, smell, and hearing, by which all our conceptions are more or less perverted and indefinite. It is through the medium of vision, that the child first acquires a just idea of colours, distance, proportion, magnitude, &c., and begins to reason and act by a comparison of his different impressions. It is through the eye alone that we appreciate the infinite variety of expression in the "human face divine," and become incited to sympathy, love, pity, charity, admiration, fear, hope, hate, anger, and other emotions; that we enjoy the beauties and sublimities of nature ; that we become acquainted with the wonders of art and science ; and, by contrasting objects with each other, that we are able to enrich our minds with whatever elevates us in dignity of being and capacities of happiness.

The eye is, perhaps, more delicate of organization, and yet, from its situation, more exposed, than any other, to external causes of disturbance. How important then that we obtain accurate ideas relative to its structure and functions, and the disorders to which it is liable, that we may be able to protect it when well, and promptly to cure it when diseased.

In our description of the diseases of the eye and its appendages, we shall adopt this classification :

First. Affections of the tunica conjunctiva, or outer covering of the eye, including—First, *acute ophthalmia;* second, *chronic ophthalmia;* third, *purulent ophthalmia ;* fourth, *gonorrhœal ophthalmia ;* fifth, *strumous or scrofulous ophthalmia ;* sixth, *granulated lids;* and, seventh, *opacity of the cornea.*

Second. Affections of the deeper seated structures of the eye, including—First, *inflammation of the cornea ;* second, *iritis ;* third, *amaurosis ;* fourth, *hydropthalmia, or dropsy of the eye ;* fifth, *cataract;* and, sixth, *fungus hœmatodes, and cancer of the eye.*

Third. Affections of the appendages of the eye, including — First, *hordeolum or stye ;* second, *entropium,* or *inversion of the eyelids ;* third, *ectropium,* or *eversion of the eyelids ;* and, fourth, *fistula lachrymalis.*

This classification is deemed sufficient for all practical purposes, and much less liable to lead to confusion than one more extended. We shall point out the prominent affections of each structure of the eye, and endeavour, in enumerating the causes, to make the reader acquainted with every thing of interest connected with each particular subject.

Ophthalmia may be *primitive* or *symptomatic,—acute* or *chronic,*—and its causes, *local* or *constitutional.* Its manifestations also may be confined to the eye itself, or sympathetic symptoms may declare themselves in the head, stomach, and other parts of the economy. These developments will depend much upon the constitution, temperament and habits of the patient, the causes which have operated to produce the malady, the severity of the inflammation, and the tissue affected. It is worthy of note, however, that when a particular tissue of one eye is diseased, the corresponding structure of the other eye is exceedingly prone to a similar morbid action, from sympathy. This may be accounted for from the fact that the eye receives its nerves and blood-vessels directly from the brain, by which the sympathetic communication between the two organs is rendered very rapid and intense.

Finally, we direct special attention to the therapeutical connection existing between morbid conditions of particular tissues, and primitive medicinal symptoms, upon the same tissues, in health. We have already a few specifics which impress certain structures only, and we trust that the time is not distant when medicines will be discovered capable of acting surely and specifically upon each separate part of the eye or its appendages. Fortunately, a few of our drugs have a wide range of action upon the visual organs, so that we shall be able, even now, to find specifics which correspond with almost any morbid symptoms that may present themselves.

SECTION II.

AFFECTIONS OF THE TUNICA CONJUNCTIVA.

ACUTE OPHTHALMIA.

Diagnosis.—One of the first *local* signs of simple inflammation of the conjunctiva, is an injection with *red blood*, of a number of the vessels which naturally admit only a *white fluid.* This gives to the eye that slight appearance of redness and distention of vessels, which characterizes the first stage of acute ophthalmia. The eye now becomes more than usually sensitive to light, smoke, and dust ; tears are easily excited ; a feeling is experienced similar to that produced by particles of sand or dust lodged under the upper eyelid, causing the patient to constantly rub the eye in order to remove what he supposes to be a foreign substance; a sense of heat, fulness, stiffness and tingling is felt in the globe and edges of the lids; and slight pains begin to shoot through the eye. At first but a part of the vessels become injected, but as the inflammation increases, the anastomosing branches become involved, until finally the whole eye presents a uniform appearance of deep redness, swelling, and turgidity. At this period of the disease, the functions of the eye are all more or less perverted; there are acute pains in the ball; great intolerance to light; a profuse secretion of scalding tears; disordered vision; agglutination of the lids in the morning from matter secreted by the meibomian glands; intense pain on moving the lids; distressing sense of distention, weight, and rigidity of the whole organ, and diminished power of motion.

The symptoms thus far detailed, are purely *local* and include all of the symptoms which are present from the commencement to the termination of many cases of simple acute ophthalmia. But in the majority of instances, the whole system sympathises with the local affection, and we are presented with the following additional train of *constitutional* or *sympathetic* symptoms: acute pains extending from the eye into the temples and anterior portion of the brain; slight chills, followed by accelerated circulation and respiration; hot and dry skin; determination of blood to the head and face; nausea; loss of appetite; lassitude; general irritability; physical weakness; and other indications of febrile excitement.

During the progress of the inflammation, a peculiar appearance is often observed above the cornea, in the form of a circular elevation termed *chemosis.* This arises from the precaution which nature has taken to protect the cornea from the injurious effects of ophthalmia, by fixing the conjunctiva more firmly upon this portion of the globe, than upon the other parts. By this peculiar construction, the distention of vessels and effusions resulting from violent inflammations, are principally manifested in the first instance, without the cornea, and thus in some measure protecting this important part from the injury it might otherwise sustain.

The severity of the symptoms will depend much upon the constitution of the patient, and the nature of the exciting cause. The disease may terminate in a cure, without any marked alteration in the appearance of the eye, or it may result in *effusion*, causing an elevation of the conjunctiva above the cornea; or in *adhesion* of some portion of the conjunctiva covering the cornea, and giving rise to those appearances known as *nebula, albugo, leucoma*, and *opacity;* or in *suppuration*, from the surface of the conjunctiva; or in *ulceration* of some part of the cornea; or in *sloughing* of the cornea. These appearances will be more particularly described in our article on *opacity of the cornea.*

Causes.—Undue exposure to intense heat or cold; inordinate use of the eyes by a glaring or dim light; the application to the eyes of irritating foreign substances; mechanical injuries; extension of contiguous inflammations to the eyes; sudden changes of temperature; metastases of gout and rheumatism.

Prognosis.—If appropriate remedies are administered in the early stage of the complaint, and before any organic lesion has taken place, we may generally predict a speedy and perfect cure. On the contrary, if effusion, ulceration, or the adhesive process of the conjunctiva over the cornea, has commenced, we must be more guarded in our prognosis, for under these circumstances the malady often ends either in impaired vision, or a total loss of sight.

Much information may be derived respecting the probable termination of the malady, by a careful examination of the causes which have been, or may still be in operation, and of the temperament and constitution of the patient. For example, an individual of an irritable and nervous temperament, and of a delicate organization, may be affected with the most violent local and constitutional symptoms for a considerable period, without endangering the integrity of the eye; while a sanguine, plethoric, and robust patient might experience no constitutional effects, and but moderate local symptoms, and yet speedily suffer from serious disorganization of one or more of the tissues. Much will also depend upon our ability to remove all causes which may have conduced to the complaint, and to enforce upon our patients the necessary restraints and attention during the treatment.

Therapeutics.—The first therapeutical indication is to confine the patient to an apartment in which the light is mostly excluded. It must be remembered that this natural stimulus of the healthy eye, becomes, during an acute inflammation of its tissues, a powerful irritant—a morbid agent capable of aggravating and perpetuating the disease. As the inflamed stomach cannot tolerate its natural stimulus, the food, so the inflamed eye cannot endure with impunity, its ordinary stimulus, the light. Perfect cleanliness should be enjoined, and an exclusion of all dust, vapours, smoke, and bright rays of light. In making applications to the eye, great care should be taken to avoid compression of the inflamed part, in order that the circulation may remain unobstructed, and that sufficient air may be admitted to the parts.

Respecting *local applications,* we entertain the most exalted opinion of *cold water.* This may be applied by means of a few folds of soft linen cloth, which may be frequently dipped in the water, and after being partly wrung out, laid loosely over the eye and the surrounding parts. This application may be persisted in at suitable intervals, until the active symptoms have subsided, and a state of sub-acute inflammation occurs, when recourse may be had, if deemed necessary, to collyria of a slightly stimulating character, like weak solutions of *zinc, nit. argenti, lead,* or *copper.* In making use of these last named articles, we should only employ a strength sufficient to create a decided *medicinal* action, and omit the application when this effect is apparent, and so long as the consequent reaction or amendment continues ; for *external* remedies, when judiciously employed, are subject to the same laws of *primary* and *secondary* action, as when administered *internally.* We shall say more upon this subject under *chronic ophthalmia.*

The medicines to which we call particular attention are, *belladonna, aconite, arsenicum, sulphur, digitalis, euphrasia, pulsatilla, arnica, spigelia, mercurius sol., graphite, lycopodium.*

Belladonna. — *External indications.* — Redness, swelling, and protrusion of the ball of the eye; chemosis; swelling of the lids; frequent discharge of hot and salt tears, or dryness of the eyes; spasmodic closure of the lids; flushed cheeks; throbbing of the carotid and temporal arteries; full and rapid pulse; hot and dry skin.

Physical sensations.—Great intolerance to light; pain, burning, and smarting in the eyes; heaviness, pressure and throbbing in the ball and lids; sharp pains in the orbits, extending into the brain; tearing pains in the eyes from within, outwards; dimness and obstruction of vision; spasmodic sensations in the eyes.

Mental and moral symptoms.—Nervousness; irritability; disinclination to mental labour.

Remarks.—*Belladonna* is suitable in ophthalmia occurring in sanguine and irritable persons, from congestions of blood to the eyes in consequence of exposure to cold, excessive use of the eyes, metastases of rheumatism and gout. It is particularly useful when constitutional symptoms show themselves in the form of acute or throbbing pains in the head and temples, hot skin, rapid pulse, flushed cheeks, dilated pupils, and perverted vision.

Aconite.—*External indications.*—Vessels of the conjunctiva injected with red blood; lids red and swollen; chemosis; dilation of the pupils; lachrymation, worse on the slightest exposure to light, dust, or smoke; photophobia; flushed cheeks; hard and rapid pulse; hot and dry skin, and other febrile symptoms.

Physical sensations.—Very great intolerance to light; pressing, stinging, burning, or exceedingly acute pains in the eyes; eyeball feels bruised, and pressed into the orbit; stinging and smarting of the lids; eyes very hot, and filled with scalding tears, or preternaturally dry; pressure, or sharp, beating, or stinging pains in the head and temples; impaired vision, as from a gauze before the eyes; general febrile disturbance.

Mental and moral symptoms.—Much mental excitement; fear and apprehension in regard to the probable result of the case.

Remarks.—This remedy is particularly called for when the local inflammation is very intense, and the constitutional symptoms run high. It operates most happily in plethoric, bilious, and sanguine individuals, who are subject to determinations of blood to the face, head, and lungs. It is appropriate in ophthalmiæ caused by colds, by the introductions of foreign substances into the eye, and by rheumatism and gout.

Arsenicum. — *External indications.* — Conjunctiva much congested, and of a dark-red colour ; œdematous swelling of the lids ; profuse lachrymation ; tears hot and corrosive to the cheeks ; lids dry and red ; eyelids partially closed from the great swelling ; nightly agglutination ; spasmodic movements of the lids, on exposure to light ; ulcers on the cornea.

Physical sensations.—Sensation as if sand had become lodged in the eye ; tearing, burning, or stinging in the ball and lids, aggravated by motion, or on exposure to light ; throbbing in the eyes when lying down ; impaired vision ; weakness, weariness, and tremour of the lids ; great intolerance to light ; constant inclination to rub the eyes.

Mental and moral symptoms.—Mind weakened, and whole system rendered nervous and irritable, by pain and suffering.

Remarks.—*Arsenicum* is applicable to those cases which arise in weakly and nervous constitutions, where the pains are severe, and the disease is unusually obstinate. In this variety of ophthalmia, the local and sympathetic symptoms are very troublesome, but there is much less danger of serious organic lesions than in most other forms of the malady. It is advised in ophthalmia arising from cold, rheumatism and gout.

Sulphur.—*External indications.*—Injection of the vessels of the conjunctiva ; redness and swelling of the lids ; lachrymation, or preternatural dryness of the eyes ; morning agglutination of the lids ; photophobia ; eyes swollen and prominent ; cornea dim ; lids œdematous ; distention of the conjunctiva from effusion.

Physical sensations.—Pressure of the eyeballs, worse on moving them ; pressure, burning, and itching of the lids ; intolerance to the rays of the sun ; twitching of the lids ; trembling of the eyes ; painful dryness of the margins of the lids; bruised feeling of the eyes, on motion; sensation of sand under the upper lid, on motion; dimness of sight.

Mental and moral symptoms.—Sensitive; despondent; out of humour.

Remarks.—*Sulphur* is adapted to lymphatic temperaments—a scrofulous or psoric dyscrasia, and may be employed in ophthalmia caused by repelled eruptions, abuse of mercury, or irritating matters introduced into the eye.

Digitalis.—*External indications.*—Intense redness of the conjunctiva; inflammation of the meibomian glands; swelling of the lids; constant and profuse lachrymation; photophobia; dryness of the nose; morning agglutination of the lids; tears hot and corrosive; countenance bloated.

Physicial sensations.—Aching, throbbing, burning, pressing, or stitching pains in the affected eyeball, worse when moving or touching it; feeling as of sand under the lids; discharge of hot and irritating tears, on exposure to the open air or to light; intolerance to light; dimness of sight; eyes constantly hot and painful; objects all appear unnatural; visions before the eyes.

Mental and moral symptoms.—The predominant mental traits are, despondency and mental languor.

Remarks.—*Digitalis* is suited to sanguine temperaments, and also to persons of a scrofulous habit. It has been successfully employed in ophthalmiæ consequent on colds, scrofula, and gout. *Euphrasia* also corresponds to most of the symptoms enumerated under *digitalis*, and may sometimes be substituted to advantage in the place of this last remedy, when the desired effect is not promptly produced.

Pulsatilla is appropriate in catarrhal or rheumatic ophthalmia, attended with pressure and burning in the eyes, as if from sand; redness and swelling of the conjunctiva and lids; coryza; profuse lachrymation in the wind or open air; burning and itching of the eyes, inducing a disposition to rub them; photophobia; inflammation, and secretion of mucus from the meibomian glands; dimness of sight; morning agglutination.

Arnica is indispensable in ophthalmic inflammations

caused by mechanical injuries of the eye, or of the parts in its vicinity. The remedy may be used both *internally* and *externally*.

Spigelia is especially adapted to rheumatic and arthritic ophthalmia; the pains are of a pressive or stitching character, and aggravated by movement; the vessels of the conjunctiva are much congested; the cornea is dim; aching pains are experienced in the eye when touched, extending deep into the orbit; the upper lids swollen and stiff.

Mercurius sol. is proper in catarrhal and rheumatic ophthalmia. Its indications are, inflammation of the eyes, attended with burning, smarting, heat, and pressure, worse in the open air; sensation as if sand were under the upper lid; profuse lachrymation; photophobia; darting pains in the eyeballs; redness and swelling of the lids; dimness of vision; pains worse when moving or touching the eye; boring pains in the eyes and surrounding parts.

Other remedies are, *graphite, lycopodium, nux vomica, calcarea carb., colocynth, rhus, cocculus, cannabis,* and *dulcamara,* to which the reader is referred.

Administration.—In very *acute* cases, we advise the third attenuation, and a repetition of the dose every two hours until the desired impression is produced. In more mild forms of the disease, we use the first or second attenuations, and repeat every six or eight hours, as long as is deemed necessary.

SECTION III.

CHRONIC OPHTHALMIA.

Chronic ophthalmia may arise in consequence of the subsidence of the active symptoms of the acute form of the disease, and the persistence of a condition of sub-acute inflammation, or from causes which operate gradually, and induce an atonic state of the parts, and a low grade of morbid action. It may continue in this chronic state for years, without causing any notable organic derangement, the only difficulty experienced, being a weak, sensitive, and irritable condition of the eyes.

Diagnosis.—When chronic ophthalmia succeeds the

acute, it will be found that a part of the vessels of the conjunctiva have recovered their tone and now circulate only the white blood, as formerly, while the larger vessels remain injected with red blood. These larger vessels, during the progress of the disorder, become so much distended by the intromission of the red globules, that a varicose dilatation often remains for a long period after the acute stage has been passed, and thus establishes the chronic malady. One of the prominent local symptoms, therefore, of chronic ophthalmia, as distinguished from the acute variety, is, the moderately congested state of the vessels, which renders the conjunctiva partly red and partly white. The eye is also much less sensitive to light, dust, and smoke; tears are not so easily excited; vision is improved; there is an absence of pain, burning, and heat; tears are not so hot and acrid; the swelling of the lids is diminished, and all febrile and sympathetic symptoms have disappeared. But the eye is more sensitive than natural to light; the edges of the lids are red or purple; nightly agglutination occurs; the patient is unable to use the eyes long at a time; objects often float before the eyes, obstructing vision; the lids itch and tingle, mostly in the morning on rising; flow of tears caused by cold air, light, wind, smoke, dust, and vapours.

Causes.—Acute inflammation; habitual intemperance; constant exposure to irritating vapours; metastases of rheumatism and gout; external injuries; repelled eruptions; protracted exposure to cold in a region of snow; excessive use of the eyes by a strong or dim light.

Prognosis.—Unless adhesions have taken place between the conjunctiva and cornea, or ulcers, cicatrixes, or effusions, have formed, so as to obstruct the rays of light, we may expect a ready cure of the disease. If, however, disorganization has already occurred, and vision has become obstructed, we may predict a cure of the morbid inflammatory action, but only a partial restoration of sight. Habitual chronic ophthalmiæ, proceeding from intemperance, constant exposure of the eyes to stimulating vapours, etc., may readily be cured by removing the exciting causes, and having recourse to the appropriate local and internal remedies.

Therapeutics.—It is in this variety of ophthalmia, that we may expect to derive most benefit from the use of stimulating collyria. The object of all remedies, as has before been observed, is to create a healthy medicinal action in the diseased part, which shall supersede the morbid action, and thus secure a cure. But we have also seen that this medicinal effect must be two-fold in order to prove curative: or, in other words, there must be a *primary* and a *secondary* effect, the former *analogous* to that of the disease, and the latter, the *reverse*, or *curative*. Whenever these two conditions result from the application of remedies, *internal* or *local*, a cure may be expected. Care, however, must always be observed, that the medicines be so adapted to the nature of the case, that the primary symptoms shall be of short duration, and succeeded by the legitimate, opposite, or curative reaction.

In deciding, therefore, respecting the proper strength of a local application to an inflamed eye, we may follow the maxims of Hahnemann, or, what will answer as well, adopt the following rule inculcated by Sir Astley Cooper, in regard to the use of collyria, viz: "To judge how far the stimulus may be carried, the criterion is exceedingly simple; if you find that a certain degree of smarting and pain is produced, which soon subsides and leaves the patient much more easy than before, you may be convinced that the collyrium is beneficial; if, on the other hand, the patient experiences a great degree of pain, which does not subside speedily, and the vessels become turgid, you may be assured that the collyrium is doing harm, and that the quantity of stimulus ought to be diminished."

The best local stimulus we ever employed, in clearly pronounced chronic inflammation of the eyes, is the wine of opium, (*vinum opii*), a single drop to be introduced into the eye once or twice in twenty-four hours, until there is a permanent reaction. When the secondary symptoms do not speedily appear after the application, we may then have recourse to a weak solution of *sulphate of zinc*, or of *nitrate of silver*. If these fail, a dilution of *aconite* may be tried.

The internal remedies are, *arsenicum, belladonna, calcarea carbonica, sulphur, rhus, silicea, nux vomica, graphite, phosphorus.*

The indications for the use of these different medicines will be found under *acute ophthalmia.* The principal difference between the two forms of the malady, consists in degree rather than in the quality of the symptoms.

Respecting the administration and repetition of doses, we prefer the first, second, and third attenuations, and advise a repetition once in twenty-four hours, until an impression is produced.

SECTION IV.

PURULENT OPHTHALMIA.

Diagnosis.—This variety of ophthalmia is more violent and destructive, and runs its course with much greater rapidity, than that which we have described. It is characterized by a profuse purulent secretion from the conjunctiva, which collects and hardens about the lids, gluing them together, and in this way acts as a constant irritant to the inflamed part. The disease commences like the simple acute ophthalmia, with itching, stinging, or burning sensations in the lids and globe, lachrymation, sensitiveness to light, redness of the conjunctiva, which soon increase to an intense villous redness, swelling of the lids, sensations as if foreign substances, like sand or sticks, were in the eye, and more or less indistinctness of vision. These symptoms augment very rapidly in intensity. The tingling sensations change to severe pains through the eye, sometimes extending to the temples, and even the brain itself; there is chemosis, the lachrymation becomes changed into a profuse secretion of pus, either yellow or greenish; the intolerance to light becomes more marked, the lids are very much swollen, and discharge much purulent matter, and there is almost a total obstruction of sight. Constitutional symptoms frequently occur, as in simple ophthalmia, in the form of headache, nausea, quick pulse, hot skin, general prostration, &c. This acute stage terminates in a short period in a sub-acute inflammation, or in ulceration and sloughing. When the former termination happens, there is a gradual subsidence of all the symptoms, and the disease remains for an indefinite period in this atonic state, after which the eye may recover its tone and healthy function. But if sloughing takes place, the destructive process may run on to a total destruction of the part, unless energetic measures are used to arrest its progress.

Causes.—Sudden alternations from heat to cold; endemic and epidemic influences; the irritation of hot sand introduced into the eyes; metastases of rheumatism, gout, scarlatina, small-pox, and measles; abuse of mercury; the morbid vaginal secretion to which the eyes of new-born children are sometimes exposed.

SECTION V.

GONORRHŒAL OPHTHALMIA.

Diagnosis.—This variety of inflammation attacks the conjunctiva also, and is attended with symptoms very similar to those of purulent ophthalmia, but of much greater intensity. This disease is supposed to be the most violent and destructive of any to which the eye is subject, and it is not uncommon so see it proceed to the entire destruction of vision, notwithstanding the most early and energetic attempts to cure it. There is especial danger, in gonorrhœal ophthalmia, of a speedy formation of ulcers of the cornea, and of rapid sloughing through the tunics of the eye. Whenever, therefore, we are called to a case of this description, with intense inflammation and redness of the eyes, greatly swollen lids, very abundant discharge of pus, or a dry and burning state of the conjunctiva and lids; excruciating pains in the eyes and head; chemosis; great intolerance to light; hot skin; nausea; thirst; and other febrile symptoms; it becomes us to exercise the utmost vigilance in our remedial measures, in order to save the eyes from ulceration and sloughing. Farther on we shall detail a method of treatment which will generally be found successful, even in the most severe cases. Nothing, however, but the strictest attention to every minute symptom of the case, and a constant watch over medicinal effects, will ensure success.

The *cause* of this affection is unquestionably the application to the eyes of *gonorrhœal matter*, and not, as some suppose, a metastasis of the disease to the eyes.

Another variety of purulent ophthalmia to which it is proper to allude, is that which occurs in infants shortly after birth. This disease is supposed to arise from the contact of the vaginal secretion of the matter with the eyes of the child during birth. The symptoms generally first make their appearance in about two weeks after birth, but they may occur before or several weeks after this period. The symptoms are similar to those of purulent ophthalmia, but, for the most part, the inflammation is less intense, and there is much less danger of the speedy supervention of ulcers of the cornea. It is quite true that ulceration and sloughing ultimately occur in these cases; but a longer time is afforded for our remedial efforts to take effect, and of course the prospect of cure thus enhanced.

SECTION VI.

STRUMOUS, OR SCROFULOUS OPHTHALMIA.

Diagnosis.—Scrofulous ophthalmia presents several symptoms which are quite characteristic, and by the aid of which we may always form a ready and accurate diagnosis. The disease occurs in subjects of a scrofulous habit, and is accompanied with the general signs peculiar to struma, in addition to the local symptoms. Indeed, these general marks will often aid materially in forming our opinion, particularly in slight cases. The light and clear complexion, blonde hair, blue eyes, tendency to glandular swellings of the neck, the tumid upper lip, eruptions during childhood behind the ears and upon the head, sensitiveness to cold, disposition to cough after colds, frequent pains and discharges from the ears, indicate the strumous dyscrasia, which often determine and develop inflammations of the scrofulous kind.

The peculiar symptoms which distinguish this inflammation are, the almost absolute intolerance to light; the violent spasmodic closure of the lids on the slightest exposure of the eyes to it, and the strumous eruptions which generally make their appearance in the neighbourhood of the eyes. The light is commonly so painful, and the dread of exposure to it is so great, that it is exceedingly difficult to make a thorough examination in children, and, as a general rule, it is better to trust to the voluntary efforts of the patient, in a moderate light, rather than resort to much violence in attempting to force open the eyes. Usually, by obtaining the confidence of the patient, we can persuade such a display of the globes as will sufficiently satisfy us in regard to the case. The vessels of the conjunctiva are generally much injected; there is a considerable discharge of purulent matter; the balls are stiff and painful; the lids swollen; vision impaired by the inflammation, or by ulcers on the cornea; one or more ulcers form on the conjunctiva covering the cornea; and, if the symptoms continue to increase, the sight is finally destroyed.

The disease varies much in its progress; is sometimes attended with but little redness of the conjunctiva, but slight pains in the globes, and but a moderate secretion of pus; at other times, during the formation of an ulcer, all these symptoms increase in intensity, until the case nearly resembles one of acute purulent ophthalmia. It is of far more common occurrence in children than in adults.

Causes.—The constitutional cause, as we have seen, is a strumous dyscrasia. The local, or exciting causes are, atmospheric vicissitudes; undue exposure to cold, light, dust, smoke, and irritating vapours; neglect of cleanliness.

Prognosis.—Severe purulent ophthalmia under the most favourable circumstances, for the application of remedies, is highly dangerous. The chief peril against which we have to guard, is ulceration of the cornea. Before this has taken place, and especially if the cornea appears bright, we may entertain hopes of a favourable termination of the case; but if these opaque specks form while the inflammation retains its intensity, we must be prepared for a partial or total loss of vision. Of the different kinds of ophthalmia, the gonorrhœal is unquestionably the most rapid in its progress, and dangerous in its character. Here, nothing but the most consummate judgment and coolness, with constant attention, can avert serious consequences. The other varieties of the malady are not quite so rapid and destructive, but they demand the most skilful and energetic efforts to ward off injurious results.

As a general rule, if we are called during the early stages of the complaint, and exhibit the appropriate specifics judiciously and boldly, little difficulty will be experienced in inducing a speedy and happy issue to either of the varieties; unfortunately, however, the physician is rarely called until the disease is so far advanced that ulceration cannot be prevented. It is evident, then, that the prognosis will depend upon the intensity of the disease, the complications which have occurred, the time it has existed, the constitution of the patient, and the remote and exciting causes.

Therapeutics.—The only local application which can be advantageously used during the acute stage of purulent ophthalmia, is pure water, either cold or tepid. This may be employed as a lotion to the parts, during the course of the acute symptoms, as the judgment of the adviser shall dictate. When the chronic stage has set in, recourse may occasionally be had to stimulating collyria, like *vinum opii*, solutions of *sulph., zinc, nitr. argenti, sulph., cuprum, acetat., plumbi*, and *aconite ;* but in regard to these applications, the same rules apply with full force here, that we have presented under the head of simple acute ophthalmia, when alluding to the use of collyria.

The following remedies will cover all of the symptoms which obtain in the different varieties of purulent ophthalmia : *arsenicum, belladonna, sulphur, rhus* photophobia; pressure and burning pains in the eye-balls, aggravated by moving the eyes; nebulous spots and ulcers on the cornea.

Belladonna is an admirable remedy in scrofulous inflammation of the eyes, with very great intolerance to light; a constant inclination to remain in the dark, or to plunge the eyes into a pillow or some other soft article; purulent discharge; great swelling of the lids; spasmodic closure of the lids on exposure to light; chemosis; tearing, throbbing, smarting, or stitching pains in the eyes; roaring in the ears; hot, dry skin; thirst; nightly agglutination; throbbing of the carotid and temporal arteries; pains in the temples and head; ulcers on the cornea; dimness of vision. We have cured several cases of purulent ophthalmia of infants, characterized by great intolerance to light, intense inflammation, throbbing of the carotid and temporal arteries, flushed cheeks, hot skin, and other indications of inordinate vascular excitement, with *belladonna*, succeeded by *mercurius*. We deem *belladonna* one of our most valuable medicines in nearly all of the acute inflammations of the eye. The effects arising from the application of a small quantity of the extract to the eyebrows or temples, are sufficient to demonstrate its marked specific action upon the structures of the eye. We have found it eminently serviceable in ophthalmia neonatorum, and in acute ophthalmia.

Sulphur is an invaluable remedy in several kinds of purulent ophthalmia. It is adapted to the *chronic* forms, with atonic distention of the conjunctival vessels; swollen and œdematous condition of the lids, with purulent discharge; suppurating ulcers on the cornea; sensation of itching, búrning, and heat in the eyes and lids; troublesome agglutination in the morning; diminished power of motion of the upper lids; pustules of the cornea; sensitiveness to the light of the sun; swollen upper lip; eruptions behind the ears, and on the scalp and face; pressure and burning pain in the eyes; impaired vision. *Sulphur* is one of those remedies which will be required more or less frequently in all varieties of ophthalmia, not only to combat those local symptoms which especially correspond with it, but to correct morbid conditions of a more general and latent character. *Sulphur* may occasionally be used with decided advantage in alternation with remedies which appear to cover all of the manifest symptoms, but which do not produce prompt impressions when given singly.

Rhus tox. is useful in *rheumatic, scrofulous,* and *catarrhal* ophthalmia, with much inflammation and swelling of the lids; redness of the balls of the eyes; profuse secretion of mucus or pus from the eyes and lids; œdematous swelling of the lids and the parts surrounding the eyes; morning agglutination, with increased redness of the eyes; pain on turning the balls; lachrymation; photophobia.

Dr. Dudgeon considers *rhus toxicodendron* one of the most important remedies in catarrhal, erysipelatous, scrofulous, and exanthematic ophthalmia. Many allopathic physicians commend the tincture of *rhus* in scrofulous ophthalmia. We can bear witness to the value of this medicine in scrofulous ophthalmia, and in chronic ophthalmia which is kept up by a dyscrasia of an erysipelatous character.

Calcarea carbonica has been successfully employed in every variety of purulent conjunctival inflammation. Its chief indications are, inflammation, redness, and purulent secretion from the eyeballs; swelling and redness of the eyelids; nightly, and sometimes daily, agglutination of the lids; great intolerance to light; nebulous specks and ulcers on the cornea; inclination to keep the eyes in darkness; scrofulous eruptions upon the face and scalp; glandular swellings of the neck; swelling of the upper lips and nostrils; pustules on the cornea; pressing or aching pains in the eyes; corrosive inflammation in the edges of the lids; acrid lachrymation; general appearance indicative of the scrofulous dyscrasia. Dr. Dudgeon expresses the opinion that *calcarea* "is one of our most important ophthalmic medicines, and is surpassed by none in its applicability to the generality of cases of scrofulous inflammation, whether of the eye itself, or its lids; and is indispensable where there is marked scrhfulous diathesis, indicated by swellings of the glands," &c.

Aconite may often precede other remedies in every variety of purulent ophthalmia, when the inflammation runs high, and gives rise to febrile symptoms. Intense redness and swelling of the affected parts; acute pains; accelerated circulation; violent photophobia; headache; hot and dry skin; thirst; flushed cheeks; throbbing of the arteries about the neck, head and face; loss of appetite; and perverted vision, point to the employment of *aconite*. In some instances it may be alternated with *belladonna* to advantage.

Mercurius sol. has proved successful in my hands in *gonorrhœal, scrofulous*, and *infantile* ophthalmia; the remedy having been preceded by *aconite*. The symptoms were, violent inflammation, and redness of the eyes; great intolerance to light; profuse acrid or purulent secretion from the balls and lids; spasmodic closure of the lids; heat in the eyes; cutting and burning pains in the parts; ulcers on the cornea; cornea dim and misty; sight impaired; frequent agglutination of the lids; gummy and scurfy matter on the edges of the lids.

Graphite is one of our best remedies in *scrofulous* ophthalmia, with excessive intolerance to light; chronic congestion of the conjunctiva; purulent secretion from the balls and lids; frequent agglutination of the lids; ulcers on the cornea; porrigo in the face; eyelids much inflamed, red, and painful; inability to open the eyes before a strong light; constant desire to keep the eyes covered; symptoms worse by day-light than by candle-light; general appearance indicative of a scrofulous diathesis.

Phosphorus is sometimes useful in obstinate and protracted cases of atonic ophthalmiæ, which have resisted the ordinary remedies. There is generally inflammation and moderate redness of the eyes; considerable secretion of viscid mucus; sensitiveness of the eyes to light; heat, burning and itching of the eyes; lachrymation during the day; frequent and sudden attacks of blindness during the day; floats before the eyes; weakness and indistinctness of vision.

Spigelia is advised in purulent inflammation, principally affecting the eyelids, with sharp pains in the lids; pressure and pain in the eyeballs during motion; distention and paralysis of the upper lids; painful ulceration of the edges of the lids; dimness of the cornea; general loss of power over the eyes. *Rummel* speaks highly of *spigelia* in rheumatic and gouty inflammations attacking the cornea.

Digitalis is recommended in conjunctival ophthalmiæ arising from colds, with acute inflammation, redness, sharp stitches, photophobia, secretion of purulent matter, and obstruction and dryness of the nose.

Nitric acid and *hepar sulph.* are the best specifics for the removal of *mercurial ophthalmia*, following the abuse of this drug in syphilis and other diseases. The symptoms are, inflammation, swelling and redness of the conjunctiva and lids; secretion of viscid mucus or pus; burning and smarting sensation in the eyes; photophobia, dark and unhealthy ulcers on the cornea; paralysis of the upper eyelids; tears easily excited; nightly agglutination; muscæ volitantes and sparks before the eyes; difficulty and pain in moving the eyes; pains in the bones and soft parts of the forehead and face.

We have employed *chininum sulph.*, at the first trituration, in several obstinate cases of strumous and chronic ophthalmia, with entire success. When the malady assumes an intermittent character, it will generally prove promptly curative.

Lobethal has employed *euphrasia* with much success in rheumatic, strumous, and catarrhal ophthalmia, where there was "considerable mucous secretion in the inflamed organ; as also in blennorrhœas of the eyes, in all which cases I employ *euphrasia* at once, internally and externally; in the former case, one drop of the pure tincture; in the latter, as a collyrium, from two to five drops in four ounces of water."

Lycopodium is well adapted to scrofulous or catarrhal ophthalmia, and in obstinate cases of ophthalmia neonatorum. Hahnemann mentions "nocturnal agglutination, and lachrymation by day," as prominent indications for the use of *lycopodium*.

We have employed *aurum* with excellent effects in several cases of mercurial and syphilitic ophthalmia.

Some authors recommend it highly in scrofulous ophthalmia.

Other remedies are, *causticum*, *sepia*, *silicea*, *staphysagria*, *china*, and *chamomilla*.

Administration.—In *acute* cases, we prefer the first, second, and third attenuations, and in the *chronic* stage, the first attenuation. The remedy should be repeated in the more violent forms of the complaint, every half hour, until we are satisfied with the impression ; but in chronic inflammations, a repetition once in twelve or twenty-four hours will suffice. During the treatment we should never neglect the external use of pure water, or milk and water, either cold or tepid.

SECTION VII.

GRANULATED LIDS.

Diagnosis.—Fleshy elevations sometimes occur on that portion of the conjunctiva which lines the eyelids, resembling in all respects granulations, and by their irritating effects upon the ball of the eye, give rise to troublesome inflammation, ulceration, and now and then to loss of sight. This affection has more frequently baffled the surgeons of the old school, than any other pertaining to the eye. Venesection, leeching, cupping, blistering, moxas, cathartics, alteratives, stimulating collyria, and caustic applications, have all been found entirely inefficient in its treatment, and the patients are generally doomed to a wretched existence, one or more years, until disorganization of the eyes, by ulceration, leaves them in perpetual darkness. By homœopathy, however, a new and healthy action can be created in the affected structure, which shall overcome and supersede the morbid action.

These morbid granulations usually arise from an acute or sub-acute inflammation of the conjunctiva occurring in individuals whose constitutions have become impaired and tainted by protracted syphilitic, gonorrhœal, psoric, or scrofulous complaints. The granulations are rough and uneven, secrete an abundance of pus, which serves to irritate and weaken the eyes, and on every motion of the lids, operate on the balls as foreign substances, thus keeping up a perpetual inflammation, and sooner or later leading to ulceration of the cornea. The disease is for the most part confined to the upper lids, although we have seen, in some instances, the conjunctiva of the lower lids rough and granulated.

Occasionally we may detect the true character of the complaint by the thickness of the lids, and their roughness and unevenness to the touch ; but the only certain method of investigation consists in turning over the lids, and thus exposing the palpebral conjunctiva to the sight.

This disease very often proceeds to a fatal disorganization of the eye, without a true knowledge on the part of the physician, respecting the nature of the case. It is usually mistaken for one of the varieties of purulent ophthalmia.

Therapeutics.—The remedies in this disease are both *local* and *constitutional.* The only local specific is the *sulphate of copper* in substance, a small piece of which is to be smoothly polished, and rubbed lightly over the granulations once or twice a day, following each application with a camel's-hair brush filled with pure water. A persevering use of this substance will, as we know from much experience in these cases, cure the most inveterate forms of the complaint.

In conjunction with the above means, we may employ one of the following medicines: *sulphur*, *calcarea carbonica*, *hepar sulph.*, *iodine*, *graphite*, and *acid nit.*, as internal remedies.

In selecting our internal remedy, regard must be had to the cause, as well as the symptoms of the disease. We advise the first attenuations, and the dose to be repeated once in twelve or twenty-four hours as long as necessary.

SECTION VIII.

OPACITY OF THE CORNEA.

Diagnosis.—Opacities or specks upon the cornea vary much in size and appearance. Various appellations have been given to these different opacities, as *nebula*, *leucoma*, *albugo*, &c., depending upon the nature of the cause, and the particular tissue affected. The opacity may consist of slight misty or opaque spots, diffused over a part or even the whole of the cornea, of a light colour, such as are caused by a perverted secretion of the inner lamina, and termed *nebula;* or of small and circumscribed spots, of a pearl colour, and entirely opaque, caused by a kind of false membrane under the conjunctiva, and termed *leucoma;* or of cicatrixes resulting from the healing of ulcers and wounds of the cornea, and termed *albugo.*

When the disease consists of a simple diffused nebulous opacity, we can distinguish through it the pupil and iris, and the rays of light pass to the retina so as to give rise to imperfect vision; but the other kinds of opacity do not permit the passage of luminous rays, and, consequently, when situated in front of the pupil, destroy or seriously impair vision.

The two first varieties are caused by purulent ophthalmia and granulated lids, and are results most to be dreaded, especially in constitutions tainted with scrofula, syphilis, psora, or mercury.

Therapeutics.—The best local stimulus is a collyrium composed of one grain of *sulphate of zinc* to four ounces of water. A few drops of this may be put into the affected eye from two to four times in twenty-four hours until the opacity begins to disappear, when we should omit it so long as amendment continues.

The internal remedies most to be relied on are, *calcarea carbonica, iodine, mercurius, sulphur, sepia, arnica, hepar sulphuris, acid nit., aurum muriaticum.*

Attenuations and repetitions the same as in *chronic ophthalmia.*

SECTION IX.

AFFECTIONS OF THE DEEPER SEATED STRUCTURES OF THE EYE.

INFLAMMATION OF THE CORNEA.

Diagnosis.—Inflammation of the cornea may exist as an independent affection, or it may occur during the progress of *iritis,* and other acute derangements of the internal textures of the eye. Soon after the inflammation sets in, a number of the serous vessels are observed to carry red blood; the cornea loses its brilliancy; the eyes become sensitive to light; a profuse secretion of tears is induced from exposure to cold air, light, dust, and smoke; tension and pains are experienced in the eye; yellow spots, composed of pus, are observed between the lamellæ of the cornea by looking obliquely through the eye; these abscesses, if the disease continues, eventually burst internally, and discharge their contents into the anterior chamber, or externally, and form those troublesome ulcers of the cornea which so often endanger sight. When these ulcers are small, and confined to the anterior portion of the cornea, they may often be cured without material injury to the eye; but when the ulceration pervades the whole lamellated structure of the cornea, it is not uncommon for the aqueous humour to escape through the opening, and even the iris itself to protrude.

SECTION X.

IRITIS.

Diagnosis.—This peculiar affection of the eye is by no means easy of detection, on account of the situation of the iris, and the small number of external symptoms which characterize the complaint. Inflammation of this texture is, however, more productive of constitutional or febrile symptoms than affections of the external tunics. This may in part be owing to the loose attachment of the conjunctiva to the eye, and the more ample scope for effusions into the subjacent cellular tissue.

Iritis commences with a dull, pressing, heavy and deep-seated pain in the orbit; contracted pupil; change of the natural colour of the iris to a dark, greenish, or reddish colour; a moderate rose-coloured blush of the conjunctiva; diminished power of vision, and considerable sensibility to light.

As the disease advances, the pains become acute, and extend from the eye into the temples and to the top of the head; the contraction is more strongly pronounced ; sparks and luminous flashes pass through and before the eyes ; the nervous system is excited ; the pulse accelerated ; the skin hot and dry ; the intestinal and urinary secretions are partially suppressed, and there are other indications of constitutional disturbance.

After these severe symptoms have continued some time, the iris presents an irregular, angular, and thickened appearance, and is covered with specks of yellow lymph. Small abscesses now form on the iris, which ultimately burst into the anterior chamber, which is afterwards usually absorbed. If extensive adhesions have formed between the iris and the capsule of the lens, or if the more deep-seated parts have become involved in the disease, an almost total loss of sight is the common result.

In some instances, the inflammation extends from the iris to the retina, the choroides, the cornea, and finally involves the whole internal structure of the eye, when the malady will present symptoms characteristic of the inflammation of these different structures. In cases of this description, the symptoms are of the most violent character, the pains are exceedingly acute and painfully throbbing, there is a very rapid contraction of the pupil, the sight is speedily extinguished, the constitutional signs are very urgent, and the patient is always in imminent danger of rapid and permanent loss of vision.

Causes.—The most common cause of iritis is the abuse of mercury. Syphilis has been often assigned as a cause of it, but, we believe, without just reason. It has often been observed during the treatment of syphilis by mercury, but, we think, never in syphilitic diseases where mercury has not been employed. Other causes are, mechanical injuries, rheumatism, gout, excessive use of the eyes over minute objects.

Therapeutics.—The most appropriate remedies are, *hepar sulphur., acid nit., muriat. aurum, cocculus, calcarea carbonica, nux vomica, belladonna, conium, lycopodium, staphysagria, arnica, aconite.*

Hepar sulphuris, acid nitric, and *aurum muriaticum,* are curative in iritis arising from abuse of *mercury,* with aching, throbbing, and tearing pains in the orbit, sometimes extending to the top of the head; pains in the bones about the eyes; fiery sparks before the eyes; intolerance to light; contracted pupil; partial or entire loss of vision; dark or greenish colour of the iris; spots of yellow lymph, or ulcers on the iris; febrile disturbance.

Cocculus, nux vomica, and *belladonna,* are indicated in arthritic and rheumatic iritis, accompanied with deep-seated, lancinating, tearing, or contractive pains in the ball, and extending to the top of the head; involuntary spasmodic movements of the globe; irregular contraction of the pupil; discoloured and puckered iris; photophobia; pains aggravated on moving the eyes, or stooping; luminous specks or dark objects float before the retina; greatly impaired vision; effusion of blood and matter into the anterior chamber of the eye; indications of gastric derangement, and of general constitutional disturbance.

Calcarea carbonica, conium, lycopodium, and *staphysagria,* are appropriate in iritic inflammations connected with a scrofulous diathesis. These remedies cover greenish or yellowish colour of the iris; pupil much contracted and distorted; ulcers which have opened internally or externally; outward distention of the iris; adhesions of the iris to the capsule of the lens; moderate participation of all the structures of the eye in the morbid action; photophobia; vision destroyed or much impaired; difficulty in distinguishing the iris from effusion of lymph and pus into the anterior chamber of the eye; great general irritability; aching, throbbing, lancinating, or pressing pains in the eye; rapid and irritable pulse; restlessness; hot skin; loss of appetite; mental and physical prostration.

Arnica is necessary when the disease can be traced to a wound, or to any other mechanical injury of the eye. It may also be properly employed in cases which proceed from sudden exposure of the eyes to an intense and glaring light.

Aconite will often be required, either alone, or in alternation with one of the other remedies, to control undue febrile excitement, and to remove the violent congestion which now and then occurs in iritis.

Administration.—The remedies may be employed at the first, second, and third attenuations, depending upon the age and susceptibility of the patient, and the violence of the inflammation. The dose should be repeated in acute cases every two hours, until we are certain of a medicinal impression upon the diseased texture. In less urgent cases, a repetition will suffice once or twice in twenty-four hours.

SECTION XI.

AMAUROSIS.

Diagnosis.—The partial or total loss of sight which particularly characterizes this disease, is principally dependent upon a diseased condition of the optic nerve and retina, although other structures occasionally participate in the disease. Amaurosis occurs at all ages, and in both sexes, but is most common at the period of the cessation of the menses in females, and at the age of forty or fifty years in males. The chief circumstances which predispose to it are, a plethoric and sanguine temperament, hereditary disposition, tendency to sanguineous congestions to the head and eyes, and an impaired constitution from abuse of drugs, stimulating drinks, and excesses in venery.

Physicians of the old school are much divided respecting the nature and treatment of amaurosis, some supposing it to be a debility requiring tonics and stimulants, while others describe it as an inflammatory affection, demanding an antiphlogistic course of treatment. In view of these discordant opinions, and empyrical methods, it is not surprising that so few amaurotic patients are cured by allopathy.

Amaurosis may be imperfect or perfect. In the former there is a partial, and in the latter a total loss of sight. In the first, the patient sees as through a gauze, or but half of the object, or double, or only when the eye is in a particular position with respect to the object; while in the last, the patient cannot distinguish day from night.

The signs of the approach of the disease are, pain in the forehead and temples, diminishing with the advance of the amaurosis, and ceasing when it has become complete; vertigo; weakness and cloudiness of vision, apparent when looking at distant or at minute objects; sparks and moats, or muscæ volitantes, float before the eyes, annoying the patient, and impairing the sight; in reading or writing, a stronger light than usual is demanded; a slight diminution in the brilliancy of the pupil.

After these precursory symptoms, the loss of vision gradually becomes more complete, until after months or years, there remains a condition of settled and more or less perfect amaurosis. In other instances, the disease advances with rapidity, and terminates in partial or total blindness in a few days. But it is not an uncommon occurrence for complete amaurosis to follow instantaneously, leaving the victim in blindness so profound that he cannot distinguish light from darkness. When either of these three conditions obtains, there are usually but few signs which indicate the presence of so serious an affection, the principal being, a dilated and immovable pupil, a loss of contractile power in the iris, and occasionally slight strabismus. But even these signs are not uniformly present, for cases of complete amaurosis are reported in which the pupil remained natural, or became preternaturally contracted and mobile on exposure to light, and in which the iris and all other visible parts of the organ were in a normal condition. The colour of the pupil in this disease is ordinarily jet black, with, perhaps, a very slight diminution of its natural brilliancy, but it sometimes presents a red, greenish, or white and cloudy appearance. Cases of this last description are often mistaken for incipient cataract, and when the loss of sight is but partial, it is not easy to distinguish between the two maladies; but the following characteristics will afford us material assistance in deciding the matter. In cataract, the dense white appearance is situated immediately behind the pupil, while in amaurosis the cloud is more deep-seated. In the former, the flame of a candle appears to be surrounded by a thin, white, diffused mist or cloud, "which increases with the distance of the light," while in the latter, "a halo or iris appears to encircle or emanate from the mist, the flame seeming to be split when at a distance."—*Stephenson.*

The shape of the pupil is usually round, but somewhat more dilated than in the normal state, thus allowing a large number of luminous rays to enter the eye. In a few cases, it loses its circular form, and becomes angular.

Amaurosis is attributed by most writers to a paralytic condition of the optic nerve, retina, or to some disease of the thalami nervorum opticorum ; but does not the peculiar immovable condition of the pupil and iris, when their natural stimulus, the light, strikes them, indicate a loss of sensibility and contractility in these structures ? And does not the partial loss of voluntary motion over the globe, which sometimes occurs during the complaint, indicate a loss of tone in the whole organ ?

We have mentioned, as one of the precursory symptoms of amaurosis, floats and muscæ volitantes before the eyes. In the imperfect form of the disease, these appearances vary much in their character, and are a source of great annoyance to the patient. Sometimes a single black speck obstructs the sight ; sometimes there is an appearance as if a dark gauze or net-work were before the eyes ; sometimes as if flies, small objects of different forms, sparks, fireballs, and various coloured lights, were moving there in various directions. The objects are more troublesome in a strong light than in dark situations, being in the former of a black or sombre colour, and in the latter, presenting themselves in the appearance of sudden flashes of light or fire.

We are occasionally presented with the disease in an intermittent form, and, in rare instances, as a temporary attendant of some particular morbid condition of the system, like pregnancy, disordered menstruation, hysteria, worms, and the irritation of indigestible food.

In addition to the symptoms already described, we sometimes observe in young and plethoric amaurotics, strongly pronounced determination of blood to the head and eyes, a constant stupifying headache, more or less redness and congestion of the eyeballs, sensitiveness of the eyes to light, a full and hard pulse, a sense of fulness, tension, and pain in the affected eye.

It is a point worthy of note, that *black* eyes are far more subject to amaurosis than *blue* or *gray* eyes. Beer supposes that where one blue or gray eye becomes affected with it, at least twenty-five or thirty black ones suffer. No satisfactory explanation has ever been suggested for this comparative exemption of blue and gray eyes.

Causes.—The causes of amaurosis may operate upon the brain itself, upon the optic nerve, or the retina. They may be divided into constitutional and local causes. In the first class we include, repeated and protracted determinations of blood to the head and eyes, by unusual physical or mental exertion; pregnancy; suppression of natural or habitual discharges; violent vomiting; excessive indulgence in venery; onanism; unbridled anger, grief, and other passions; abuse of stimulants; large doses of opium, lead, belladonna, hyoscyamus, stramonium; abuse of bitter medicines, as quassia, cinchona, chamomela, chicory, &c.; exercise in a hot sun; general debility; derangement of the digestive organs; the depressing emotions; the pressure of tumours upon the vessels of the neck in such a manner as to prevent the return of blood from the brain.

We include in the second class, morbid growths within the orbit; mechanical injuries of the eye; sudden transitions from darkness to a brilliant light; lightning; frequent use of optical instruments, like the telescope and microscope; exostoses within the cranium; sanguineous effusion upon the brain; injuries of the head.

Prognosis.—When the disease is dependent on some cause which can be readily removed, if recent, and the patient is young and healthy, we may predict a favourable termination. If, however, the cause has been long in operation, the loss of sight has been very gradual, the constitution is much impaired, and the cause cannot be speedily removed, the prognosis must be unfavourable. Amaurosis depending on morbid growths within the orbit or cranium, may be considered incurable; but when it depends upon a slight effusion upon the brain, or the pressure of a tumour upon the jugular vein of the neck, we may often effect a cure by causing the effused fluid to be absorbed or removed by an operation, or the extraction of the offending tumour. We once cured a case of several months' duration, by removing from the neck a tumour of the size of an orange, and thus renewing the free course of blood from the head. The sight returned almost immediately after the operation. The loss of sight which sometimes accompanies pregnancy and intermittent diseases, often subsides spontaneously on the birth of the infant, or the cure of the disease. A favourable prognosis may commonly be entertained in those recent cases which depend on congestion of the optic nerve, retina, or thalami nervorum opticorum, arising from general plethora, suppressed menstruation, or hæmorrhoids. The effects also of mechanical injuries, lacerations, contusions and blows upon the eye, may frequently be cured.

Therapeutics.—The specifics for the different forms of amaurosis are, *belladonna, nux vom., china, phosphorus, ruta grav., stramonium, sulphur, euphrasia, arnica, cannabis, hyoscyamus.*

Belladonna.—External indications.—Pupil dilated and immovable; strabismus; pupil black and round or angular; partial or total loss of vision; listless expression.

Physical sensations.—Power of vision diminished or extinct; sensation of weight and pressure in the eyeball; throbbing or stupifying headache; objects appear double, or wrong side up, or half concealed, or blurred, or surrounded by a fog or mist; dark, fiery and red bodies float before the eyes; bright flashes before the eyes; the candle seems surrounded by a halo of different colours, but in which the *red* predominates.

Mental and moral symptoms.—Mood generally irritable, but high spirits alternating with despondency.

Remarks.—This remedy is called for in amaurotics of full and plethoric habits, and where the malady has been caused by inflammation or congestion of the optic nerve, retina, or some part of the brain.

Nux vomica.—External indications.—Pupils contracted, sometimes dilated; spasmodic motions of the eyeball; photophobia.

Physical sensations.—Intermittent obscuration of vision; black or gray moats before the eyes; stupifying headache; weakness of sight, worse in the light of day; luminous vibrations on the side of the eye; vertigo.

Mental and moral symptoms.—Disposition melancholic and hypochondriacal.

Remarks.—*Nux* is applicable in amaurotic complaints arising from excess of study and abuse of stimulants and opium. It is also indicated for temporary loss of sight, which sometimes accompanies intermittent diseases.

China.—*External indications.*—Pupils dilated and insensible, or slightly contracted; a white cloud deep within the eye; photophobia.

Physical sensations.—Indistinct and confused vision; muscæ volitantes; sudden obscurations of sight; only the outlines of objects can be discerned; general debility; irritability; morbid sensitiveness of the whole system.

Mental and moral symptoms.—Disposition cheerful and languid.

Remarks.—*China* will apply when the disease is of a purely atonic character, and has originated from excessive loss of blood or pus, or from protracted chronic or acute diseases.

Phosphorus.—*External indications.*—Pupils and eyes natural.

Physical sensations.—Sudden attacks of blindness during the day; distant objects appear to be enveloped in smoke or mist; black spots before the eyes; diminished vision; he sees as through a net-work or gauze; sparks before the eyes in the dark; tremulous vision; luminous vibrations before the eyes; the flame of a candle seems to be surrounded by a green halo.

Mental and moral symptoms.—Spirits gloomy, dejected, and without any cheerful reaction.

Remarks.—In amaurosis consequent upon onanism, loss of animal fluids, and in impoverished old people, *phosphorus* is an excellent remedy.

Ruta grav.—*External indications.*—Pupils contracted; involuntary movements of the balls of the eyes; spasms of the lids.

Physical sensations.—Sense of weight and pressure in the eyeballs; weakness of the eyes; inclination to read or write by a very strong light; muscæ volitantes; red halo surrounding the flame of a candle; cloudy vision; weariness of the eyes.

Mental and moral symptoms.—Indifferent, irresolute and peevish.

Remarks.—Amaurotic complaints arising from abuse of the eyes with optical instruments, in reading fine print, or working at small objects, and also from contusions, and other mechanical injuries, will require the use of *ruta.*

Stramonium.—*External indications.*—Pupils dilated and immovable; eyes staring, and somnolent or glistening.

Physical sensations.—Sense of weight and tension in the eyes; obscuration of sight; objects appear small or double; black colours appear gray; sparks and specks float before the eyes; objects seem surrounded with a red or light border; cloudy vision; vertigo; headache.

Mental and moral symptoms.—Disposition irritable and touchy; hysterical and cataleptic.

Remarks.—*Stramonium* is suitable in paralytic affections of the optic nerve and retina, connected with deranged menstruation, hysteria, epilepsy, and catalepsy.

In incipient amaurosis, and frequent and sudden and short attacks of blindness, we may refer to *sulphur, euphrasia, arnica, cannabis, hyoscyamus, conium, aurum, digitalis.*

Administration.—We are in the habit of employing from the first to the sixth attenuations. Repetitions should not be made more than once or twice in the twenty-four hours. As soon as an impression is apparent, we should await the result before administering again.

SECTION XII.

HYDROPHTHALMIA, OR DROPSY OF THE EYE.

Diagnosis.—This disorder proceeds from the formation of a preternatural quantity of the aqueous or the vitreous humours, while the absorbent vessels convey into the circulation only their customary amount of these secretions; or the humours may be formed as usual, but owing to some defect or loss of power of the absorbents, the natural quantity is not taken up and carried into the circulation. But it is highly probable, in most cases, that the disease is dependent on a morbid condition of both the secerning and absorbent vessels, and that the normal equilibrium between secretion and absorption becomes thereby destroyed. This idea receives confirmation from the fact, that most dropsies of the eye can be traced to previous inflammation of the internal textures of the organ.

The unnatural accumulation may be confined to the aqueous humour in the anterior chamber, or to the vitreous humour in the posterior chamber, or both humours may be affected at the same time. When the aqueous humour is alone involved, the disease may be recognised by the following marks: dimensions of the cornea larger than natural; increased size of the anterior chamber of the eye; turbid appearance of the aqueous humour; partial or total loss of motion of the iris; pupil natural and immovable; iris less brilliant than natural; sense of weight and tension in the eyeball; weakness of sight; perversion of vision, either in the form of presbyopia or myopia; general loss of voluntary motion over the ball; partial or total loss of vision.

When there is a preternatural accumulation of the vitreous humour, the enlargement of the globe is more deep-seated; the ball assumes a conical shape; the cornea is unusually prominent; the pupil is contracted; there is a diminution of vision; myopia; deep-seated pains; tension and heaviness; impaired motion of the eyeball; and eventually, total blindness.

When the disease consists of an unnatural accumulation of both humours, we shall have a combination of symptoms including nearly all described under the aqueous and vitreous varieties of dropsy. After the vitreous humour has been for some time affected, its character is changed, and it acquires a soft and usually a watery appearance.

In many cases, the eye attains a size so enormous

as to protrude far from the orbit, and it is thus rendered quite impossible to close the lids over it. In this condition the patient has a frightful appearance, and the organ itself, from its exposure, is constantly irritated and inflamed.

Causes.—The immediate cause of dropsies of the eye, is an undue action in the arteries which secrete the humours, and a diminished action of the absorbent vessels; or, sometimes, an inordinate aqueous or vitreous secretion, with a normal action of the absorbents.

Hydrophthalmia is generally supposed to depend upon some constitutional cause, like general dropsy, hydrocephalus, chlorosis, or secondary syphilis; but as a general rule, it may be traced to some previous inflammation of the internal structures of the eye. In infants and young children, it is often exceedingly difficult to discover the real cause, especially when the external indications are obscure, and, on this account, the earlier history of the case can rarely be ascertained; but in adults, we shall often be able to discover previous sub-acute inflammation in the internal structures.

Prognosis.—The allopathists deem this disease, when fully formed, *incurable*. They find that no shedding of blood, no punishment of the stomach, bowels, salivary glands, skin, or other inoffensive parts of the body, can cure or palliate it. That the prognosis is unfavourable, we do not deny; but we believe the disease may often be cured in its early stages. I have treated but two cases homœopathically; and but one with a favourable result. This was of six months' standing, confined to the aqueous humour, and with but moderate distention of the cornea: the other case involved both humours, had continued more than a year, and had arrived at the condition termed "ox eye," when the treatment was commenced. In this instance paracentécis became necessary, and the patient ultimately lost the eye.

So long as the disease is confined to its incipient stage, and even after the unnatural accumulation has commenced, provided no serous disorganization has taken place in the important tissues of the eye, we may predict a favourable result; but if organic lesions have occurred, and the accumulation in the anterior or posterior chamber is considerable, with total loss of sight, our prognosis must be unfavourable.

Therapeutics.—If the dropsy depends upon a constitutional fault, our remedies must be addressed to the remote difficulties. So long as these continue, mere local means will be inadequate to accomplish our object; but constitutional and local remedies may be used in alternation with probable advantage. If the eye be much distended, and medicines do not act with sufficient promptness and energy, the operation of paracentesis may be made to evacuate the superabundant humours, after which, the remedies will generally prove sufficiently powerful.

We believe the following to be the best at present known: *belladonna, china, pulsatilla, mercurius, hyoscyamus, stramonium, conium, nux vom., arsenicum, plumbum, aconite, sepia, sulphur.*

It is doubtful whether either of these exercises a positively specific influence upon the secretory and absorbent vessels affected in hydrophthalmia, but they are capable of acting upon the generally morbid condition upon which the local disorder depends, and thus aid in arresting its progress, and occasionally in effecting cures.

Administration.—In the same manner as advised in *amaurosis.*

SECTION XIII.

CATARACT.

Diagnosis.—Strictly speaking, this disease belongs to the province of surgery rather than that of medicine; but as homœopathy promises results somewhat important in a medicinal point of view, we take the liberty of writing a few words respecting the malady in this place.

By the term cataract is understood, an opacity of the chrystalline lens, or its capsule, which causes an obscuration, or a total loss of vision. Authors recognise and describe several varieties, both of the lenticular and capsular cataract, and amongst these, the most common are—

First. The *firm* or *hard cataract*, peculiar to old people, and recognised by its amber colour, small size, and by its density and hardness. Vision is never totally destroyed in these cases, and the structures of the eye retain their natural contractility.

Second. The *fluid* or *milky cataract*, caused by a change of the lens into a white and semi-fluid mass, of so large a size as to nearly obliterate the posterior chamber, impair the motions of the pupil, and prevent the admission of rays of light.

Third. The *soft* or *caseous cataract*, which presents an appearance somewhat similar to the last variety, with the lens much enlarged, of a cheesy consistence, and of a light gray or sea-green colour, obliteration of the posterior chamber, impaired motion of the pupil and iris, and either partial or total blindness. The lens, in this variety, always presents an appearance of more firmness and consistence than in the milky cataract, and the dark irregular spots or lines which sometimes traverse it, remain the same in all positions of the head, while those which are now and then observed in the milky variety, change their location with every motion of the eyes.

Fourth. *Capsular cataract*, consisting of an opacity of the capsule of the chrystalline lens. The opacity commences at the margin of the pupil, in the form of " distinct, white, shining points, specks or streaks; its colour, therefore, is always very light, and never altogether uniform, even when the disease is completely formed."—*Beer*. When this kind of cataract occurs in children at or soon after birth, it is called *congenital cataract*.

The capsular cataract does not generally continue for a long period before the lens becomes involved also in the opacity. When the disease has been preceded by a good deal of inflammatory action, we may find cohesions of the anterior capsule of the lens with the urea; or of the posterior layer of the capsule with the membrana hyaloidea; or of the whole of the capsule with the lens; or all the three species of adhesion may exist together."—*Beer*, p. 318.

Cataract is sometimes complicated with amaurosis. This complication is not always easy of detection, on account of the symptoms of these diseases bearing so close a resemblance. When the lens or its capsule are alone affected, the opacity is immediately behind the pupil, the iris and pupil possess some degree of *mobility*, and there is some little appreciation of light; but when amaurosis is conjoined with cataract, we have the same appearance of the lens or capsule, but a *dilated* and *immovable* pupil, an insensible and immovable state of the iris, and an absolute loss of vision.

The first intimation we have of a forming cataract, is defective vision when attempting to read fine print, or to look at minute objects. As the disease advances, all objects appear indistinct; a mist is constantly before the affected eye; a strong light is required to read or write; a small speck now commences just behind the centre of the pupil, and continues to extend until the opacity entirely obstructs the passage of rays of light to the eye; when the opacity is complete, a black ring is seen around the edge of the pupil, and the sight continues to diminish until blindness results.

Causes.—Frequent and long-continued use of the eyes in reading fine print, writing, or looking at minute objects by a strong light; congestion of blood to the eyes, from exercise in a hot sun, in furnaces, and other places where hot and bright fires are kept up; exposure of the eyes to irritating fumes and vapours, like sulphurous acid, chlorine and other gases, and the vapours of sulphuric ether, alcohol, nitric, sulphuric and muriatic acids, hereditary predisposition, mechanical injuries, wounds of the capsule or lens.

Prognosis.—When the cataract is confined to the lens, or to its capsule, and no complications exist from unnatural adhesions, from amaurotic symptoms, or from serious constitutional disturbance, a favourable issue may be expected. On the other hand, a dilated pupil, an immovable iris, a profound blindness, which has been disproportionate to the gradually forming opacity, unnatural adhesions of the capsule, and an irritable and vitiated constitution, will render our prognosis unfavourable.

Therapeutics.—Before resorting to the operation of *couching*, or *extraction*, as is so often done by the old school surgeons, we should always give our medicines a fair trial. It is quite true that we have but few remedies which simulate this affection in their pathogenesis, yet the successful results which have been observed from the use of medicines in a few cases, render it incumbent on us to avail ourselves of them on all proper occasions.

After a thorough trial with medicines, if there is no prospect of amendment, the patient should be turned over to the surgeon for the necessary operation.

In a few cases of incipient cataract, much benefit has followed the local employment of sulphuric ether vapour to the eye, and should our internal remedies prove fruitless, there can be no objection to a trial of this substance.

As internal remedies, we suggest, *conium, pulsatilla, magnesia carb., sulphur, cannabis, phosphorus, digitalis, spigelia, euphrasia.*

Conium and *cannabis* may be exhibited when the cataract has arisen from a wound, or other injury to the eye.

Magnesia carb., pulsatilla, digitalis, and *phosphorus,* have proved curative in capsulo-lenticular cataract, either with or without abnormal adhesions, also in opacity of the lens or capsule alone. These remedies are useful when the disease has been accompanied with ophthalmia.

Sulphur is appropriate in those cases which seem to be connected with a scrofulous or psoric diathesis. It has also been found curative in cataract complicated with amaurosis. *Euphrasia* or *spigelia* may sometimes be alternated with *sulphur* with benefit.

Administration.—The same as in *amaurosis.*

SECTION XIV.

FUNGUS HÆMATODES, AND CANCER OF THE EYE.

Diagnosis.—*Fungus hæmatodes* has always been confounded with *scirrhus*, or *cancer*, until Burns, Hey, and Abernethy pointed out the characteristics of the two diseases, both in respect to their formation and development, as well as their pathology. They possess several qualities in common, like malignancy, inevitable tendency to the destruction of the affected parts, the power of contaminating the whole system, and giving rise ultimately to fatal constitutional symptoms; but in other respects, they are entirely dissimilar. Fungus hæmatodes is not usually attended with the severe stinging and lancinating pains of cancer; its texture is spongy and elastic, and is soft and apparently fluctuating under the touch, while the scirrhus is hard and stony. When fully formed, the fungous tumour is of the consistence of brain, is of a dark and livid hue, and bleeds on the slightest touch, while the substance of cancer is hard, fibrous, and cartilaginous; at its commencement, and during its development, the fungus is knotty and unequal, and thus affords a sign which distinguishes it from cancerous and other tumours. Fungus is more prone to occur in young subjects, while cancer is for the most part confined to persons past the middle age. Fungus of the eye commences in the posterior chamber, while cancer of the eye attacks primarily the conjunctiva or lachrymal gland. The progress of fungus is more rapid and destructive than that of cancer.

The first symptom observed in fungus hæmatodes, is defective vision, and, on looking into the eye, a small shining spot is perceived at the bottom of it. This nucleus of the disease commences in the retina and optic nerve, is traversed by branches of the central artery of the retina, and progresses from within outwards through the vitreous humour, absorbing it in its course, until it arrives near the iris, when it presents a dark amber or greenish hue, and is apt to be mistaken for cataract. As the enlargement increases, the ball of the eye becomes prominent, irregular, and knotty, the cornea ulcerates, and the disease displays itself externally in the form of a soft, medullary, and purple fungus, bleeding at the least touch. The pupil becomes dilated and immovable in the early part of the complaint, and also somewhat changed in colour, which becomes a strongly pronounced amber or brown when the swelling arrives at the iris. The sclerotica soon acquires a dark blue colour, is crossed by dilated veins, and is sometimes attacked by the malady as well as the cornea. After the fungus has shown itself externally, the absorbent glands of the jaw and neck become affected with a medullary degeneration; the countenance assumes a sallow and cadaverous appearance; general debility and nervous irritation occur; loss of appetite; impaired digestion; nausea; irritable stomach; restlessness, and the usual symptoms of hectic fever terminate the patient's existence.

Cancer of the eye, as we have before remarked, generally attacks persons advanced in life. This disease, unlike fungus hæmatodes, commences in the conjunctiva, caruncula lachrymalis, or lachrymal gland, in the form of a hard warty excrescence, which continues for an indefinite period, sometimes attended with twinging and lancinating pains, at other times free from all uneasy feelings, until finally its interior structure becomes altered in texture, an ichorous matter forms within the swelling, which gradually makes its way to the surface, and thus develops the first stage of ulceration. When arrived at this point, vision is destroyed, an irregular fungous mass shoots up from the ulcerated point, highly vascular, of a red, brown, or livid colour, and easily excited to hæmorrhage. As the mass increases, the tissues of the eye become distended; the ulceration and sloughing advance; severe lancinating pains dart through the globe; the appetite is impaired; the patient loses flesh, strength, and courage; sleep is disturbed; the countenance assumes an anxious, distressed, and sallow appearance; hectic fever sets in, and the sufferer speedily yields to the last result.

Hitherto the diseases under consideration have usually been deemed incurable by internal remedies, and on this account surgeons have advised the early extirpation of all suspected tumours, hoping in this way to eradicate the affection while it is local, and before the mass of blood becomes contaminated. But it must be admitted, even when the operation has been resorted to early, and under the most favourable circumstances, that a lamentable want of success has, for the most part, followed all surgical measures. Stealthy and insidious at their commencement, they gradually glide along, depositing in all surrounding textures their destructive and fatal poison, until disorganization begins, when the livid, foul, and destructive phenomena appear in their hideousness, rapidly communicating their influence through the whole organism, and baffling all efforts of the physician and surgeon.

But though experience has so little of promise, we cannot admit that there are no remedies in the whole range of the materia medica capable of counteracting this morbid influence. We may yet find some medicine sufficiently specific to cure these diseases during their forming stage. We believe, indeed, that homœopathy will, ere long, accomplish all that we require in this matter. Only a limited number of well authenticated homœopathic cures of true medullary fungus, or of cancer, have been reported; but the results in these few cases should inspire us with some confidence of success, especially during the early period of the maladies.

Causes.—The *immediate* cause of medullary fungus and of cancer is involved in doubt. Some have suggested the operation of animalculæ, others of a subtle poison, and others of a kind of unhealthy inflammation caused by some constitutional defect. Sir Astley Cooper supposes the morbid degeneration always to be "preceded by a disposition in the constitution to its production."

There is unquestionably a *specific morbid action* in the tumour itself, but whether this is owing to some poison which acts *specifically* upon the *particular* part alone, or to some constitutional vice, we are undecided. That there are drugs capable of neutralizing this morbid influence, whether it be constitutional or local, we entertain no doubt.

The *exciting* causes are blows, contusions, obstructions of blood from pressure, and mechanical injuries generally, although the disease often originates without any apparent or traceable cause.

Prognosis.—In our present state of knowledge, the prognosis must be generally unfavourable; but not many years will elapse before this state of things will change, and we shall be able to meet the complaint with sure and efficient specifics.

Therapeutics.—Having had but little personal experience in regard to the homœopathic treatment of these affections, we shall simply allude to the medicines which appear to us most appropriate, and refer the reader to the reports of cases which have been cured by other practitioners.

Belladonna has cured malignant disease of the eye, attended with violent pains in the eyeball; a red shining point in the posterior chamber; pupils dilated and immovable; loss of vision; unusual hardness of the substance of the eye; iris of a dark colour, and covered with injected bloodvessels.

Malignant affections of the eye have also been cured by *conium, carbo vegetabilis, arsenicum, mercurius, acid nit., calcarea carbonica,* and *iodine.*

Administration.—The same as in *amaurosis.*

SECTION XV.

AFFECTIONS OF THE APPENDAGES OF THE EYE.

HORDEOLUM.—STYE.

Diagnosis.—This is a small boil-like swelling in the edge of the eyelid, resembling in size and general appearance a barleycorn. It generally commences in the follicles of Meibomius, near the angle of the eye, soon assumes a dark red or purple colour, and becomes quite painful from the violence of the accompanying inflammation. The inflammation sometimes confines itself to the cellular membrane, and advances very slowly to the suppurative stage, thus causing not only highly troublesome local pains, but a considerable degree of febrile disturbance. In these cases, gangrene and sloughing of the cellular membrane is apt to occur, and either protract the cure, or leave the part in a condition liable to take on a renewed morbid action from the smallest exciting cause. In other instances, suppuration occurs speedily, the abscess bursts and discharges itself freely, and a prompt cure results.

Causes.—Use of highly spiced, fat, and stimulating food; disordered stomach and bowels; abuse of the eyes in reading, writing, or sewing by gas-lights; scrofulous, psoric, and other impurities of the blood.

Therapeutics.—The appropriate remedies are, *sulphur, pulsatilla, staphysagria, sepia, lycopodium.* We usually employ the third attenuation, and administer a dose twice daily until the swelling and inflammation disappear.

SECTION XVI.

ENTROPIUM.—INVERSION OF THE EYELIDS.

Diagnosis.—This affection consists of an unnatural turning inwards of the whole or a portion of the tarsus and eyelashes, in such a manner as to keep up a constant irritation of the globe, and thus generate a troublesome chronic ophthalmia. If the disease is allowed to continue for any length of time, the cornea loses its brilliancy, its vessels become injected, and ulcers form ; there is continual lachrymation ; partial or entire loss of vision ; great pain and annoyance from the presence of the offending eyelashes.

Causes.—Cicatrices arising from previous ulceration of the tarsi ; chronic ophthalmias ; relaxation and paralysis of the lids ; ulceration of the ciliary glands.

ECTROPIUM.—EVERSION OF THE EYELIDS.

Diagnosis.—Eversion of the lids may be caused by a swelling and relaxation of the lining membrane of the eyelid, which presses the edge of the lid forward until it becomes everted, or by a contraction of the skin of the lid, in consequence of the healing of wounds, ulcers, carbuncles, burns, boils, etc. The consequences of eversion are, constant exposure of the globe to external irritating causes ; chronic inflammation of the eye ; frequent discharge of tears ; dryness of the ball ; photophobia ; nebulous spots and ulcers of the cornea.

Causes.—The principal causes of eversion in consequence of swelling of the lining membrane of the lid, are, protracted chronic ophthalmias of a scrofulous nature ; relaxation from intemperance or old age ; a diseased state of the follicles of Meibomius ; morbid growths in the part. Other causes of eversion are, cicatrices on the skin of the lid arising from incisions, burns, ulcers, smallpox pustules, and carbuncles.

Therapeutics.—The medicines which have been commended in these affections are, *hepar sulphur, mercurius sol., calcarea carb., digitalis, borax.*

Should these remedies disappoint our expectations, a portion of the lid should be *excised,* in such a manner, and in such a situation that the healing cicatrix will restore the displaced tarsi and cilia to their normal position. The operation is simple, unattended with danger, and quite efficient. If opacity or ulceration of the cornea has already commenced when we are first called to the case, it will be advisable to have recourse to the operation without delay, and correct all local or constitutional faults afterwards, with suitable medicines.

The attenuations and repetitions of doses the same as in *amaurosis.*

SECTION XVII.

FISTULA LACHRYMALIS.

Diagnosis.—Under this head authors generally include, obstruction of the puncta lachrymalis and of the lachrymal canals, inflammation and suppuration of the lining membrane of the lachrymal sac, and inflammation, thickening, and obstructions of the membrane lining the ductus ad nasum.

In the most simple form of the complaint, there will be merely an obstruction of the puncta, arising from disease of the Meibomian glands, or of the eyelids, and a consequent interruption to the passage of tears to the lachrymal sac. The manifest symptoms in this instance will be, a continual watering of the eye and overflow of tears upon the cheek, weakness of vision, and an undue dryness of the nostril of the affected side.

Another form of the complaint commences in the lachrymal sac, manifesting itself in the form of a small, hard, and circumscribed swelling, apparently within the sac. This swelling is quite tender to the touch, and gradually increases in size until suppuration occurs, when the parts over and around the tumour acquire a red and shining appearance, not unlike erysipelas. During the early period of the inflammation, the puncta are closed, and tears are forced over upon the cheek. The inflammation also extends down the nasal canal, causing a degree of tenderness, dryness, and obstruction in the duct and nostril. If the suppurative process continues unchecked, the sac, after becoming much distended, bursts, and gives gradual exit to the enclosed pus, thus reducing the swelling, and developing a *fistula of the lachrymal sac.* During the suppurative process, the inflammatory action frequently extends to the external textures of the eye, and if the patient be scrofulous or highly irritable, some constitutional disturbance may be present.

If the disease is permitted to increase, or if injudicious surgical interference has seriously injured the affected tissues, we may expect adhesive inflammation between the walls of the membrane of the nasal duct, and permanent obstruction to the passage of tears to the nostril, and also a closure of the lachrymal canals. When this state of things happens, the tears run over the cheek as fast as formed, and we are presented with the disease termed *stillicidium lachrymarum.*

Still another form of the malady consists in a primary inflammation and thickening of the membrane of the ductus ad nasum, which gives rise to a partial or total obstruction to the passage of the tears, and their consequent accumulation in the lachrymal sac. This undue lachrymal accumulation induces distention of the part, and, after a time, inflammation of its lining membrane, and the other consequences which we have before enumerated. This form of fistula is dependent upon some disease of the nostril, like syphilitic, scrofulous, mercurial, and cancerous ulcerations, or inflammation of the nasal membrane from other causes.

When the malady is fully developed, it is difficult to decide in which particular structure the inflammation originated; but our diagnosis will always be facilitated by carefully considering the causes of the affection, and the previous inflammations. In whatever part it commences, the inflammation is certain to extend, sooner or later, to the contiguous structures.

Causes.—Scarpa advanced the idea, that all forms of fistula lachrymalis were attributable to a disease of the minute glands of Meibomius, or an inflammation of the lining membrane of the eyelid. This idea has been partially refuted by several eminent oculists, but there is, notwithstanding, much truth in the theory. According to our own observations, those forms of fistula which have originated in the puncta, or lachrymal sac, have been preceded by an inflammation of the Meibomian glands, or of the conjunctiva of the eyelids; but where the disease has originated in the ductus ad nasum, it may generally be traced to a previous inflammation, ulceration, or injury to the mucous membrane of the nostril.

The remote causes which predispose to the affection are, a scrofulous, syphilitic, or mercurial taint; general debility and tendency to membranous inflammations; caries of the nasal bones; fractures and other injuries in the region of the lachrymal sac and nasal duct; chronic ophthalmia; pressure of tumours against the lachrymal sac and the puncta.

Prognosis.—Previous to suppuration of the sac, and if there is only a partial obstruction in the lachrymal canals, we may anticipate a prompt cure by internal remedies. But if the puncta and nasal duct be entirely closed, and the suppurative stage in the sac is far advanced, our prognosis must be unfavourable or evasive. Much, however, must always depend upon the condition of the system, and the causes and complications which influence each particular case.

Therapeutics.—Various methods have been proposed by surgeons for the cure of fistula lachrymalis, but they have proved for the most part unsatisfactory. The different surgical means which have been most commended are, the introduction of a tube or style into the nasal duct; the injection of the sac and nasal canal, through the puncta, by means of Anel's syringe, and the introduction of quicksilver. That cures have now and then followed each of these methods, we do not deny; but the numerous instances of permanent aggravation of the malady by their employment, render it probable that there has been altogether more injury than benefit from their introduction into surgical practice. The same opinion is at this time entertained by several distinguished ophthalmic surgeons. It therefore becomes us to investigate all of the causes and accompanying symptoms of each particular case, that we may better select remedies, and thus combat with a prospect of success the *remote* as well as the *immediate* symptoms.

The following medicines have been found curative in the various forms and stages of the complaint: *calcarea carb., acid nit., hepar sulph., silicia, aurum, petroleum, belladonna, iodine, digitalis, lachesis, lycopodium, kali carb., natrum carb.*

The lower attenuations are always to be preferred, and the dose repeated every twelve or twenty-four hours until the disordered tissues are suitably impressed.

THE END.

INDEX.

www.ingramcontent.com/pod-product-compliance
Lightning Source LLC
LaVergne TN
LVHW021055110826
845150LV00001B/83

* 9 7 8 1 4 2 5 5 6 7 1 8 7 *